AF214139

Debonding and Fixed Retention in Orthodontics

Debonding and Fixed Retention in Orthodontics

An Evidence-Based Clinical Guide

Edited by

Theodore Eliades
DDS, MS, Dr Med Sci, PhD, DSc, FIMMM, FRSC, FInstP, FDS RCS(Ed)
Professor and Director, Clinic of Orthodontics and Pediatric Dentistry, Center of Dental Medicine, University of Zurich, Switzerland

Christos Katsaros
DDS, Dr med dent, Dr hc, Odont Dr/PhD
Professor and Chair, Department of Orthodontics and Dentofacial Orthopedics, School of Dental Medicine/Medical Faculty, University of Bern, Switzerland

WILEY Blackwell

This edition first published 2024

Registered Offices
John Wiley & Sons, Inc., 111 River Street, Hoboken, NJ 07030, USA
John Wiley & Sons Ltd, The Atrium, Southern Gate, Chichester, West Sussex, PO19 8SQ, UK

For details of our global editorial offices, customer services, and more information about Wiley products visit us at www.wiley.com.

Wiley also publishes its books in a variety of electronic formats and by print-on-demand. Some content that appears in standard print versions of this book may not be available in other formats.

Library of Congress Cataloging-in-Publication Data
Names: Eliades, Theodore, editor. | Katsaros, Christos, editor.
Title: Debonding and fixed retention in orthodontics : an evidence-based clinical guide / edited by Theodore Eliades, Christos Katsaros.
Description: Hoboken, NJ : Wiley-Blackwell, 2024. | Includes bibliographic references and index.
Identifiers: LCCN 2022059886 (print) | LCCN 2022059887 (ebook) | ISBN 9781119623953 (hardback) | ISBN 9781119623960 (adobe pdf) | ISBN 9781119623977 (epub)
Subjects: MESH: Dental Debonding–methods | Dental Debonding–adverse effects | Orthodontic Appliances, Fixed | Dental Enamel
Classification: LCC RK521 (print) | LCC RK521 (ebook) | NLM WU 192 | DDC 617.6/43–dc23/eng/20230429
LC record available at https://lccn.loc.gov/2022059886
LC ebook record available at https://lccn.loc.gov/2022059887

Cover Design: Wiley
Cover Image: © Dr. Andreas Karamouzos, Dr. Effimia Koumpia and Dr. Anastasios A. Zafeiriadis

Set in 9.5/12.5pt STIXTwoText by Straive, Pondicherry, India
Printed and bound by CPI Group (UK) Ltd, Croydon, CR0 4YY

C9781119623953_140823

Contents

List of Contributors

María Arregui
Department of Odontology
Faculty of Dentistry
Universitat Internacional de Catalunya
Sant Cugat del Valles
Barcelona, Spain

Georgios N. Belibasakis
Department of Dental Medicine
Karolinska Institutet
Huddinge, Sweden

Christoph Bourauel
Department of Oral Technology
School of Dentistry
University Hospital Bonn
Bonn, Germany

T. Gerald Bradley
School of Dentistry
University of Louisville
Louisville, Kentucky, USA

William Brantley
Division of Restorative and Prosthetic Dentistry
College of Dentistry
The Ohio State University
Columbus, OH, USA

Christian J. Day
Department of Orthodontics
Bristol Dental School
University of Bristol
Bristol, UK

Theodore Eliades
Clinic of Orthodontics and Pediatric Dentistry
Center of Dental Medicine
University of Zürich
Zürich, Switzerland

Teresa Flores
Department of Orthodontics
Faculty of Dentistry
Universitat Internacional de Catalunya
Sant Cugat del Valles
Barcelona, Spain

Lluís Giner-Tarrida
Department of Odontology
Faculty of Dentistry
Universitat Internacional de Catalunya
Sant Cugat del Valles
Barcelona, Spain

Angélica Iglesias
Department of Orthodontics
Faculty of Dentistry
Universitat Internacional de Catalunya
Sant Cugat del Valles
Barcelona, Spain

Masahiro Iijima
Division of Orthodontics
and Dentofacial Orthopedics
Department of Oral Growth and Development
Health Sciences University of Hokkaido
Ishikari, Tobetsu, Hokkaido, Japan

Anthony J. Ireland
Department of Orthodontics
Bristol Dental School
University of Bristol, Bristol, UK

Andreas Karamouzos
Department of Orthodontics
Faculty of Dentistry
School of Health Sciences
Aristotle University of Thessaloniki
Thessaloniki, Greece

Christos Katsaros
Department of Orthodontics and Dentofacial Orthopedics,
School of Dental Medicine/
Medical Faculty
University of Bern
Bern, Switzerland

Katerina Kavvadia
Department of Dentistry
School of Medicine
European University Cyprus
Nicosia, Cyprus

Dimitrios Kloukos
Department of Orthodontics and Dentofacial Orthopedics,
School of Dental Medicine/
Medical Faculty
University of Bern
Bern, Switzerland

Despina Koletsi
Clinic of Orthodontics and Pediatric Dentistry
Center of Dental Medicine
University of Zürich
Zürich, Switzerland

Effimia Koumpia
Department of Orthodontics
Faculty of Dentistry
School of Health Sciences
Aristotle University of Thessaloniki
Thessaloniki, Greece

Thaleia Kouskoura
Department of Pediatric Oral Health and Orthodontics
University Center for Dental Medicine, University of Basel
Basel, Switzerland

Spyridon N. Papageorgiou
Clinic of Orthodontics and Pediatric Dentistry
Center of Dental Medicine
University of Zürich
Zürich, Switzerland

Pawel Pazera
Department of Orthodontics and Dentofacial Orthopedics,
School of Dental Medicine/ Medical Faculty
University of Bern
Bern, Switzerland

Andreu Puigdollers
Department of Orthodontics
Faculty of Dentistry
Universitat Internacional de Catalunya
Sant Cugat del Valles
Barcelona, Spain

Jonathan R. Sandy
Department of Orthodontics
Bristol Dental School
University of Bristol
Bristol, UK

Iosif Sifakakis
Department of Orthodontics
School of Dentistry
National and Kapodistrian University of Athens
Athens, Greece

Eser Tüfekçi
Department of Orthodontics
School of Dentistry
Virginia Commonwealth University
Richmond, VA, USA

Anastasios A. Zafeiriadis
Department of Orthodontics
Faculty of Dentistry
School of Health Sciences
Aristotle University of Thessaloniki
Thessaloniki, Greece

dictated by the bias of the supervising instructor for postgraduate students or the content of relevant weekend courses – the sort that have saturated the professional community – rather than the result of an evidence-based approach.

The objective of this textbook is to provide succinic and clinically relevant information on the underlying mechanisms of success or failure for these two fundamental phases of treatment. The book is structured around two axes: debonding and resin grinding, and fixed retainer placement.

The first section covers aspects of the topic that have not yet been found in relevant texts, including methods of appliance removal, cutting efficiency of burs, grinding and enamel effects, complicated interfacial characteristics of attachments with enamel and aligners, airborne pathogens and aerosol produced during resin grinding, and future materials utilizing biomimetic approaches for bonding, among others.

The second section provides an analysis of the materials utilized in fixed retainer bonding, with emphasis on resin, wires, their effect on material deformation during mastication or placement, and release of bisphenol-A from fixed retainer resin adhesives, as well as clinical effectiveness and unwanted effects of fixed retainers on tooth position.

We hope the book will serve as a source of information serving education and practice alike.

Theodore Eliades
Christos Katsaros

Section A

Debonding

1

Cutting with Rotating Instruments and Cutting Efficiency of Burs

María Arregui[1], Lluís Giner-Tarrida[1], Teresa Flores[2], Angélica Iglesias[2], and Andreu Puigdollers[2]

[1] *Department of Odontology, Faculty of Dentistry, Universitat Internacional de Catalunya, Sant Cugat del Valles, Barcelona, Spain*
[2] *Department of Orthodontics, Faculty of Dentistry, Universitat Internacional de Catalunya, Sant Cugat del Valles, Barcelona, Spain*

1.1 Introduction

The retention phase is a crucial part of orthodontic treatment. Its importance keeps increasing since patients look for a long-lasting 'perfect' result for aesthetic reasons, even though some degree of relapse is always expected. For this reason, life-long retention is more commonly advised every day by clinicians (Padmos et al. 2018).

Many studies have analysed the retention phase in terms of stability, retention material, adhesion, clinician and patient preference and hygiene (Al-Moghrabi et al. 2018; Eroglu et al. 2019; Gugger et al. 2016; Sifakakis et al. 2017), but none of the literature has focused on the consequences of retention on the enamel. Unlike bracket debonding, the detachment of lingual retainers is usually accidental and may be caused by excessive force, adhesive material wear or retainer rupture. The enamel could be altered due to the applied load that caused the rupture in the adhesive interphase or the removal of remaining adhesive or retainer materials (Ryf et al. 2012).

Debonding and Fixed Retention in Orthodontics: An Evidence-Based Clinical Guide, First Edition. Edited by Theodore Eliades and Christos Katsaros.

Cleaning and polishing procedures for remnants of adhesive materials are as variable as retention protocols. No consensus has been reached on the ideal protocol for adhesive removal (Janiszewska-Olszowska et al. 2014). The various techniques include using hand instruments, rotatory instruments (high- and low-speed), sandblasting, ultrasound and bur and disc materials including tungsten carbide burs, diamond burs, composite burs, rubber burs and Sof-Lex discs (Eliades 2019; Janiszewska-Olszowska et al. 2015; Shah et al. 2019). This is a critical moment, as the aim is to remove the material with no or minimal damage to the enamel structure and without overheating the pulp due to friction caused by the instruments. To do so, it is extremely important to carefully select the burs and rotary instruments to be used. For this reason, it is important to have a good understanding of the cutting efficiency of the burs, which type of bur is most suitable, the bur's longevity and the maximum number of uses due to loss of effectiveness. It is also important to take into account the characteristics of the rotating instruments: rotational speed, torque or power, water spray coolant, etc., to avoid damaging the tooth.

In this chapter, we will discuss aspects of the retention phase concerning enamel preservation and the consequences of temporarily adhesive procedures, such as appliances bonding, on the enamel surface. We will analyse the repercussions of adhesive procedures for retention materials, especially considering that life-long retention may require one or more rebonding procedures (Jin et al. 2018). We will also deal with the correct selection of burs for the removal of cement from brackets and fixed retainers; the subsequent final finishing with polishing tools to help recover the enamel aesthetics; and the most advisable protocol for removing fixed retainers, whether for final removal or for a rebonding procedure.

1.2 Enamel Surface and Damage Associated with Debonding Techniques: Burs and Polishing

Thanks to advanced microscopy technology and mineral property analysis techniques, the composition of enamel and its properties before and after adhesive treatments have been widely studied. The vast majority of studies are based on the vestibular surface because there is significant concern about enamel preservation due to aesthetic concerns. However, more aggressive bonding techniques are often used on the lingual surface because this surface does not have aesthetical importance. Such studies are usually done on labial surfaces; it is not common to do them on lingual surfaces.

An *in vitro* study using a scanning electron microscope (SEM) found an important difference between the two enamel surfaces. The lingual surface appears to be smoother, with smaller micropores and a less pronounced wavelike appearance after conditioning, which resulted in less mechanical interlocking in the enamel-bonding interphase and, thus, lower shear bond strength (SBS) values and greater tooth damage compared to the buccal side (Brosh et al. 2005). This interesting data is rarely discussed when adhesion protocols for retainers or lingual brackets are presented.

Sufficient bonding strength, easy debonding and limited damage to the enamel surface are critical factors in orthodontics (Shinya et al. 2008). A lower enamel Adhesive Remnant Index (ARI) after cleaning of residual adhesive corresponds to less damage to the enamel surface (David et al. 2002; Fjeld and Ogaard 2006). Removal systems are important not only for enamel preservation after appliance removal but also in lingual retention: the polishing phase is crucial for patient comfort because studies show that patients' tongues can detect changes in surface roughness (SR) of less than 1 μm (Jones et al. 2004). Furthermore, the smoother surface helps reduce the amount of bacterial plaque deposited.

Before selecting instruments, some basic concepts related to burs must be considered: cutting, grinding, and finishing and polishing actions. *Cutting* is a unidirectional action related to instruments with blades, such as tungsten carbide burs. Depending on the number of blades, the bur will have more of a cutting or polishing function. Also, if we use a low-speed handpiece, by allowing a change of rotation, we can obtain a greater polishing effect rather than cutting. It has been seen that tungsten carbide burs can leave a regular pattern on the enamel structure (Figure 1.1). The *grinding* action is responsible for removing small particles from the surface by the effect of abrasive wear, and their action is unidirectional. Diamond burs are an example (Figure 1.2). Different types of diamond burs are available depending on the size of the component particles. During the *finishing and polishing* phase, the use of tungsten carbide burs with more blades or diamond burs with fine grit is

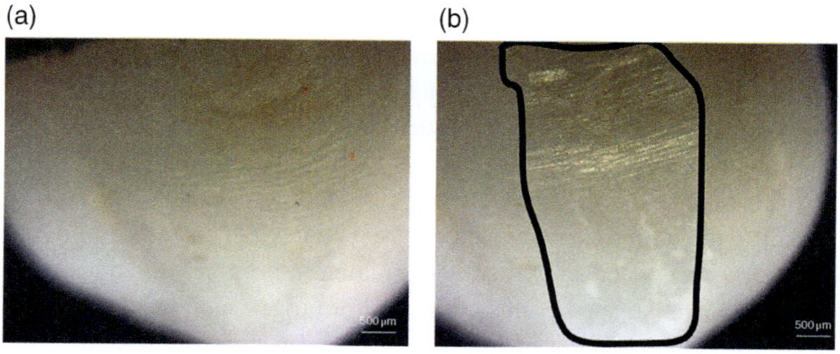

Figure 1.1 (a) Natural tooth; (b) tooth ground with a carbide bur.

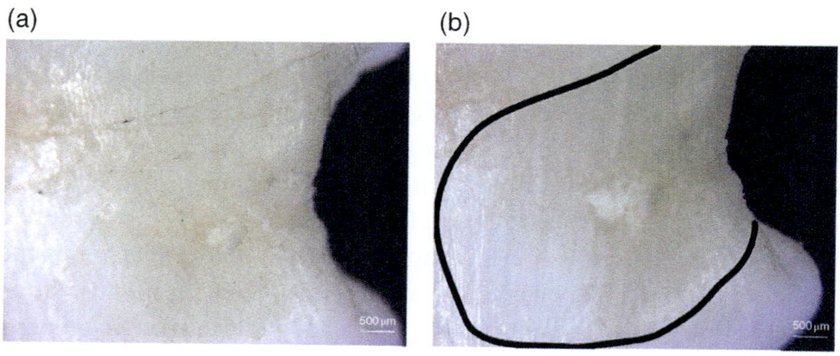

Figure 1.2 (a) Natural tooth; (b) tooth ground with a diamond bur.

indicated to give the final texture to the surface. Polishing gives a gloss to the enamel, which regains its usual brightness after the cement is removed and becomes smooth and homogeneous. This final part of the polishing process is usually carried out with abrasive instruments such as rubber cups, discs, strips and fine-grained polishing pastes (Anusavice 2013).

To remove cement properly, it is important to take into account the *cutting efficiency* of the burs, which is defined as the maximum capacity to remove dental tissue with the minimum effort during a specific period of time (Choi et al. 2010). It is measured and evaluated by calculating the amount of substrate removed (by weight or length of the cut) in a given time. Many studies have observed a reduction in cutting efficiency after repeated use of burs (Bae et al. 2014).

This reduction of cutting efficiency is associated with factors such as (i) wear of the burs due to use and friction, (ii) debris clogging the bur surface, and (iii) the procedures for cleaning, disinfecting and sterilizing the burs. Some studies have determined that cutting efficiency decreases between the first and the sixth sterilization cycles (Bae et al. 2014; Emir et al. 2018; Regev et al. 2010). Firoozmand et al. (2008) determined that the lifetime of a bur is five uses, since after that it is difficult to guarantee a proper and efficient cut. These results were confirmed by Emir et al. (2018).

1.2.1 Design and Type of Burs

1.2.1.1 Diamond Burs

The selection of diamond burs should focus on constant cutting efficiency throughout their life span because studies have shown that these burs tend to lose their efficiency due to use (Bae et al. 2014; Emir et al. 2018; Prithviraj et al. 2017). One of the factors related to the reduction in cutting efficiency is the pull-out of diamond chips (Bae et al. 2014; Pilcher et al. 2000; Prithviraj et al. 2017) (Figure 1.3).

Manufacturers use various methods to adhere abrasive particles to the bur shaft, such as electrodepositing a nickel coating on diamond chips (Ben-Hanan et al. 2008; Siegel and Anthony Von Fraunhofer 1998), electrodepositing a chrome-nickel coating (Regev et al. 2010; Siegel and Anthony Von Fraunhofer 1998), sintering, microabrasion (Prithviraj et al. 2017; Siegel and Anthony Von Fraunhofer 1998; Siegel and Von Fraunhofer 1996) and chemical vapour deposition (Jackson et al. 2004). The quality of diamond burs is based on the concentration of abrasive particles and the capacity of the adhesive system to retain the diamond particles during continuous use.

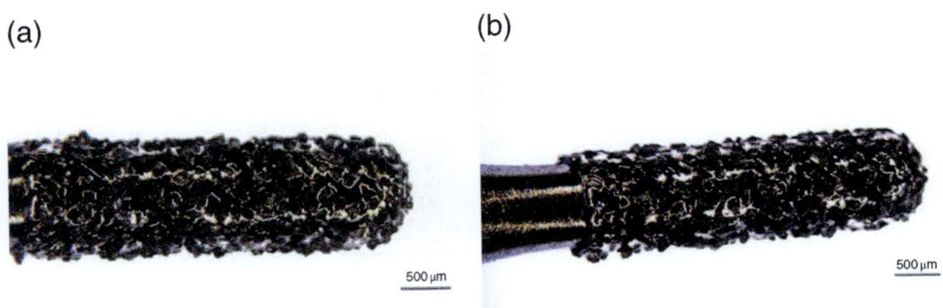

Figure 1.3 (a) Diamond bur before use; (b) diamond bur after use.

The diamond particles used in burs vary between manufacturers, and the primary characteristics are (i) whether the diamonds are natural or synthetic, (ii) their size and shape, and (iii) the individual features of burs. Natural diamonds have more irregular shapes than synthetic ones, which facilitates their deposition in a nickel or chrome-nickel coating matrix. The size of the diamond chips determines the thickness and category of the burs: ultrafine, fine, medium or coarse (Siegel and Anthony Von Fraunhofer 1998). In cutting efficiency studies, medium grit (120–140 μm) or coarse grit (150–160 μm) burs are generally used. Fine and ultra-fine grit burs are not usually evaluated in the literature, as their use is more indicated for finishing and polishing.

The cutting and grinding actions of diamond burs are caused by friction. Every movement of the bur in both directions removes tissue with the abrasive action of the sharp edges of the diamond chips (Figure 1.4).

1.2.1.2 Tungsten Carbide Burs

Tungsten carbide burs are composed of 8 to 40 blades (Figure 1.5); the most frequently used have 8, 12, 20 or 40 blades and are indicated for contouring and smoothing various dental materials and structures (Jefferies 2007). These burs generally are characterised by their hardness and cutting edge, but they wear out with each use and are also fragile and susceptible to fracture (Di Cristofaro et al. 2013).

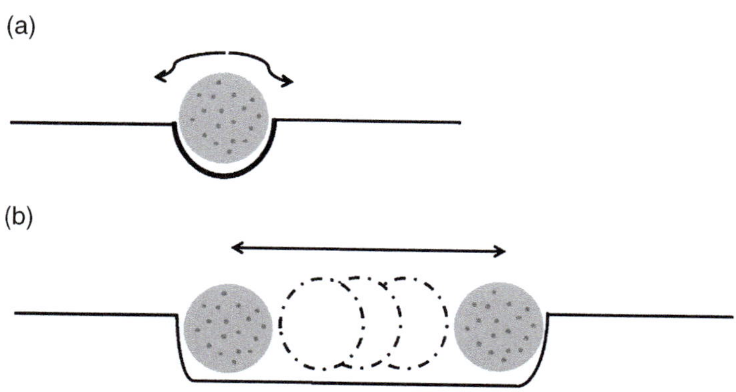

Figure 1.4 Grinding action by diamond burs. (a) During the first step in the grinding process, the bur starts to remove tissue. (b) Every movement of the bur in both directions removes tissue by abrasive action.

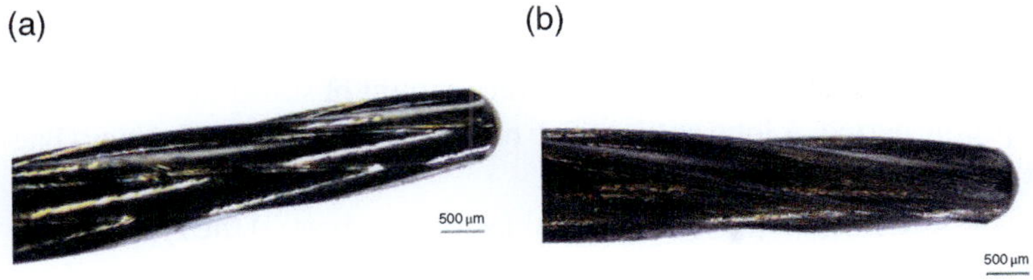

Figure 1.5 (a) Carbide bur before use; (b) carbide bur after use.

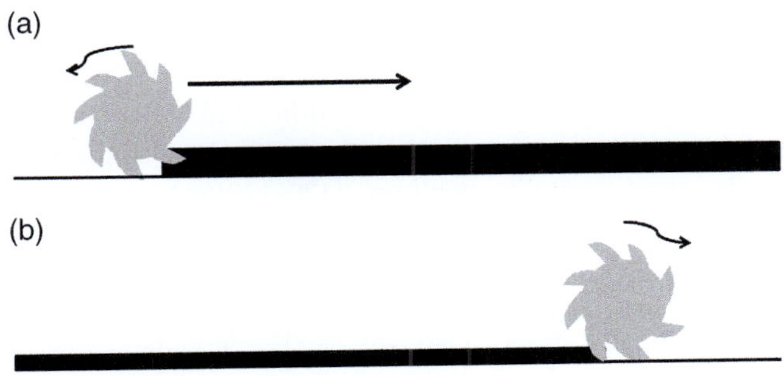

Figure 1.6 (a) Cutting action in a clockwise direction; (b) polishing action in a counterclockwise direction.

Tungsten carbide burs have a bidirectional cut so that when the burs are rotated in a clockwise direction, they have a cutting action. In a counterclockwise direction, they have a polishing action such that a regular pattern is observed on the tooth structure, corresponding to the ordered arrangement of the blades on the bur (Figure 1.6).

Burs with fewer blades are normally used for cutting and grinding, while those with more blades are used to finish polishing and provide texture, as they have a less aggressive effect on the enamel surface.

Carbide burs are considered the gold standard in the literature for removing orthodontic cement during the debonding procedure because they are faster and more effective than other tools that can be used in this stage. But there is always a risk of removing part of the enamel and altering the external surface, in which case the enamel will not recover its original external roughness (Bosco et al. 2020).

1.2.2 Cutting Efficiency

Cutting efficiency can be defined as the amount of substrate removed in a specific period. A long cutting time means lower cutting efficiency (Bae et al. 2014).

This efficiency depends on several factors, such as (i) the type of burs used (diamond or carbide); (ii) the cutting instrument, which may be a turbine or an electric motor handpiece; (iii) the water flow (to remove debris that is clogging the burs and control the intra-pulp temperature); (iv) the force applied by the operator; and (v) the substrate.

1.2.2.1 Diamond and Carbide Burs

Studies usually compare carbide burs with each other and with diamond burs. Diamond burs are also compared with each other, comparing different particle sizes, usually medium (120–140 μm) or coarse (150–160 μm) grit, with different designs (channelled or conventional) and shapes (chamfered or thin taper).

In general, carbide burs have good cutting efficiency; it is greater in burs with deep angles and sharp edges (Di Cristofaro et al. 2013). Another factor that improves cutting efficiency is a negative cutting angle: it makes the bur more effective because it reduces debris that clogs the bur and interferes with cutting and speed. Some studies observe that carbide burs are faster and more effective than diamond burs (Ercoli et al. 2009); this may be due to their hardness and cutting edge compared to the hardness of the metal that acts as a binder for diamond chips. However, other publications consider diamond burs to have a higher cutting efficiency than carbide burs (Emir et al. 2018).

All diamond burs exhibit similar behaviour: the greatest loss of efficiency occurs between the first and second cuts, after which it decreases progressively (Bae et al. 2014; Pilcher et al. 2000). This is due to wear of the burs during use.

The cutting performance of this type of burs primarily depends on the diamonds. Natural diamonds have irregular shapes with sharper edges, so the most effective burs have a higher proportion of natural diamonds (Prithviraj et al. 2017; Siegel and Von Fraunhofer 1996, 1999). Other factors are the size and diameter of the diamond chips. Larger grit means the bur has greater cutting efficiency. However, studies show that burs with medium and coarse grit often do not differ in their cutting efficiency. This may be because manufacturers assign a category to their burs, such as medium grit; then, when studies analyse the burs with a SEM and measure the diamond chips, the diamonds are observed to be larger and correspond more closely to the coarse size described by the ISO standard (Bae et al. 2014; Prithviraj et al. 2017). In general, these differences between manufacturer classifications and the analysis during studies may be due to the filters used in the manufacturing process to standardise the grit allowing a range of sizes to pass through, so that sometimes particles with greater diameters are introduced.

Cutting efficiency is compromised when diamond chips are pulled out of the binder with which they are attached to the bur shaft rather than by the wear of the diamond cutting edge (Bae et al. 2014; Ben-Hanan et al. 2008; Emir et al. 2018; Prithviraj et al. 2017). The extent to which diamonds can be pulled out is associated with the properties of the metal used as a binder (Bae et al. 2014) or the system used to bond the diamonds to the bur. The chips are less likely to be detached when the binder is more powerful and has higher adhesion properties, and therefore the bur has greater cutting efficiency. It has also been seen that burs that use nickel electroplating have lower cutting efficiency than burs that use a proprietary brazing system (PBS) (Prithviraj et al. 2017). SEM studies of burs processed by means of electrodeposition with nickel have observed that spaces are left by detached diamond chips; in addition, some diamond chips are embedded too far into the metal matrix, leaving fewer cutting edges exposed and providing less area for cutting (Prithviraj et al. 2017). Another factor that can affect cutting efficiency is a secondary effect of spaces left by diamonds when they are clogged with debris. This effect reduces the effective work of the burs, which is why it is important to cool them properly during grinding or polishing so the water removes this debris (Ben-Hanan et al. 2008).

The design and shape of diamond burs also influence their cutting efficiency. Some studies have compared chamfered and thin-taper burs and observed that burs with a larger diameter (chamfered) have a larger cutting area, greater peripheral speed, and higher cutting efficiency than thinner burs (Bae et al. 2014). However, it has been observed that chamfered burs produce a larger temperature increase due to greater friction. Other studies have compared conventional and channelled burs and observed that conventional burs have a higher cutting efficiency than channelled burs (Funkenbusch et al. 2016). It has been seen that grooved burs allow a better distribution of water along the bur between the grooves, providing constant cleaning and reducing clogging debris in the bur, and also achieve faster heat dissipation (Galindo et al. 2004), but no statistically significant differences were observed compared to conventional burs (Ercoli et al. 2009).

The effect of cleaning, disinfecting and sterilisation on the cutting efficiency of burs has also been studied, and some studies concluded that these procedures do not directly affect cutting efficiency (Bae et al. 2014). However, other authors have observed that cleaning and sterilising burs that are used repeatedly improved their cutting behaviour because debris is eliminated during the cleaning procedure (Rotella et al. 2014).

Some studies have evaluated whether bur wear affects the SR the burs cause on the tooth structure or materials as well as cutting efficiency. It seems that the more worn the bur is, the lower the cutting efficiency and SR. The loss of roughness may be heterogeneous, but it can affect the bonding process (Emir et al. 2018). When studying different materials, it is observed that the cutting efficiency of burs used to cut zirconium or lithium disilicate or metals is reduced more rapidly since those materials have harder surfaces than the tooth structure (Emir et al. 2018; Galindo et al. 2004; Nakamura et al. 2015; Siegel and Von Fraunhofer 1996).

In summary, the cutting efficiency of carbide burs is reduced due to wear and tear on the blades (Di Cristofaro et al. 2013). On the other hand, in diamond burs, the factors that influence wear and cutting efficiency are (i) diamond chips being pulled out, (ii) wear of the cutting edges of the diamond chips, (iii) debris clogging the cutting areas, and (iv) wear of the material that acts as a binding agent for the diamond chips on the shank (Ben-Hanan et al. 2008).

1.2.2.2 Rotating Instruments: Turbines and Electric Motor Handpieces

For more than 50 years, turbines have been used in dentistry to grind or polish dental structures and materials because of their performance: (i) they are ergonomic and lightweight, (ii) they are reasonably priced, and (iii) they can quickly remove tooth structure. On the other hand, turbines have these disadvantages: (i) vibration and noise, (ii) the release of aerosols, and (iii) low torque, which causes them to slow down when too much force is detected and decreases cutting capacity – a turbine can even get stuck and stop (Choi et al. 2010; Eikenberg 2001; Ercoli et al. 2009; Kenyon et al. 2005; Rotella et al. 2014) (Figure 1.7).

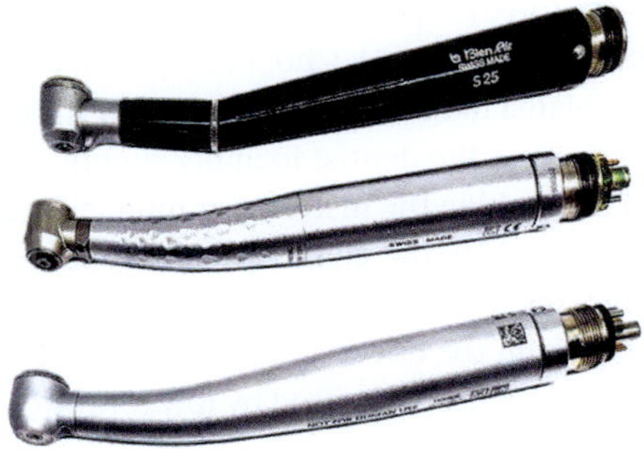

Figure 1.7 Different types of turbines.

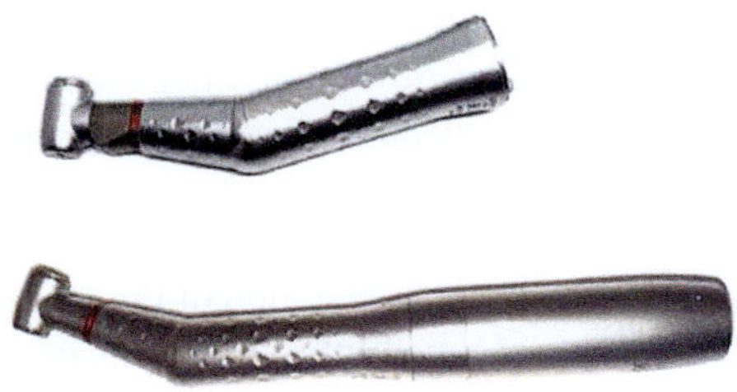

Figure 1.8 Electric motor handpieces.

Electric motor handpieces were developed 20 or 30 years ago. They are characterised by their variable power and higher torque than turbines and therefore maintain their rotation speed with less risk of getting stuck when more force is applied than usual. Other positive aspects of these instruments are that (i) they are quieter and have less vibration; (ii) they release fewer aerosols, reducing the risk of cross-contamination; and (iii) they provide more precise and concentric cuts than turbines. On the other hand, electric motor handpieces weigh more, making them less ergonomic than turbines (Choi et al. 2010; Eikenberg 2001; Ercoli et al. 2009; Kenyon et al. 2005; Rotella et al. 2014) (Figure 1.8).

Studies have been carried out to compare cutting efficiency depending on the cutting instrument used: turbine or electric motor handpiece. All the studies came to the same conclusion – that the electric motor handpiece had a higher cutting efficiency than the turbine – although no statistically significant differences were observed (Choi et al. 2010; Eikenberg 2001; Ercoli et al. 2009; Rotella et al. 2014). All the authors believe the reason is the difference in torque: the high torque of the electric motor handpiece means its rotational speed is not reduced when more force is applied (Choi et al. 2010; Eikenberg 2001; Ercoli et al. 2009; Rotella et al. 2014). Choi et al. (2010) even add that the difference could be related to the increased weight of the electric motor handpiece, which may cause the dentist to apply slightly more force (without being aware of it), making the instrument more efficient.

Not only is the electric motor handpiece more efficient than the turbine, but a smoother surface is obtained. In contrast, rough marks can be seen from the effect of a turbine, which may be related to loss of speed and possible stall caused by low torque (Geminiani et al. 2014).

1.2.2.3 Other Factors Related to Cutting Efficiency

As previously mentioned, various factors reduce cutting efficiency, including water flow, which depends on the instruments, and applied force, which depends on both the instrument and the dentist.

Water flow is a very important factor since it removes debris that may remain attached to the bur and avoids iatrogenic injury caused by heat generated during preparation of the tooth (most of the energy that is not used is transformed into heat). The amount of heat transmitted to the tooth usually depends on the type of bur, applied force, cutting time and rate, cooling technique, speed, and torque of the instrument (Galindo et al. 2004).

Most studies that have measured the effect of water flow on the temperature inside the pulp chamber have observed that grinding does not affect the pulp chamber because the water-flow coolant helps to decrease the temperature and prevent the pulp from reaching a critical temperatures. The water flow indicated in these studies to prevent an increase in pulp temperature is between 25 and 50 ml/min, regardless of whether the bur is made of diamond or carbide. More water is always better to cool the tooth preparation (Ercoli et al. 2009; Galindo et al. 2004; Siegel and von Fraunhofer 2000; Siegel and Patel 2016; Von Fraunhofer and Siegel 2000).

The importance of water flow is based on the number and distribution of water outlets on the instruments (Ercoli et al. 2009; Siegel and Von Fraunhofer 2002). Earlier turbines (and some of today's turbines) had only one water port at the base of the head, so the bur was not fully cooled. Today, electric motor handpieces and modern turbines have three or four water ports (Figure 1.9), increasing the water flow of the entire bur. This allows control over the temperature, increases the

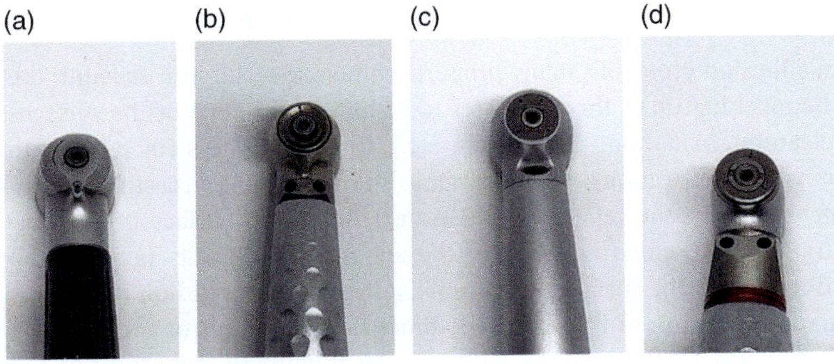

Figure 1.9 (a) Turbine with one water port; (b) turbine with three water ports; (c) turbine with four water ports; and (d) electric motor handpiece with three water ports.

removal of debris, and therefore increases cutting efficiency. Studies have compared the efficiency of dry and wet cutting and concluded that wet cutting increases the cutting rate and removes three times more tissue than dry cutting (Ercoli et al. 2009).

The last important factor related to cutting efficiency is the force applied when preparing the tooth. Different authors have conducted studies with dentists to determine the force they apply. Elias et al. (2003) determined that the force varied between 0.66 and 2.23 N, and Siegel et al. (Siegel and Von Fraunhofer 1997, 1999) concluded that the most effective force for medium-grit burs is 0.92 N. Most literature considers that dentists exert a force between 50 and 150 g when preparing a tooth (Eikenberg 2001; Galindo et al. 2004; Siegel and Von Fraunhofer 1997, 1999). Elias et al. (2003) concluded that the magnitude of the force depends more on the power of the rotating instrument than on the speed of the instrument or outside force applied by the operator. On the other hand, Funkenbusch et al. (2016) consider that greater force applied by the operator generally increases cutting efficiency, so we can observe that there is no consensus about whether force depends more on the instrument or the operator. In summary, all studies consider that as the burs wear out and cutting efficiency is reduced, the force applied by the operator increases, leading to a risk of raising the temperature if there is not proper water flow (Emir et al. 2018; Pilcher et al. 2000; Rotella et al. 2014; Siegel and Von Fraunhofer 1996).

1.2.3 Effect of the Debonding Technique on the Enamel

In adhesion protocols, many properties must be taken into account: the chemical nature of the substrates to be joined, the state of the surfaces (cleaning, oxidation, passivation, etc.), their roughness (in relation to previous preparations such as carving, milling, roughing, casting, micro-etching, etc.), the relationship between the energy surface of the substrate to be bonded and that of the adhesive, wettability between the adhesive and the surface or substrate, adhesive viscosity, liquid transformation, strength of the adhesive, dimensional changes of the adhesive during this transformation, strength and toughness (cohesion) of the cured adhesive and film thickness of the adhesive agent.

When fixed lingual retention is selected, many of these variables must be considered. For example, a smoother lingual surface may require a more aggressive pretreatment or a longer acid-etching exposure to ensure mechanical porosity and greater resistance to debonding.

Another important aspect of fixed retention is the increasing preference of clinicians for life-long retention, which will also affect the bonding procedure. Since adhesion in orthodontics is almost always temporary, when looking for definitive bonding, some aspects of the protocol must be revised.

Regarding the retainer itself, there is no consensus among practitioners about adequate stiffness or properties of the material. These are influenced by the clinician's experience, training and beliefs. However, most agree about the use of a fluid composite resin with an acid-etching-priming procedure for adhesion.

The consequences of a permanent adhesive technique become evident when rupture, debonding or fracture of the interphase of the retainer occurs. In this case, we encounter damage from the mechanical removal of adhesive remnants and additional chemical damage from the rebonding procedure.

Disruption of the demineralization/remineralization balance in teeth can lead to irreversible structural damage, as adult enamel cannot self-regenerate (Yamaguchi et al. 2006). Removal of lingual retainer, orthodontic brackets and residual cement causes inevitable enamel loss that is irreversible by biological mechanisms (Pus et al. 1980). This loss can be minimised by carefully selecting less aggressive removal processes. However, any enamel repair must be induced by external methods

(Eisenburger et al. 2001), which should be instituted as soon as possible after orthodontic appliance removal.

Reported amounts of enamel loss after bracket debonding and cleaning are highly variable, ranging from 5–10 μm (Zachrisson and Arthun 1979) to 29.5–41.2 μm (Pus et al. 1980). This high variability may be attributed to differences in the methods used for remnants, bracket bonding (self-etching versus conventional etching cement and direct versus indirect bonding) (Flores et al. 2015; Iglesias et al. 2020; Mielczarek and Michalik 2014) or analysis (weight comparison, surfometry [Hosein et al. 2004], profilometry [Pus et al. 1980], SEM [Fjeld and Ogaard 2006]). A significant loss of enamel volume is observed in premolars subjected to simulated orthodontic treatment compared to untreated enamel. Enamel loss can be reversed, but not completely recovered, by remineralization with toothpaste. This finding may be attributable to the rapid decrease in fluoride release over time (Hahnel et al. 2014).

Recently, research done at the Orthodontics Department of Universitat Internacional de Catalunya compared different removal techniques (specifically after retention debonding) and found higher levels of rugosity (Sa, Sq, Sz) of the enamel in samples to which a high-speed white stone was applied (Figure 1.10). Tungsten burs were also tested at high and low

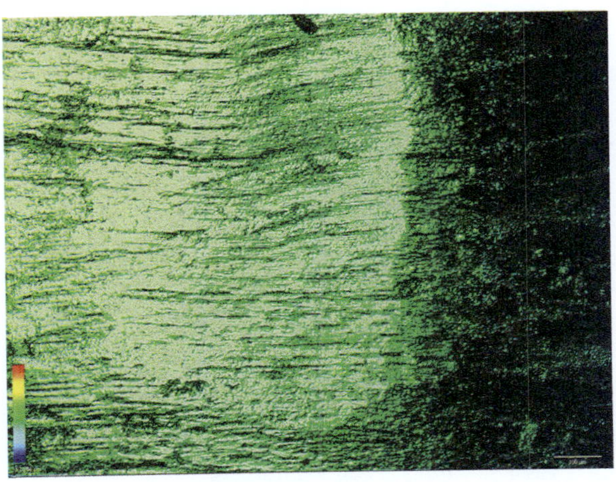

Figure 1.10 Enamel appearance after debonding and polishing with white stone using a high-speed handpiece.

speeds (Figures 1.11 and 1.12), with 15-blade burs, and the results showed less damage of the enamel when using a tungsten bur at low speed. This protocol of low-speed tungsten bur and posterior polishing with rubber cups was applied in accordance with other studies that analysed similar parameters after bracket debonding (Ireland et al. 2005).

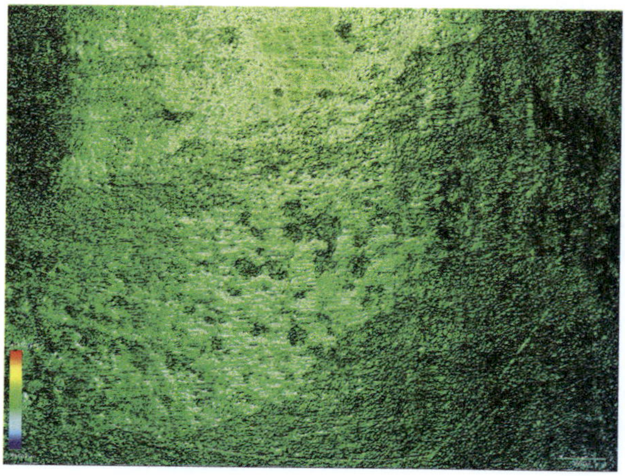

Figure 1.11 Enamel appearance after debonding and polishing with a tungsten carbide bur using a high-speed handpiece.

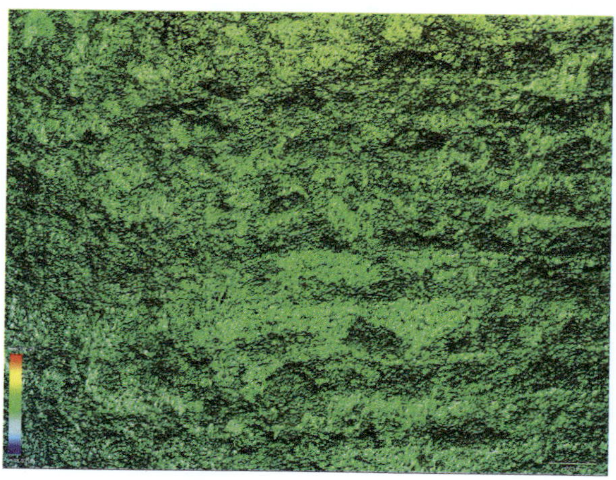

Figure 1.12 Enamel appearance after debonding and polishing with a tungsten carbide bur using a low-speed handpiece.

1.3 Preservation and Remineralization

Researchers have examined the potential use of toothpaste containing surface (S) prereacted glass-ionomer (PRG) filler (Flores et al. 2017; Ikemura et al. 2008) based on calcium phosphate (Cochrane et al. 2010) or a novel fluoride-containing bioactive glass (Coceska et al. 2016) for inhibiting demineralization and recovering enamel loss (Fujimoto et al. 2010). In aqueous environments, PRG forms a stable glass-ionomer phase via a reaction between polyacrylic acid and fluoride-containing glass (Ikemura et al. 2008). The buffering action of S-PRG reduces the acidity of the oral environment (Fujimoto et al. 2010; Iijima et al. 2014; Ikemura et al. 2008). Furthermore, S-PRG filler releases strontium and fluorine ions, which improve the acid resistance of teeth by reacting with hydroxyapatite (Featherstone et al. 1983). More novel investigations have focused on the study of biometric hydroxyapatite toothpaste as a preventive measure in remineralization cases (Bossù et al. 2019; Memarpour et al. 2019).

Nanometric techniques permit three-dimensional data to be obtained with minimum sample preparation (Hashimoto et al. 2013). Reports of nanometric studies of healthy and affected enamel have described the enamel topography and SR.

SR affects the aesthetic properties, bacterial adhesion and plaque formation of enamel by altering the pathogenic environment (Elkassas and Arafa 2014; Kaga et al. 2014). Researchers have analysed the enamel SR using atomic force microscopy (AFM) and SEM as nanometric techniques. In contrast to SEM, AFM does not dehydrate the surface enamel during sample preparation (Bitter 1998; Keszthelyi and Jenei 1999). Similar to AFM, confocal microscopy (CFM) and profilometry are non-invasive nanometric techniques that enable the quantification of SR parameters with high measurement sensitivity and without altering the enamel surface quality (Poggio et al. 2012).

In a recent study (Iijima et al. 2014), toothpaste containing 5 or 30% S-PRG offered greater enamel remineralization than NaF-containing toothpaste, as indicated by the improved surface hardness and elastic modulus values. Remineralization was primarily determined by the toothpaste's strontium- and fluorine-releasing capacities rather than the fraction of S-PRG filler. Using SR and microhardness analyses, Elkassas and Arafa (2014) demonstrated the superior remineralizing efficacy of fluoride varnish compared to fluoride toothpaste, which they attributed to the greater fluoride content of the varnish. However, toothpaste may yield better long-term results because fluoride varnish is only intended for use over one year.

Kaga et al. (2014) reported that the buffering effect of S-PRG filler inhibits enamel demineralization. An aqueous solution containing S-PRG filler exhibited a rapid increase in pH at one day, a gradual increase over six days, and the lowest Ca ion concentration among remineralization solutions. Although human saliva can harden the enamel surface, calcifying solutions may have greater remineralizing potential due to their higher concentrations of calcium and phosphate (Reynolds 1997; Reynolds et al. 2003). Calcium phosphate precipitates on the enamel surface as an amorphous precursor that undergoes rapid transformation to apatite crystals (Shen et al. 2001). Lippert et al. (2004) observed no enamel hardening due to saliva.

A previous study reported higher SR values after remineralization with 70 wt% S-PRG compared to untreated enamel. The improvement could have been due to an increasing number of filler particles on the enamel surface (Hahnel et al. 2014). Fluoride toothpaste can reportedly restore the surface of lesions (Gjorgievska et al. 2013; Mielczarek and Michalik 2014), indicating its potential utility in cases with an elevated risk of caries, such as orthodontic patients (Gjorgievska et al. 2013).

1.4 Clinical Considerations

Due to the stability of the enamel composition and its poor ability to restore itself once its structure has been damaged, it is vital to create protocols that produce the least possible iatrogenesis. Among them, the use of different, less-aggressive burs for removing residual cement accompanied by a remineralization protocol that can help reconstitute damaged enamel should be incorporated into any debonding protocol. It is important to minimise the structural damage previously discussed in all temporary bonding procedures and in fixed retentions.

Given that it is impossible to avoid changing the surface structure of the enamel even if the most appropriate and least invasive protocols are followed, the systematic use of post-treatment remineralizing agents should be practically mandatory after treatment to remove residual cement. These parameters should remain a vital focus of study, as we have yet to find a non-harmful method.

References

Al-Moghrabi, D., Johal, A., O'Rourke, N. et al. (2018). Effects of fixed vs removable orthodontic retainers on stability and periodontal health: 4-year follow-up of a randomized controlled trial. *Am. J. Orthod. Dentofacial Orthop.* 154 (2): 167–174.e1.

Anusavice, S.R. (2013). Materials and processes for cutting, finishing, and polishing. In: *Phillip's Science of Dental Materials* (ed. S.R. Anusavice), 231–253. Elsevier Ltd.

Bae, J.H., Yi, J., Kim, S. et al. (2014). Changes in the cutting efficiency of different types of dental diamond rotary instrument with repeated cuts and disinfection. *J. Prosthet. Dent.* 111 (1): 64–70.

Ben-Hanan, U., Judes, H., and Regev, M. (2008). Comparative study of three different types of dental diamond burs. *Tribol. Mater. Surf. Interfaces* 2 (2): 77–83.

Bitter, N. (1998). A scanning electron microscope study of the long-term effect of bleaching agents on the enamel surface in vivo. *Gen. Dent.* 46 (1): 84–88.

Bosco, E., Iancu Potrubacz, M., Arrizza, L. et al. (2020). Enamel preservation during composite removal after orthodontic debonding comparing hydroabrasion with rotary instruments. *Dent. Mater. J.* 39 (3): 367–374.

Bossù, M., Saccucci, M., Salucci, A. et al. (2019). Enamel remineralization and repair results of biomimetic hydroxyapatite toothpaste on deciduous teeth: an effective option to fluoride toothpaste. *J. Nanobiotechnol.* 17 (1): 1–13.

Brosh, T., Strouthou, S., and Sarne, O. (2005). Effects of buccal versus lingual surfaces, enamel conditioning procedures and storage duration on brackets debonding characteristics. *J. Dent.* 33: 99–105.

Choi, C., Driscoll, C.F., and Romberg, E. (2010). Comparison of cutting efficiencies between electric and air-turbine dental handpieces. *J. Prosthet. Dent.* 103 (2): 101–107.

Coceska, E., Gjorgievska, E., Coleman, N.J. et al. (2016). Enamel alteration following tooth bleaching and remineralization. *J. Microsc.* 262 (3): 232–244.

Cochrane, N.J., Cai, F., Huq, N.L. et al. (2010). Critical review in oral biology & medicine: new approaches to enhanced remineralization of tooth enamel. *J. Dent. Res.* 89 (11): 1187–1197.

David, V.A., Staley, R.N., Bigelow, H.F., and Jacobsen, J.R. (2002). Remnant amount and cleanup for 3 adhesives after debracketing. *Am. J. Orthod. Dentofacial Orthop.* 121 (2): 291–296.

Di Cristofaro, R.G.R., Giner, L., and Mayoral, J.R. (2013). Comparative study of the cutting efficiency and working life of carbide burs. *J. Prosthodont.* 22 (5): 391–396.

Eikenberg, S.L. (2001). Comparison of the cutting efficiencies of electric motor and air turbine dental handpieces. *Gen. Dent.* 49 (2): 199–204.

Eisenburger, M., Addy, M., Hughes, J.A., and Shellis, R.P. (2001). Effect of time on the remineralization of enamel by synthetic saliva after citric acid erosion. *Caries Res.* 35 (3): 211–215.

Eliades, T. (2019). Orthodontic applications of biomaterials. *J. Chem. Inf. Model.* 53: 230.

Elias, K., Amis, A.A., and Setchell, D.J. (2003). The magnitude of cutting forces at high speed. *J. Prosthet. Dent.* 89 (3): 286–291.

Elkassas, D. and Arafa, A. (2014). Remineralizing efficacy of different calcium-phosphate and fluoride based delivery vehicles on artificial caries like enamel lesions. *J. Dent.* 42 (4): 466–474.

Emir, F., Ayyildiz, S., and Sahin, C. (2018). What is the changing frequency of diamond burs? *J. Adv. Prosthodont.* 10 (2): 93–100.

Ercoli, C., Rotella, M., Funkenbusch, P.D. et al. (2009). In vitro comparison of the cutting efficiency and temperature production of 10 different rotary cutting instruments. Part I: turbine. *J. Prosthet. Dent.* 101 (4): 248–261.

Ercoli, C., Rotella, M., Funkenbusch, P.D. et al. (2009). In vitro comparison of the cutting efficiency and temperature production of ten different rotary cutting instruments. Part II: electric handpiece and comparison with turbine. *J. Prosthet. Dent.* 101 (5): 319–331.

Eroglu, A.K., Baka, Z.M., and Arslan, U. (2019). Comparative evaluation of salivary microbial levels and periodontal status of patients wearing fixed and removable orthodontic retainers. *Am. J. Orthod. Dentofacial Orthop.* 156 (2): 186–192.

Featherstone, J.D.B., Shields, C.P., Khademazad, B., and Oldershaw, M.D. (1983). Acid reactivity of carbonated apatites with strontium and fluoride substitutions. *J. Dent. Res.* 62 (10): 1049–1053.

Firoozmand, L., Faria, R., Araujo, M.A. et al. (2008). Temperature rise in cavities prepared by high and low torque handpieces and Er:YAG laser. *Br. Dent. J.* 205 (1): E1.

Fjeld, M. and Ogaard, B. (2006). Scanning electron microscopic evaluation of enamel surfaces exposed to 3 orthodontic bonding systems. *Am. J. Orthod. Dentofacial Orthop.* 130: 575–581.

Flores, T., Mayoral, J., Giner, L., and Puigdollers, A. (2015). Comparison of enamel-bracket bond strength using direct- and indirect-bonding techniques with a self-etching ion releasing S-PRG filler. *Dent. Mater. J.* 34 (1): 41–47.

Flores, T., Mayoral, J.R., Artés, M. et al. (2017). Increase in enamel volume of premolars by remineralization with s-prg filler containing toothpaste following debonding of lingual buttons: an in-vitro nanometric study. *Int. J. Sci. Res.* 7: 539–541.

Fujimoto, Y., Iwasa, M., Murayama, R. et al. (2010). Detection of ions released from S-PRG fillers and their modulation effect. *Dent. Mater. J.* 29 (4): 392–397.

Funkenbusch, P.D., Rotella, M., Chochlidakis, K., and Ercoli, C. (2016). Multivariate evaluation of the cutting performance of rotary instruments with electric and air-turbine handpieces. *J. Prosthet. Dent.* 116 (4): 558–563.

Galindo, D.F., Ercoli, C., Funkenbusch, P.D. et al. (2004). Tooth preparation: a study on the effect of different variables and a comparison between conventional and channeled diamond burs. *J. Prosthodont.* 13 (1): 3–16.

Geminiani, A., Abdel-Azim, T., Ercoli, C. et al. (2014). Influence of oscillating and rotary cutting instruments with electric and turbine handpieces on tooth preparation surfaces. *J. Prosthet. Dent.* 112 (1): 51–58.

Gjorgievska, E.S., Nicholson, J.W., Slipper, I.J., and Stevanovic, M.M. (2013). Remineralization of demineralized enamel by toothpastes: a scanning electron microscopy, energy dispersive X-ray analysis, and three-dimensional stereo-micrographic study. *Microsc. Microanal.* 19 (3): 587–595.

Gugger, J., Pandis, N., Zinelis, S. et al. (2016). Retrieval analysis of lingual fixed retainer adhesives. *Am. J. Orthod. Dentofacial Orthop.* 150 (4): 575–584.

Hahnel, S., Wastl, D.S., Schneider-Feyrer, S. et al. (2014). Streptococcus mutans biofilm formation and release of fluoride from experimental resin-based composites depending on surface treatment and S-PRG filler particle fraction. *J. Adhes. Dent.* 16 (4): 313–321.

Hashimoto, Y., Hashimoto, Y., Nishiura, A., and Matsumoto, N. (2013). Atomic force microscopy observation of enamel surfaces treated with self- etching primer. *Dent. Mater. J.* 32 (1): 181–188.

Hosein, I., Sherriff, M., and Ireland, A.J. (2004). Enamel loss during bonding, debonding, and cleanup with use of a self-etching primer. *Am. J. Orthod. Dentofacial Orthop.* 126: 717–724.

Iglesias, A., Flores, T., Moyano, J. et al. (2020). In vitro study of shear bond strength in direct and indirect bonding with three types of adhesive systems. *Materials (Basel)* 13 (11).

Iijima, M., Ito, S., Nakagaki, S. et al. (2014). Effects of immersion in solution of an experimental toothpaste containing S-PRG filler on like-remineralizing ability of etched enamel. *Dent. Mater. J.* 33 (3): 430–436.

Ikemura, K., Tay, F.R., Endo, T., and Pashley, D.H. (2008). A review of chemical-approach and ultramorphological studies on the development of fluoride-releasing dental adhesives comprising new Pre-Reacted Glass ionomer (PRG) fillers. *Dent. Mater. J.* 27 (3): 315–339.

Ireland, A.J., Hosein, I., and Sherriff, M. (2005). Enamel loss at bond-up, debond and clean-up following the use of a conventional light-cured composite and a resin-modified glass polyalkenoate cement. *Eur. J. Orthod.* 27: 413–419.

Jackson, M.J., Sein, H., and Ahmed, W. (2004). Diamond coated dental bur machining of natural and synthetic dental materials. *J. Mater. Sci. Mater. Med.* 15 (12): 1323–1331.

Janiszewska-Olszowska, J., Szatkiewicz, T., Tomkowski, R. et al. (2014). Effect of orthodontic debonding and adhesive removal on the enamel – current knowledge and future perspectives – a systematic review. *Med. Sci. Monit.* 20: 1991–2001.

Janiszewska-Olszowska, J., Tandecka, K., Szatkiewicz, T. et al. (2015). Three-dimensional analysis of enamel surface alteration resulting from orthodontic clean-up -comparison of three different tools. *BMC Oral Health* 15 (1): 1–7.

Jefferies, S.R. (2007). Abrasive finishing and polishing in restorative dentistry: a state-of-the-art review. *Dent. Clin. N. Am.* 51: 379–397.

Jin, C., Bennani, F., Gray, A. et al. (2018). Survival analysis of orthodontic retainers. *Eur. J. Orthod.* 40 (5): 531–536.

Jones, C.S., Billington, R.W., and Pearson, G.J. (2004). The in vivo perception of roughness of restorations. *Br. Dent. J.* 196 (1): 42–45.

Kaga, M., Kakuda, S., Hashimoto, M. et al. (2014). Inhibition of enamel demineralization by buffering effect of S-PRG filler-containing dental sealant. *Eur. J. Oral Sci.* 122: 78–83.

Kenyon, B.J., Van Zyl, I., and Louie, K.G. (2005). Comparison of cavity preparation quality using an electric motor handpiece and an air turbine dental handpiece. *J. Am. Dent. Assoc.* 136 (8): 1101–1105.

Keszthelyi, G. and Jenei, A. (1999). An atomic force microscopy study on the effect of bleaching agents on enamel surface. *J. Dent.* 27: 509–515.

Lippert, F., Parker, D.M., and Jandt, K.D. (2004). In vitro demineralization/remineralization cycles at human tooth enamel surfaces investigated by AFM and nanoindentation. *J. Colloid Interface Sci.* 280: 442–448.

Memarpour, M., Shafiei, F., Rafiee, A. et al. (2019). Effect of hydroxyapatite nanoparticles on enamel remineralization and estimation of fissure sealant bond strength to remineralized tooth surfaces: an in vitro study. *BMC Oral Health* 19 (1): 1–13.

Mielczarek, A. and Michalik, J. (2014). The effect of nano-hydroxyapatite toothpaste on enamel surface remineraliztion. An in vitro study. *Am. J. Dent.* 27: 287–290.

Nakamura, K., Katsuda, Y., Ankyu, S. et al. (2015). Cutting efficiency of diamond burs operated with electric high-speed dental handpiece on zirconia. *Eur. J. Oral Sci.* 123 (5): 375–380.

Padmos, J.A.D., Fudalej, P.S., and Renkema, A.M. (2018). Epidemiologic study of orthodontic retention procedures. *Am. J. Orthod. Dentofacial Orthop.* 153 (4): 496–504.

Pilcher, E.S., Tietge, J.D., and Draughn, R.A. (2000). Comparison of cutting rates among single-patient-use and multiple-patient-use diamond burs. *J. Prosthodont.* 9: 66–70.

Poggio, C., Dagna, A., Chiesa, M. et al. (2012). Surface roughness of flowable resin composites eroded by acidic and alcoholic drinks. *J. Conserv. Dent.* 15 (2): 137–140.

Prithviraj, D.R., Saraswat, S., Sounderraj, K. et al. (2017). Cutting efficiency and longevity of differenty manufactured dental diamond rotary points – an in vitro study. *J. Appl. Dent. Med. Sci.* 3 (1): 8–14.

Pus, M.D. and Way, D.C. (1980). Enamel loss due to orthodontic bonding with filled and unfilled resins using various clean-up techniques. *Am. J. Orthod. Dentofacial Orthop.* 77 (3): 269–283.

Regev, M., Judes, H., and Ben-Hanan, U. (2010). Wear mechanisms of diamond coated dental burs. *Tribol. Mater. Surf. Interfaces* 4 (1): 38–42.

Reynolds, E.C. (1997). Remineralization of enamel subsurface lesions by casein phosphopeptide-stabilized calcium phosphate solutions. *J. Dent. Res.* 76 (9): 1587–1595.

Reynolds, E.C., Cai, F., Shen, P. et al. (2003). Retention in plaque and remineralization of enamel lesions by various forms of calcium in a mouthrinse or sugar-free chewing gum. *J. Dent. Res.* 82 (3): 206–212.

Rotella, M., Ercoli, C., Funkenbusch, P.D. et al. (2014). Performance of single-use and multiuse diamond rotary cutting instruments with turbine and electric handpieces. *J. Prosthet. Dent.* 111 (1): 56–63.

Ryf, S., Flury, S., Palaniappan, S. et al. (2012). Enamel loss and adhesive remnants following bracket removal and various clean-up procedures in vitro. *Eur. J. Orthod.* 34 (1): 25–32.

Shah, P., Sharma, P., Goje, S.K. et al. (2019). Comparative evaluation of enamel surface roughness after debonding using four finishing and polishing systems for residual resin removal – an in vitro study. *Prog. Orthod.* 20 (1): 18. https://doi.org/10.1186/s40510-019-0269-x.

Shen, R., Cai, F., Nowicki, A. et al. (2001). Remineralization of enamel subsurface lesions by sugar-free chewing gum containing casein calcium phosphate. *J. Dent. Res.* 80 (12): 2066–2071.

Shinya, M., Shinya, A., Lassila, L.V.J. et al. (2008). Treated enamel surface patterns associated with five orthodontic adhesive systems — surface morphology and shear bond strength. *Dent. Mater. J.* 27 (1): 1–6.

Siegel, S.C. and Anthony Von Fraunhofer, J. (1998). Dental cutting: the historical development of diamond burs. *J. Am. Dent. Assoc.* 129 (6): 740–745.

Siegel, S.C. and Patel, T. (2016). Comparison of cutting efficiency with different diamond burs and water flow rates in cutting lithium disilicate glass ceramic. *J. Am. Dent. Assoc.* 147 (10): 792–796.

Siegel, S.C. and Von Fraunhofer, J.A. (1996). Assessing the cutting efficiency of dental diamond burs. *J. Am. Dent. Assoc.* 127 (6): 763–772.

Siegel, S.C. and Von Fraunhofer, J.A. (1997). Effect of handpiece load on the cutting efficiency of dental burs. *Mach. Sci. Technol.* 1 (1): 1–13.

Siegel, S.C. and Von Fraunhofer, A. (1999). Dental cutting with diamond burs: heavy-handed or light-touch? *J. Prosthodont.* 8 (1): 3–9.

Siegel, S.C. and von Fraunhofer, J.A. (2000). Cutting efficiency of three diamond bur grit sizes. *J. Am. Dent. Assoc.* 131 (12): 1706–1710.

Siegel, S.C. and Von Fraunhofer, J.A. (2002). The effect of handpiece spray patterns on cutting efficiency. *J. Am. Dent. Assoc.* 133 (2): 184–188.

Sifakakis, I., Zinelis, S., Patcas, R., and Eliades, T. (2017). Mechanical properties of contemporary orthodontic adhesives used for lingual fixed retention. *Biomed. Tech.* 62 (3): 289–294.

Von Fraunhofer, J.A. and Siegel, S.C. (2000). Enhanced dental cutting through chemomechanical effects. *J. Am. Dent. Assoc.* 131 (10): 1465–1469.

Yamaguchi, K., Miyazaki, M., Takamizawa, T. et al. (2006). Effect of CPP – ACP paste on mechanical properties of bovine enamel as determined by an ultrasonic device. *J. Dent.* 34: 230–236.

Zachrisson, B.U. and Arthun, J. (1979). Enamel surface appearance after various debonding techniques. *Am. J. Orthod.* 75 (2): 121–127.

2

Debonding Protocols

Eser Tüfekçi[1] *and William Brantley*[2]

[1] *Department of Orthodontics, School of Dentistry, Virginia Commonwealth University, Richmond, VA, USA*
[2] *Division of Restorative and Prosthetic Dentistry, College of Dentistry, The Ohio State University, Columbus, OH, USA*

2.1 Introduction

At the end of orthodontic treatment, fixed appliances and residual resin are removed, and the enamel surface is restored as closely as possible to its pretreatment condition. When removing fixed appliances, orthodontists must closely follow the recommended debonding protocols to minimize possible iatrogenic damage to the enamel surface. If not properly carried out, bracket removal procedures may cause enamel cracks and fractures (Fischer-Brandies et al. 1993; Naini and Gill 2008; Strobl et al. 1992).

Throughout orthodontic treatment, fixed appliances need to remain attached to tooth surfaces. According to Reynolds (1975), a shear bond strength of 60–80 kg/cm^2 (6–8 MPa) is appropriate for brackets to withstand occlusal and orthodontic forces while allowing safe bracket and resin removal. (The units for bond strength and alternative use of debonding force are discussed in this chapter's appendix.) Otherwise, frequent bracket failures may affect the progression and outcome of orthodontic treatment (Beckwith et al. 1999; Stasinopoulos et al. 2018).

In the literature, shear bond strength levels well beyond the recommended optimal range of 6–8 MPa have been reported (Rix et al. 2001; Romano

Debonding and Fixed Retention in Orthodontics: An Evidence-Based Clinical Guide, First Edition. Edited by Theodore Eliades and Christos Katsaros.

et al. 2009). The high bond strength of new-generation orthodontic adhesives is mainly attributed to advances in dental materials (Gange 2015; Zhang et al. 2016). Previous studies have shown that stress levels greater than 13 MPa may cause significant enamel damage during the removal process (Retief 1974; Rix et al. 2001).

2.2 Bond Failure Locations during Debonding

The location of a bond failure is important when removing fixed appliances from tooth surfaces. The adhesive remnant index (ARI), a technique to assess the mode of failure between enamel and a bracket base, was first introduced by Artun and Bergland in 1984. Evaluation of the adhesive remaining on the tooth surface plays a role in enamel cleaning procedures following debonding to remove resin and restore the enamel surface as closely as possible to its pretreatment condition. The following scoring system is used to determine the amount of adhesive remaining on the tooth surface:

Score 0 = No adhesive left on the tooth
Score 1 = Less than half of the adhesive left on the tooth
Score 2 = More than half of the adhesive left on the tooth
Score 3 = All adhesive left on the tooth, with a distinct impression of the bracket mesh

Bond failures can occur at the bracket–tooth and bracket–adhesive interfaces (*adhesive failures*) or within the adhesive (*cohesive failures*) (Bishara and Trulove 1990b; Swartz 1988). In general, adhesive bond failure at the bracket–adhesive interface is the most desirable type because it has the least potential to damage the enamel during bracket removal (Ødegaard and Segner,1988). However, adhesive failure at the enamel–adhesive interface is not desirable as it may result in enamel cracks, especially if the shear bond strength levels are well above the optimal 6–8 MPa (Jerioudi 1991; Leão Filho et al. 2015).

The ideal location of bond failure is the subject of ongoing controversy. According to some clinicians, it is preferable to have a failure within the resin (cohesive failure) to decrease the risk of enamel fracture. However, with more resin left on the tooth surface, cohesive failure results in more extensive resin cleanup and chairside time at the debonding appointment than adhesive failure. Also, using a bur for a long time to remove the resin may negatively affect the enamel surface. Because of these drawbacks with cohesive resin failure, other clinicians prefer adhesive failure, which leaves less resin on the tooth surface.

2.3 Protocols for Bracket Removal

The protocols for the removal of brackets include mechanical, ultrasonic, electrothermal and laser debonding. Of these, mechanical debonding is the most popular technique for removing metal brackets: special pliers such as debonding or Howe pliers are used to apply force in a shear, tensile or torsional mode to break the bond at the bracket–resin interface. The force can be applied at the bracket base in a mesial-distal or occlusal-gingival direction. Debonding can also be achieved by squeezing the bracket wings in a mesial-distal direction while lifting the bracket off in a peeling mode. This technique is generally considered safe for removing metal brackets, even on enamel with increased brittleness, such as endodontically treated teeth.

When removing metal brackets, damage to the enamel is not of much concern due to the ductility of the metal (Kusy 1988; Reddy et al. 2013; Swartz 1988). However, when working with ceramic brackets, extra attention is needed during the debonding procedure because of the high bond strength and low fracture toughness of ceramics (Kusy 1988; Scott Jr. 1988; Swartz 1988). The high bond strength of ceramics is attributed to mechanical and chemical bonds (Gwinnett 1988; Kocadereli et al. 2001; Reddy et al. 2013). Unlike ductile metal brackets, the brittle nature of ceramic brackets makes them less flexible and more challenging to peel away from tooth surfaces (Flores et al. 1990; Gwinnett 1988; Kocadereli et al. 2001). Therefore, while enamel damage is rare when removing metal brackets, it is a valid concern with ceramic brackets.

The early ceramic bracket systems using silane coupling for adhesion to bonding agents exhibited excessively high bond strength, causing damage to the enamel at the time of debonding. The nature of the bond between the bracket and adhesive plays a role in the location of bond failure. Mechanical retention usually causes failure at the bracket–adhesive interface, which is preferable to minimize enamel damage. Metal brackets with a mesh base (mechanical) leave more adhesive on the tooth surface than ceramic brackets with chemical retention. Because the chemical bond between the ceramic and adhesive is stronger than the bond between the bracket and enamel, removing these types of brackets usually does not leave resin on the tooth surface, which creates a risk for enamel damage.

Because of this problem, to facilitate ceramic bracket debonding, manufacturers have incorporated a metal part into the bracket design to allow the base to flex and peel off during removal. Modified ceramic brackets with a vertical metal slot or a ball base have been shown to provide easy and safe bracket removal (Bishara and Trulove 1990a,b; Mundstock et al. 1999).

Studies comparing the shear bond strength of metal and ceramic brackets showed that the bond is stronger between the ceramic–adhesive interface than between the metal–adhesive interface (Mirzakouchaki et al. 2012; Ødegaard and Segner 1988). Furthermore, ARI revealed that the location of bond failure is mainly between the enamel and adhesive with ceramic brackets. On the other hand, with metal brackets, bond failure was located between the bracket and the adhesive. In contrast, Mirzakouchaki et al. (2012) reported that teeth with ceramic brackets had more adhesive left on their surfaces than teeth with metal brackets when examined optically at 10X magnification.

Modified ceramic brackets have been shown to exhibit shear bond strength levels and ARI scores similar to metal brackets (Bishara and Trulove 1990a; Ødegaard and Segner 1988). According to previous *in vitro* studies, the most common ARI score is 3, indicating that bond failure frequently occurs between the adhesive and metal brackets (Mundstock et al. 1999; Ryf et al. 2012; Suliman et al. 2015). Similarly, in an *in vivo* study, Bonetti et al. (2011) observed that bond failure took place most frequently at the metal bracket–adhesive interface, with 100% of the resin remaining on tooth surfaces. None of the samples had a score of 0 indicating a failure at the enamel–adhesive interface. The analyses were conducted at 35X magnification.

Bishara and Fehr (1993) evaluated debonding forces during ceramic bracket removal. The debonding force was applied to both sides of the adhesive by placing the plier blades near the enamel surface but within the resin. This method created a crack in the resin, and once the crack was initiated, the force transmitted to the enamel was expressed at much lower levels compared to loading in a shear mode applied at only one side (Gwinnett 1988; Maskeroni et al. 1990). The same study investigated the effect of plier blade width on the debonding force generated during bracket removal. The findings indicated that narrow blades produced a 20% decrease in force levels compared to wider blades. Bishara and Fehr (1993) concluded that this significant reduction in debonding force minimizes the risk of enamel damage.

Sinha et al. (1995) reported that debonding with sharp-edged pliers that apply a bilateral force at the bracket base–adhesive interface was the most effective method for debonding polycrystalline alumina orthodontic brackets.

Arici and Minors (2000) examined various debonding methods for ceramic bracket removal and concluded that the contact area between the plier tips and the adhesive plays an important role in the initial debonding force level. The use of pliers with pointed and sharp tips and the application of force in a diagonal direction were recommended for efficient and safe bracket removal. They found no enamel damage or bracket fracture when these methods were used for ceramic bracket removal.

Su et al. (2012) investigated the effect of three debonding techniques on the enamel surface after bracket removal using stereomicroscopy at 25X magnification. Pliers like Howe and Weingart (the squeezing debracketing technique) and lift-off instruments (the tensile debracketing technique) were shown to leave at least 85% of the resin on tooth surfaces. However, the shearing debracketing technique exhibited low ARI scores (6–12% resin), indicating a high risk of enamel cracks or fractures.

A recent clinical study by Pithon et al. (2015) assessed the level of discomfort in patients during bracket removal with four different debonding pliers. The instruments used were a lift-off debonding instrument, a straight cutter plier that applied pressure to the bracket base in the mesial–distal direction, a Howe plier that deformed the bracket base by applying pressure to the mesial and distal wings, and a bracket removal plier. After debonding, the amount of orthodontic resin remaining on tooth surfaces was also evaluated using a portable microscope to determine the most comfortable debonding technique with the least enamel damage. Although statistically significant differences were not observed among the four techniques, clinical observation revealed that the straight cutter instrument had the lowest ARI scores. Therefore, the authors reported that an adhesive bond failure at the resin–enamel interface could indicate a greater possibility of enamel damage than the other methods. In addition, the straight cutter instrument was noted to cause the highest level of discomfort, while the lift-off plier was found to be the most comfortable debonding tool.

2.4 Ultrasonic Debonding

Another approach for bracket removal uses an ultrasonic device with special tips. Previous studies have reported reduced debonding forces with an ultrasonically employed chisel tip for ceramic bracket removal (Bishara and Trulove 1990b; Boyer et al. 1995; Chen et al. 2015). Bishara and Trulove (1990b) determined that 38–50 seconds of debonding time were needed with the ultrasonic method instead of 1 second with the mechanical approach. In a similar study, Boyer et al. (1995) determined that about 16 seconds were needed to debond brackets ultrasonically. The authors of both studies concluded that although the forces to debond the brackets were much less than for conventional mechanical debonding, the long removal time and need for relatively moderate levels of debonding forces would make this method uncomfortable for patients. Excessive and rapid wear of the expensive ultrasonic tips and the need for water cooling during ultrasonic debonding were additional disadvantages of this method (Bishara and Trulove 1990b). Therefore, despite promising results, ultrasonic bracket removal has never become the method of choice for debonding.

2.5 Electrothermal Debonding

Electrothermal debonding is another recommended method for ceramic bracket removal. It was first described by Sheridan et al. (1986a, b). This technique uses a special heating element to transfer heat to the adhesive (Bishara and Trulove 1990b; Brouns et al. 1993). The heat softens the adhesive resin, allowing removal of the ceramic bracket with low levels of debonding force at the adhesive interface. Electrothermal debonding is reported to decrease debonding forces by 50% (Rueggeberg and Lockwood 1990). The advantages of this technique include decreased ceramic bracket failure, decreased debonding time and minimal potential enamel damage (Bishara and Trulove 1990a).

One concern with electrothermal debonding is the temperature increase in the pulp chamber. Histologic studies on cellular changes in the pulp structures exhibited no pathosis or other abnormal findings (Sheridan et al. 1986b). This finding was later confirmed by Kraut et al. (1991) in a clinical study that evaluated patient comfort level, histologic changes in pulp cells and enamel damage. Debonding was carried out in orthodontic patients whose premolars were scheduled for extraction. Electrothermal debonding was reported to be less traumatic when compared to the conventional debonding method. Furthermore, the histological and enamel surface analyses of the extracted teeth showed no pulpal anomalies or enamel damages. Therefore, the study concluded that electrothermal debonding is a good alternative to mechanical debonding.

Stratmann et al. (1996) compared conventional mechanical and thermal debonding methods for ceramic bracket removal. These authors reported that using a thermal debonding unit to heat the slots of the ceramic brackets provided an efficient means of bracket removal. The site of bond failure was usually at the resin–bracket interface instead of the resin–enamel interface found with the mechanical debonding method. Debonding time was reported to be 2 ± 1 seconds per bracket.

A clinical study by Dovgan et al. (1995) evaluated the time it took to debond brackets with electrothermal debonding along with patient acceptance and pulp changes. It took about two seconds to remove brackets, and patients reported a positive experience. Also, the histological examinations did not reveal pulp necrosis but did find slight odontoblastic disruption. Later studies on the effect of heat on the pulp indicated that electrothermal debonding does not significantly increase intrapulpal temperatures and therefore is safe to use (Jost-Brinkmann et al. 1997; Kailasam et al. 2014).

2.6 Use of Lasers for Debonding

The use of lasers to debond ceramic brackets has been introduced for the prevention of possible enamel cracks and fractures (Ghazanfari et al. 2016; Strobl et al. 1992; Tocchio et al. 1993). Carbon dioxide (CO_2), neodymium-doped yttrium aluminium garnet (Nd:YAG) and erbium-doped yttrium aluminium garnet (Er:YAG) lasers have gained popularity for bracket removal by softening the adhesive. This method is similar to the electrothermal debonding technique, as bracket removal is achieved primarily by softening the orthodontic adhesive with a heat source (Tocchio et al. 1993). However, in contrast to the thermal technique, when using a laser, the heat can be more easily controlled to prevent overheating (Bishara and Fehr 1993; Ma et al. 1997; Mimura et al. 1995; Strobl et al. 1992). In addition to thermal softening, lasers also work with thermal ablation and photoablation mechanisms that cause a rapid increase in the resin temperature, allowing easy removal of the bracket. With thermal ablation, the rapidly increased temperature causes the resin to vaporize. With photoablation, very high-energy laser light interacts with the adhesive (Willenborg 1989). All of these methods allow quick, safe removal of ceramic brackets.

Strobl et al. (1992) evaluated the use of CO_2 and Nd:YAG lasers to debond ceramic brackets. Both types of lasers were reported to provide a safe and efficient means of bracket removal. Ma et al. (1997) reported safe bracket removal with the use of the CO_2 laser. The debonding time was about five seconds, and the force required to debond the brackets was significantly reduced. Similarly, Feldon et al. (2010) reported a decrease in debonding force with the use of diode lasers. Furthermore, the authors noted that when removing monocrystalline ceramic brackets with this type of laser, there was no significant increase in the pulp temperature. Ahrari et al. (2012) evaluated the removal of chemically and mechanically retained ceramic brackets using CO_2 or the conventional method. When brackets were removed with pliers, there was a higher incidence of bracket failure for chemically retained brackets than mechanically retained brackets (45% vs. 15%). However, there were no fractures in either type of brackets when the laser was used for debonding. Furthermore, the authors reported favourable ARI scores (high scores, such as 3) and no pulpal damage.

Oztoprak et al. (2010) have shown that within seconds, using the Er:YAG laser, high bond strength levels may be efficiently decreased to low levels for the safe removal of polycrystalline ceramic brackets. The study showed that as the force levels to debond the bracket decreased, the amount of adhesive remaining on the tooth surface increased (high ARI scores). Furthermore, teeth in the laser group had more adhesive on their surfaces than those in the control group. Therefore, high adhesive retention in the laser group resulted in less or no enamel damage. Mundethu et al. (2014) also showed that brackets can be safely removed with a pulsed laser. Alakus-Sabuncuoglu and Ersahan (2016) have also reported a safe method of removing ceramic brackets using the Er:YAG laser.

Oztoprak et al. (2010) reported that the Er:YAG laser has less of a thermal effect on the bonding agent, with little heat conduction to the pulp. Similarly, other studies on the laser effects of intrapulpal heating and pulpal damage indicated that, if well-controlled, Er:YAG and CO_2 lasers may be safely used (Nalbantgil et al. 2011, 2014). Otherwise, the heat source may be harmful to the pulp because of the high temperatures generated by such lasers (Ma et al. 1997; Wigdor et al. 1993). Yassaei et al. (2015) investigated the efficiency of the diode laser in ceramic bracket debonding. These authors concluded that with its low voltage and low current properties, a diode laser offers an excellent alternative to other laser types without risk to the enamel or pulp. In everyday orthodontic practice, the high cost of lasers is the main drawback.

Hayakawa (2005) reported that using a high-peak-power Nd:YAG laser effectively debonded monocrystalline and polycrystalline ceramic brackets with significantly lower force levels than the conventional method. In contrast, Nasiri et al. (2019) noted that the Nd:YAG laser did not decrease the shear bond strength when removing metal brackets. The laser was also thought to be harmful, as it could significantly increase the pulpal temperature. Therefore, it was concluded that the laser was unsuitable for removing metal brackets.

Overall, when using lasers for bracket debonding, the time spent to remove ceramic brackets, the force levels and the risk of enamel damage are less than with conventional mechanical debonding using pliers (Ghazanfari et al. 2016).

2.7 Guidelines from Manufacturers

Today, orthodontic companies provide debonding guidelines specific to their ceramic brackets. In certain cases, pliers are designed to remove particular bracket brands. According to a recent survey (Ngan et al. 2020), the most common technique for ceramic bracket removal is mechanical debonding. In that survey, most respondents indicated that they were using specially designed bracket-removing pliers from the bracket manufacturer. Interestingly, these clinicians were unaware of ultrasonic, laser and electrothermal debonding methods. Previously, Zachrisson et al. (1980) reported that the ideal way to remove brackets was mechanical debonding, and applying a light force to squeeze the bracket at the base was a simple and efficient means of debracketing. The Ngan et al. (2020) survey results indicate that mechanical debonding is still the preferred method of bracket removal among orthodontists after four decades.

2.A Appendix: Units for Debonding Stress and Consideration of Debonding Force

As previously noted, the adhesive bond strength of the bracket base to tooth enamel is traditionally measured as the shear bond strength, in which some loading member applies a compressive force at the bracket base–enamel interface to cause a sliding motion that results in debonding. While the shear bond strength may represent better clinically relevant conditions, some investigators have alternatively measured the tensile bond strength for the adhesive, using a special loading arrangement to pull the resin-bonded bracket from the tooth surface. Generally, extracted teeth are employed for these *in vitro* bond strength measurements.

The bond strength is usually reported in units of MPa (megapascals), which implies that the debonding stress is relatively uniform across the bracket base and interface exposed to shear or tensile loading. In reality, localized stress concentrations occur during these bond strength tests, and the adhesive resin failure is expected to begin at an area of stress concentration where a defect exists in the resin microstructure. A more appropriate measurement in tests of adhesive bond quality would be the debonding force in grams, which has a more direct meaning to the clinician performing the debonding than an abstract bond strength value in megapascals. These matters and concerns have been discussed in detail by Eliades and Brantley (2000).

References

Ahrari, F., Heravi, F., Fekrazad, R. et al. (2012). Does ultra-pulse CO(2) laser reduce the risk of enamel damage during debonding of ceramic brackets? *Lasers. Med. Sci.* 27: 567–574. https://doi.org/10.1007/s10103-011-0933-y. Epub 2011 Jun 11. PMID: 21667137.

Alakus-Sabuncuoglu, F. and Ersahan, E.E. (2016). Debonding of ceramic brackets by ER: YAG laser. *J. Istanbul. Univ. Fac. Dent.* 50 (2): 24–30.

Arici, S. and Minors, C. (2000). The force levels required to mechanically debond ceramic brackets: an in vitro comparative study. *Eur. J. Orthod.* 22: 327–334.

Artun, J. and Bergland, S. (1984). Clinical trials with crystal growth conditioning as an alternative to acid-etch enamel pretreatment. *Am. J. Orthod.* 85: 333–340. https://doi.org/10.1016/0002-9416(84)90190-8. PMID: 6231863.

Beckwith, F.R., Ackerman, R.J. Jr., Cobb, C.M., and Tira, D.E. (1999). An evaluation of factors affecting duration of orthodontic treatment. *Am. J. Orthod. Dentofacial. Orthop.* 115: 439–447.

Bishara, S.E. and Fehr, D.E. (1993). Comparison of effectiveness of pliers with narrow and wide blades in debonding ceramic brackets. *Am. J. Orthod. Dentofacial. Orthop.* 103: 253–257.

Bishara, S.E. and Trulove, T.S. (1990a). Comparisons of different debonding techniques for ceramic brackets: part I. Background and methods. *Am. J. Orthod. Dentofacial. Orthop.* 98: 145–153.

Bishara, S.E. and Trulove, T.S. (1990b). Comparisons of different debonding techniques for ceramic brackets: an in vitro study. Part II. Findings and clinical implications. *Am. J. Orthod. Dentofacial. Orthop.* 98: 263–273.

Bonetti, G.A., Zanarini, M., Parenti, S.I. et al. (2011). Evaluation of enamel surfaces after bracket debonding: An in-vivo study with scanning electron microscopy. *Am. J. Orthod. Dentofacial Orthop.* 140: 696–702.

Boyer, D.B., Engelhardt, G., and Bishara, S.E. (1995). Debonding orthodontic ceramic brackets by ultrasonic instrumentation. *Am. J. Orthod. Dentofacial. Orthop.* 108: 262–266.

Brouns, E.M.M., Schopf, P.M., and Kocjancic, B. (1993). Electrothermal debonding of ceramic brackets. An in vitro study. *Eur. J. Orthod.* 15: 115–123.

Chen, Y.L., Chen, H.Y., Chiang, Y.C. et al. (2015). Effect of the precrack preparation with an ultrasonic instrument on the ceramic bracket removal. *J. Formos. Med. Assoc.* 114: 704–709. https://doi.org/10.1016/j.jfma.2013.06.006.

Dovgan, J.S., Walton, R.E., and Bishara, S.E. (1995). Electrothermal debracketing: patient acceptance and effects on the dental pulp. *Am. J. Orthod. Dentofacial. Orthop.* 108: 249–255.

Eliades, T. and Brantley, W.A. (2000). The inappropriateness of conventional orthodontic bond strength assessment protocols. *Eur. J. Orthod.* 22: 13–23.

Feldon, P.J., Murray, P.E., Burch, J.G. et al. (2010). Diode laser debonding of ceramic brackets. *Am. J. Orthod. Dentofacial. Orthop.* 138: 458–462.

Fischer-Brandies, H., Kremers, L., Reicheneder, C. et al. (1993). Uber die Schmelzchädigung in Abhängigkeit von der Methode der Bracketentfernung [Enamel damage depending on the method of bracket removal]. *Fortschr Kieferorthop* 54: 64–70. [German].

Flores, D.A., Caruso, J.M., Scott, G.E., and Jeiroudi, M.T. (1990). The fracture strength of ceramic brackets: a comparative study. *Angle. Orthod.* 60: 269–276.

Gange, P. (2015). The evolution of bonding in orthodontics. *Am. J. Orthod. Dentofacial. Orthop.* 147 (4 Suppl): S56–S63.

Ghazanfari, R., Nokhbatolfoghahaei, H., and Alikhasi, M. (2016). Laser-aided ceramic bracket debonding: a comprehensive review. *J. Lasers Med. Sci.* 7: 2–11.

Gwinnett, A.J. (1988). A comparison of shear bond strengths of metal and ceramic brackets. *Am. J. Orthod. Dentofacial. Orthop.* 93: 346–348.

Hayakawa, K. (2005). Nd: YAG laser for debonding ceramic orthodontic brackets. *Am. J. Orthod. Dentofacial. Orthop.* 128: 638–647. https://doi.org/10.1016/j.ajodo.2005.03.018.

Jerioudi, M.J. (1991). Enamel fracture caused by ceramic brackets. *Am. J. Orthod. Dentofacial. Orthop.* 99: 97–99.

Jost-Brinkmann, P.G., Radlanski, R.J., Artun, J., and Loidl, H. (1997). Risk of pulp damage due to temperature increase during thermodebonding of ceramic brackets. *Eur. J. Orthod.* 19: 623–628.

Kailasam, V., Valiathan, A., and Rao, N. (2014). Histological evaluation after electrothermal debonding of ceramic brackets. *Ind. J. Dent. Res.* 25: 143–146.

Kocadereli, I., Canay, S., and Akça, K. (2001). Tensile bond strength of ceramic orthodontic brackets bonded to porcelain surfaces. *Am. J. Orthod. Dentofacial. Orthop.* 119: 617–620.

Kraut, J., Radin, S., Trowbridge, H.I. et al. (1991). Clinical evaluations on thermal versus mechanical debonding of ceramic brackets. *J. Clin. Dent.* 2: 92–96.

Kusy, R.P. (1988). Morphology of polycrystalline alumina brackets and its relationship to fracture toughness and strength. *Angle. Orthod.* 58: 197–203.

Leão Filho, J.C., Braz, A.K., de Araujo, R.E. et al. (2015). Enamel quality after debonding: evaluation by optical coherence tomography. *Braz. Dent. J.* 26: 384–389.

Ma, T., Marangoni, R.D., and Flint, W. (1997). In vitro comparison of debonding force and intrapulpal temperature changes during ceramic orthodontic bracket removal using a carbon dioxide laser. *Am. J. Orthod. Dentofacial. Orthop.* 111: 203–210.

Maskeroni, A.J., Meyers, C.E., and Lorton, L. (1990). Ceramic bracket bonding: a comparison of bond strength with polyacrylic acid and phosphoric acid enamel conditioning. *Am. J. Orthod. Dentofacial. Orthop.* 97: 168–175.

Mimura, H., Deguchi, T., Obata, A. et al. (1995). Comparison of different bonding materials for laser debonding. *Am. J. Orthod. Dentofacial. Orthop.* 108: 267–273.

Mirzakouchaki, B., Kimyai, S., Hydari, M. et al. (2012). Effect of self-etching primer/adhesive and conventional bonding on the shear bond strength in metallic and ceramic brackets. *Med. Oral. Patol. Oral Cir. Bucal.* 1 (17): e164–e170. https://doi.org/10.4317/medoral.17024.

Mundethu, A.R., Gutknecht, N., and Franzen, R. (2014). Rapid debonding of polycrystalline ceramic orthodontic brackets with an ER:YAG laser: an in vitro study. *Lasers. Med. Sci.* 29: 1551–1556.

Mundstock, K.S., Sadowsky, P.L., Lacefield, W., and Bae, S. (1999). An in vitro evaluation of a metal reinforced orthodontic ceramic bracket. *Am. J. Orthod. Dentofacial. Orthop.* 116: 635–641.

Naini, F.B. and Gill, D.S. (2008). Tooth fracture associated with debonding a metal orthodontic bracket: a case report. *World. J. Orthod.* 9 (3): e32–e36.

Nalbantgil, D., Oztoprak, M.O., Tozlu, M., and Arun, T. (2011). Effects of different application durations of ER:YAG laser on intrapulpal temperature change during debonding. *Lasers Med. Sci.* 26: 735–740.

Nalbantgil, D., Tozlu, M., and Oztoprak, M.O. (2014). Pulpal thermal changes following Er-YAG laser debonding of ceramic brackets. *Sci. World J.* https://doi.org/10.1155/2014/912429.

Nasiri, M., Mirhashemi, A.H., Etemadi, A. et al. (2019). Evaluation of the shear bond strength and adhesive remnant index in debonding of stainless steel assisted with Nd:YAG laser irradiation. *Front. Dent.* 16: 37–44. https://doi.org/10.18502/fid.v16i1.1107.

Ngan, A.Y., Bollu, P., Chaudry, K. et al. (2020). Survey on awareness and preference of ceramic bracket debonding techniques among orthodontists. *J. Clin. Exp. Dent.* 12: e656–e662.

Ødegaard, J. and Segner, D. (1988). Shear bond strength of metal brackets compared with a new ceramic bracket. *Am. J. Orthod. Dentofacial. Orthop.* 94: 201–206. https://doi.org/10.1016/0889-5406(88)90028-5.

Oztoprak, M.O., Nalbantgil, D., Erdem, A.S. et al. (2010). Debonding of ceramic brackets by a new scanning laser method. *Am. J. Orthod. Dentofacial. Orthop.* 138: 195–200.

Pithon, M.M., Santos Fonseca Figueiredo, D., Oliveira, D.D., and Coqueiro Rda, S. (2015). What is the best method for debonding metallic brackets from the patient's perspective? *Prog. Orthod.* 16 (17): https://doi.org/10.1186/s40510-015-0088-7.

Reddy, Y.G., Sharma, R., Singh, A. et al. (2013). The shear bond strengths of metal and ceramic brackets: an in-vitro comparative study. *J. Clin. Diagn. Res.* 7: 1495–1497.

Retief, D.H. (1974). Failure at the dental adhesive-etched enamel interface. *J. Oral Rehabil.* 1: 265–284.

Reynolds, I.R. (1975). A review of direct orthodontic bonding. *Brit. J. Orthod.* 2: 171–178.

Rix, D., Foley, T.F., and Mamandras, A. (2001). Comparison of bond strength of three adhesives: composite resin, hybrid GIC, and glass-filled GIC. *Am. J. Orthod. Dentofacial. Orthop.* 119: 36–42.

Romano, F., Correr, A., and Sobrinho, L. (2009). Shear bond strength of metallic brackets bonded with a new orthodontic composite. *Braz. J. Oral. Sci.* 8: 76–80.

Rueggeberg, F.A. and Lockwood, P.E. (1990). Thermal debracketing of orthodontic resins. *Am. J. Orthod. Dentofacial. Orthop.* 98: 56–65.

Ryf, S., Flury, S., Palaniappan, S. et al. (2012). Enamel loss and adhesive remnants following bracket removal and various clean-up procedures in vitro. *Eur. J. Orthod.* 34: 25–32. https://doi.org/10.1093/ejo/cjq128.

Scott, G.E. Jr. (1988). Fracture toughness and surface cracks – the key to understanding ceramic brackets. *Angle. Orthod.* 58: 5–8.

Sheridan, J.J., Brawley, G., and Hastings, J. (1986a). Electrothermal debracketing. Part 1. An in vitro study. *Am. J. Orthod.* 89: 21–27.

Sheridan, J.J., Brawley, G., and Hastings, J. (1986b). Electrothermal debracketing. Part II. An in vivo study. *Am. J. Orthod.* 89: 141–145.

Sinha, P.K., Rohrer, M.D., Nanda, R.S., and Brickman, C.D. (1995). Interlayer formation and its effect on debonding polycrystalline ceramic orthodontic brackets. *Am. J. Orthod. Dentofacial. Orthop.* 108: 455–463.

Stasinopoulos, D., Papageorgiou, S.N., Kirsch, F. et al. (2018). Failure patterns of different bracket systems and their influence on treatment duration: a retrospective cohort study. *Angle. Orthod.* 88: 338–347.

Stratmann, U., Schaarschmidt, K., Wegener, H., and Ehmer, U. (1996). The extent of enamel surface fractures. A quantitative comparison of thermally debonded ceramic and mechanically debonded metal brackets by energy dispersive micro- and image-analysis. *Eur. J. Orthod.* 18: 655–662.

Strobl, K., Bahns, T.L., Wiliham, L. et al. (1992). Laser-aided debonding of orthodontic ceramic brackets. *Am. J. Orthod. Dentofacial. Orthop.* 101: 152–158.

Su, M.Z., Lai, E.H., Chang, J.Z. et al. (2012). Effect of simulated debracketing on enamel damage. *J. Formos. Med. Assoc.* 111: 560–566. https://doi.org/10.1016/j.jfma.2011.12.008.

Suliman, S.N., Trojan, T.M., Tantbirojn, D., and Versluis, A. (2015). Enamel loss following ceramic bracket debonding: a quantitative analysis in vitro. *Angle. Orthod.* 85: 651–656. https://doi.org/10.2319/032414-224.1.

Swartz, M.L. (1988). Ceramic brackets. *J. Clin. Orthod.* 22: 82–88.

Tocchio, R.M., Williams, P.T., Mayer, F.J., and Standing, K.G. (1993). Laser debonding of ceramic brackets. *Am. J. Orthod. Dentofacial. Orthop.* 103: 155–162.

Wigdor, H., Abt, E., Ashrafi, S., and Walsh, J.T. Jr. (1993). The effect of lasers on dental hard tissues. *J. Am. Dent. Assoc.* 124: 65–70.

Willenborg, G.C. (1989). Dental laser applications: emerging to maturity. *Lasers Surg. Med.* 9: 309–313. https://doi.org/10.1002/lsm.1900090402.

Yassaei, S., Soleimanian, A., and Nik, Z.E. (2015). Effect of diode laser debonding of ceramic brackets on enamel surface and pulpal temperature. *J. Contemp. Dent. Pract.* 16: 270–274.

Zachrisson, B.U., Skogan, O., and Höymyhr, S. (1980). Enamel cracks in debonded, debanded, and orthodontically untreated teeth. *Am. J. Orthod.* 77: 307–319.

Zhang, Z.C., Qian, Y.F., Yang, Y.M. et al. (2016). Bond strength of metal brackets bonded to a silica-based ceramic with light-cured adhesive. *J. Orofacial. Orthop. (Fortschritte der Kieferorthopädie)* 77: 366–372.

3

Bonding and Debonding Considerations in Orthodontic Patients Presenting Enamel Structural Defects

Despina Koletsi[1], *T. Gerald Bradley*[2], *and Katerina Kavvadia*[3]

[1] *Clinic of Orthodontics and Pediatric Dentistry, Center of Dental Medicine, University of Zurich, Zurich, Switzerland*
[2] *School of Dentistry, University of Louisville, Louisville, Kentucky, USA*
[3] *Department of Dentistry, School of Medicine, European University Cyprus, Nicosia, Cyprus*

3.1 Introduction

Developmental defects of tooth structure, mainly represented by amelogenesis imperfect (AI), enamel hypoplasia, molar incisor hypomineralisation (MIH), and enamel fluorosis, create a challenging clinical dilemma for the dentist and the orthodontist – the latter particularly when the requirements for fixed appliance orthodontic treatment are profound. Routine procedures such as bonding and debonding strategies at the beginning and/or end of treatment, as well as during therapy, with potential rounds of rebracketing, impose the greatest burden of caution and risk for (additional) tooth damage.

Much of the knowledge about these developmental defects originates from research in restorative, operative and paediatric dentistry and dental materials. Such defects occur during the development of the enamel and can be qualitative and/or quantitative. Due to challenges encountered in the adhesion of restorative materials, efficient bonding of orthodontic brackets may be impaired. The minimum bond strength of orthodontic brackets suggested to withstand normal orthodontic forces is between 6 and 8 MPa. However, the bond strength for hypocalcified,

Debonding and Fixed Retention in Orthodontics: An Evidence-Based Clinical Guide, First Edition. Edited by Theodore Eliades and Christos Katsaros.

hypoplastic and fluorotic teeth is compromised. Furthermore, upon debonding, detachment of the brackets and removal of the bonded adhesion material has been associated with additional loss of dental tissue. The enamel tears or cracks in a way that the thin, fragile and friable defective enamel in patients presenting enamel developmental defects may chip away more easily. Enamel microcracks in debonded teeth can cause plaque stagnation areas with increased staining and therefore are at higher risk for the development of caries (Zachrisson et al. 1980). Increasing bond strength, however, can make detachment and debonding of orthodontic appliances more laborious, thus risking greater enamel damage. It has been reported that fractures occur more frequently when bond strength exceeds a certain threshold. A gold standard must be achieved between effective bond strength for bonding and effective and efficient debonding in order to avoid irreversible damage to the enamel (Bishara et al. 1993).

The aim of this chapter is to map the evidence regarding enamel preparation challenges in bonding and debonding of fixed orthodontic appliances for the management of cases with enamel structural defects, as well as to propose relevant considerations for clinical practice.

3.2 General Considerations and Challenges of Bonding and Debonding Strategies

Enamel preparation and acid-etching come first in consideration of orthodontic bonding. The mechanism of enamel etching has been well described through the years, while for orthodontic bonding, orthophosphoric acid in concentrations less than 37% and/or less time, compared to etching for restorative purposes, has been proposed (Eliades 2006).

Given the interactions of the etching agent with the enamel structure (Buonocore 1981), loss of superficial layers of tissue varying between 20 and 50 μm after conditioning has been reported, which concurrently enables resin tags from the adhesive of the bracket base surface during bonding to penetrate the enamel layers (Silverstone et al. 1975). Thus, sufficient bracket bond strength is anticipated analogously with enamel bonding with restorative materials. Notwithstanding, this mostly standard process of enamel preparation, which takes place in a relatively sound tooth substance, poses certain implications and considerations when teeth with developmental defects are treated. The ultimate bonding outcome depends on intrinsic factors related to the extent and severity of the developmental defect and also on the management approach. The bracket–enamel interface is the key. For intact enamel, it has been shown that bonding and debonding rounds during the course of treatment may induce surface structural changes, especially in areas where thinner enamel layers are located, while in general, the mechanical properties of the tissue are not altered (Ioannidis et al. 2018). No evidence exists for enamel with developmental defects; however, it has been reported that tissues with mineral loss and more brittle conformations have reduced hardness and fracture more easily (van Dorp et al. 1990; Faria-e-Silva et al. 2011).

Enamel breakdown and variations in porosity and hardness of the tooth substance are likely to affect the success of bonding restorative materials (Lagarde et al. 2020) while also affecting the bond strength of fixed orthodontic appliances (Shahabi et al. 2014). Efforts have been instigated to identify potential conditioning agents to demineralise the enamel prior to bracket bonding to create a specific environment for enhanced bond strength to the tooth surface.

One of the most commonly studied parameters is the application of self-etching primers, since they exhibit shorter resin tags within the enamel, as evidenced by scanning electron microscopy studies, and simultaneously present acceptable levels of bonding retention (Kanemura et al. 1999). As such, one might consider the method more suitable for cases where enamel defects exist and minimal destruction of the tissue is required (Eliades 2006). *In vitro* evidence from hypoplastic teeth presenting AI has suggested comparable tensile bond strength values between teeth prepared with self-etching and etchant-rinse adhesive systems; conditioning practices with self-etching primer have been associated with the creation of a rougher and more grooved enamel surface (Yaman et al. 2014). A recent systematic review of MIH-affected teeth made similar findings regarding the use of self-etching adhesives. Investigation of conditioning agents such as sodium hypochlorite to produce deproteinisation of the enamel substrate has also been considered (Lagarde et al. 2020). The latest evidence from restorative research has suggested that deproteinisation after conventional etching and rinse practices is beneficial with regard to bond strength of MIH-affected teeth

(Lagarde et al. 2020; Sönmez and Saat 2017). Research on other developmental defects such as AI-affected teeth also supports a beneficial effect of deproteinisation (Ahmed et al. 2019), and evidence of null effects of the deproteinising agent stems from experimental animal studies (Pugach et al. 2014).

Nonetheless, debonding strategies to protect the integrity and structure of the compromised enamel structure have not been widely studied, and evidence is scarce to date. The destructive potential and effects of debonding in conjunction with the inevitable side effects of the etching stage prior to bonding have long been recognised with regard to previously intact enamel (Eliades 2006). However, there is evidence that the structural conformation and optical properties of the enamel are affected even in non-etching mediated bonding, i.e. upon utilisation of glass ionomer bonding cement (Eliades et al. 2004). It has been speculated that the debonding process imposes the greatest burden of damage on the enamel substrate, rather than the procedures involved in the preparation of the tissue for bonding (Eliades 2006; Øgaard et al. 2004). In addition, the type of fixed appliances and use of brackets have also been investigated for increased risk of enamel surface damage, with ceramic brackets being 20% more likely to produce enamel cracks and enamel structure damage following debonding (Dumbryte et al. 2015). As such, caution should be exhibited when treating teeth affected with developmental defects, and the treatment modalities and adjuncts should be carefully selected.

There is currently no empirical report on the most effective strategy for adhesive-resin cleanup after debonding when an enamel defect exists. Knowledge in the field may be retrieved from classic evidence related to cutting instrumentation in practice (Siegel and von Frauhofer 1999a,b). In this respect, the selection of a tungsten bur may be preferred versus a diamond cutting bur due to the mode of action: the tungsten bur follows a plastic flow cutting process and is more suitable for effectively cutting ductile substrates like composites, using great caution on the interface between the defected enamel and adhesive remnants. On the other hand, diamond burs generate significant tensile stress and chip formation, leading to the propagation of cracks in the material that may continue within the enamel (Eliades and Koletsi 2020).

Currently, novel cutting instrumentation materials – fibre-glass or fibre-reinforced composite burs – are under investigation for achieving smoother composite removal. After resin cleanup, these materials have been reported to produce enamel surfaces with minimal roughness that resemble intact natural enamel (Shah et al. 2019).

3.3 Enamel Structural Defects

Amelogenesis imperfecta (AI) represents a group of developmental conditions, genomic in origin, which affect the structure and clinical appearance of enamel and may be associated with morphologic or biochemical changes elsewhere in the body, affecting general health status. AI prevalence varies from 1:700 to 1:14.000 (conditional on the population under study) and presents with four distinct enamel phenotypes (Witkop 1989), as seen in Table 3.1. The enamel may present as hypoplastic (HPAI), hypocalcified (HCAI), hypomineralised (HMAI), or hypocalcified and hypomineralised (HCMAI); and affected teeth may be discoloured, sensitive or prone to disintegration (Pires Dos Santos et al. 2008; Seow 2014). Diagnosis is based on the family history, pedigree plotting and detailed clinical observation of the phenotype. Inheritance patterns may be autosomal dominant, autosomal recessive, sex-linked and sporadic. Recent evidence shows mutations in one of the genes AMEL, ENAM, FAM83H, WDR72, KLK4 and MMP20 known to affect enamel formation and associated with half of the AI phenotypes. In the other half, the genes involved are currently unknown (Seow 2014). Regarding orthodontic considerations, children with AI may exhibit a greater prevalence of anterior open bite malocclusion and accelerated tooth eruption than the unaffected population (Chen et al. 2013). Bracket failure has also been reported as a prevalent situation.

Applying fixed appliances for AI patients presents a challenge to achieve satisfactory adhesion to the defective enamel in bonding and to determine whether the enamel surface and structure are capable of withstanding both the forces applied during the active phase of orthodontic treatment and the bracket removal stress during debonding (Alachioti et al. 2014; Arkutu et al. 2012). Often the bonding capacity of conventionally and acid-etched brackets is compromised, leading to multiple bond failures during treatment and the need to step back to handle the treatment of individual teeth, thus increasing treatment duration (Arkutu et al. 2012). For patients with defective enamel, such as those with AI, the risk of fractures of the fragile enamel at the

Table 3.1 Enamel defects and orthodontics: amelogenesis imperfecta.

	AI oral phenotype	Enamel findings	Radiographic findings	Type of enamel defect	Enamel defects and tooth development	Bonding considerations
Amelogenesis imperfecta (AI) (Witkop 1989) Prevalence is 1 : 700 to 1 : 14000 depending on the population studied.	Hypoplastic (HPAI) 60–73% of AI 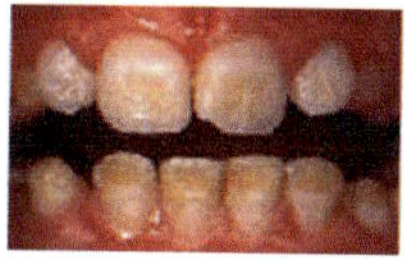	Enamel of reduced thickness. Surface smooth, rough, pitted or grooved	Enamel contrasts normally from dentin. 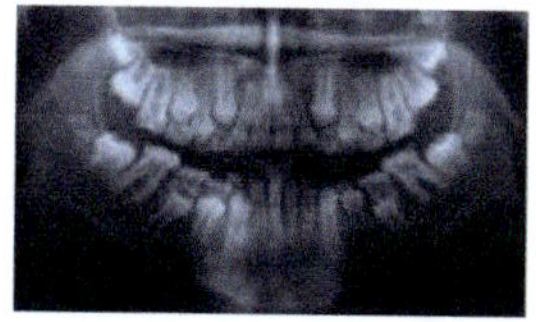	Quantitative	Aposition	Smooth – Pitted + Debonding concerns
	Hypomaturation (HMAI) 20–40% of AI 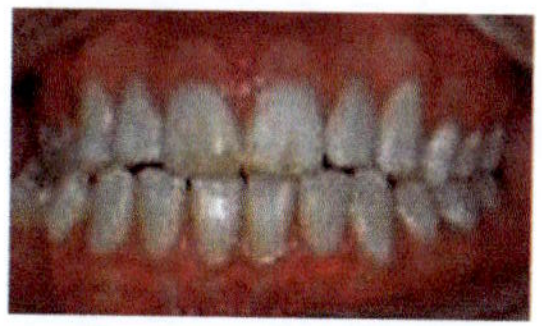	Normal thickness of enamel, moulted appearance, soft, chips away Calculus formation	Enamel has same radiopacity as dentin.	Qualitative	Pre-eruptive maturation	Bonding and debonding concerns Alternative orthodontic methods

Hypocalcified (HCAI) 7% of AI 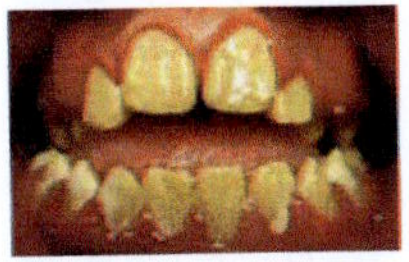	Normal thickness of enamel, friable, soft, rapidly disintegrating, orange-yellow at eruption Tooth sensitivity, staining and calculus formation	Enamel less radiopaque than dentin 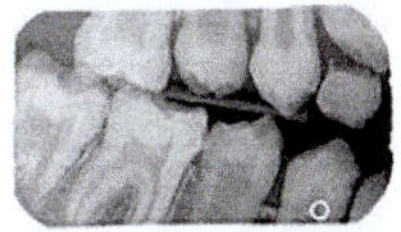	Qualitative	Calcification	NaOCl 5% deproteinisation (Ahmed et al. 2019; Saroğlu et al. 2006; Venezie et al. 1994) Debonding concerns
Hypoplastic and hypomaturation 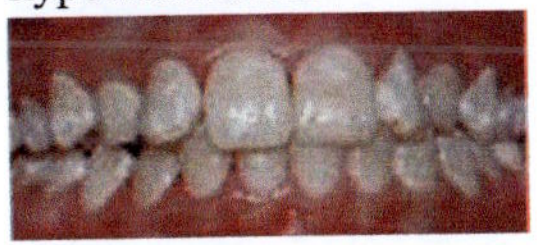	Enamel has moulted appearance, white, yellow, brown, pitted Thin hypomaturation areas that may be softer	Enamel with same radiopacity as dentin Molar taurodontism	Quantitative and qualitative	Aposition Pre-eruptive maturation	Debonding concerns Alternative orthodontic methods

bracket–tooth interface may dramatically increase during bond failures within the treatment course or at the debonding stage.

3.3.1 Bonding/Debonding Considerations for AI Subtypes

Although the challenges of orthodontic bonding in AI patients have been previously reported (Arkutu et al. 2012; Chen et al. 2013), evidence from clinical research is limited. The evidence for managing bonding considerations comes from reports of cases of orthodontic bonding in HCAI patients (Venezie et al. 1994), from extrapolation of ex vivo studies on primary teeth with HCAI on bonding for restorative procedures in general (Ahmed et al. 2019; Saroğlu et al. 2006) and from a systematic review of the subject (Dashash et al. 2013). For HMAI cases, there is practically no evidence in the literature regarding bonding management procedures in orthodontic patients.

Diagnosis of the specific AI phenotype is considered important to decide on the appropriate orthodontic management approach and bonding technique (Arkutu et al. 2012; Chen et al. 2013). In patients with HPAI, the enamel defect appears quantitative but otherwise normal. This means the enamel–adhesion material interaction during bonding may be done using customary bonding procedures and materials, with extra caution during the acid etching stage and application of reduced-concentration orthophosphoric acid for a limited time. Nevertheless, concerns exist about debonding procedures for HPAI teeth due to the thin enamel.

In patients with HCAI, the defect is qualitative: the enamel is more porous and has lower mineral content than sound enamel. It consists of a poorly calcified matrix that disintegrates rapidly and leaves the dentin largely exposed. The enamel is weaker and is practically insufficient for bonding, and fractures may be anticipated during debonding. Earlier studies have reported high failure rates of resin-bonded restorations to HCAI-affected teeth (Koruyucu et al. 2014), mostly attributed to alterations in the enamel surface and its high protein content. Since bonding between enamel and adhesive restorations is largely dependent on the retentive capacity of the enamel, strategies to achieve optimum adhesion have been described and may be framed under the clinical decisions to remove the excess organic matter and acquired pellicle prior to acid etching (Ahmed et al. 2019). Deproteinisation of the enamel with sodium hypochlorite

(NaOCl; household bleach) has been proposed in HCAI enamel to overcome this problem. The first attempt at this approach was described in 1994 by Venezie et al. in an HCAI patient, where 5% NaOCl was applied for one minute prior to etching with phosphoric acid. The technique resulted in a bracket successfully bonded to a tooth affected by HCAI, followed by a clinically successful acid etch pattern, with no further complications reported. Sodium hypochlorite is known to be an excellent protein denaturant, acting by removing organic material and excess protein surrounding the enamel crystals to improve the quality of the etch and bond strength in AI cases (Saroğlu et al. 2006; Venezie et al. 1994). It has been used in AI, but only in hypocalcified teeth. Various protocols of NaOCl 5% application (one minute use) have been investigated, both as a pretreatment, i.e. before etching (Ahmed et al. 2019), and after acid etching (Saroğlu et al. 2006), resulting in significant improvement of the etching pattern and greater shear bond strength, respectively.

In cases of hypomaturation AI (HMAI), the enamel defect is qualitative; the enamel contains excessive organic material with small, disorganised enamel crystals that become porous over time. It is softer, stains easily and chips away, leaving exposed dentin; thus, bonding and debonding may be challenging. There is no previous evidence regarding bonding in HMAI. Restoring HMAI is usually recommended before restorative material placement to remove all defective enamel and apply bonding directly to the dentine (Ahmed et al. 2019). However, for bracket bonding, removing enamel prior to bracket placement is considered utterly destructive. NaOCl pretreatment of the enamel is not recommended for HMAI cases, as this would probably add to the destruction of the enamel and remove large portions of enamel protein. The enamel mineral content of HMAI teeth may be extremely low and make any effort to apply bracket bonding directly to the hypomaturated enamel unsuitable. Moreover, for combined HMCAI cases, material adhesion and bonding may be further complicated and disrupted by rapid and excessive calculus formation (Venezie et al. 1994).

Overall, to date, a number of alternative methods have been proposed to reduce the risk of enamel destruction upon bonding and/or debonding and offer increased retention and stability of appliances – plastic brackets, glass ionomer cement base adhesives, and traditional banded appliances – however, the evidence is weak. Plastic brackets may be used instead of metal or ceramic brackets when there are greater aesthetic demands, as they can easily be removed with a handpiece plier at debonding and minimise the risk of enamel damage (Arkutu et al. 2012). However, material properties should be carefully examined to ensure the use of an effective bracket system for successful tooth movement. Plastic brackets may experience significant creep deformation upon torsional loading, leading to considerations for specific types of tooth movement (Eliades 2007).

Traditional banded appliances are old-fashioned and generally out of clinical use for teeth other than molars. However, such appliances may be used selectively for specific teeth (i.e. premolars that are beyond the aesthetic zone) to overcome some adhesion and debonding problems. Furthermore, in cases of minimal clinical crown height where standard banding is not possible, the use of preformed stainless steel crowns with welded tubes or brackets is recommended. Using such coverage crowns may help prevent an excessive decrease in tooth height as a result of the developmental defect and may also enable bite raising following orthodontic treatment to aid restoration placement. However, these techniques may have shortcomings related to the availability of chair time for the clinician and patient and aesthetic considerations (Chen et al. 2013). Using removable appliances also constitutes a viable treatment option in certain cases requiring minimal and specific orthodontic tooth movement strategies, with no involvement of any fixed adjunct (Eliades and Koletsi 2020).

In summary, orthodontic considerations and perspectives for AI cases should be based on the type of developmental defect. HPAI cases should be managed through customary bonding/debonding procedures, while in HCAI cases, one may proceed with deproteinisation by applying NaOCl either before or after etching. For HMAI and/or HMCAI cases, any bonding/debonding of fixed appliances must consider the increased risk for further enamel damage, and fixed appliance application should be avoided if possible. In addition, for the latter, evidence is weak or non-existent.

3.3.2 Enamel Hypoplasia and Molar Incisor Hypomineralisation

Enamel hypoplasia is a quantitative defect presenting as reduced enamel thickness including pits, grooves and/or irregular areas of missing enamel. Clinically, hypoplasia may show great variation in the number of teeth affected and is rarely of regular shape (Table 3.2). The borders of the hypoplastic enamel lesions are mostly regular and

Table 3.2 Enamel defects and orthodontics: molar incisor hypomineralisation (MIH), enamel hypoplasia and fluorosis.

	Oral phenotype	Enamel findings	Type of enamel defect	Tooth development stage	Bonding considerations
MIH	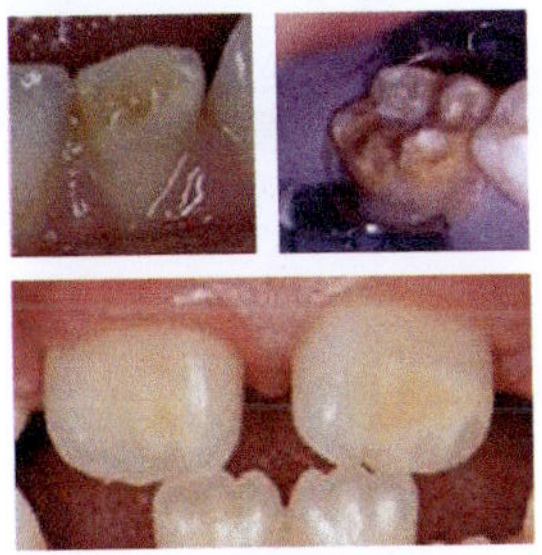	Demarcated enamel opacities, white or brown, with or no enamel breakdown, irregular apatite and porous enamel structure	Qualitative	Calcification	Bond strength does not seem to be affected.
Enamel hypoplasia	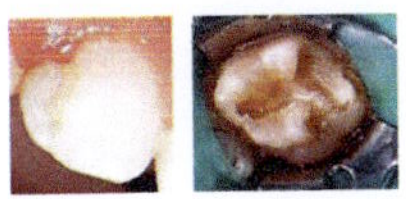	Thinner layer of enamel	Quantitative	Aposition	Enamel restoration prior to bracket placement

(*Continued*)

Table 3.2 (Continued)

	Oral phenotype	Enamel findings	Type of enamel defect	Tooth development stage	Bonding considerations
Fluorosis	Mild 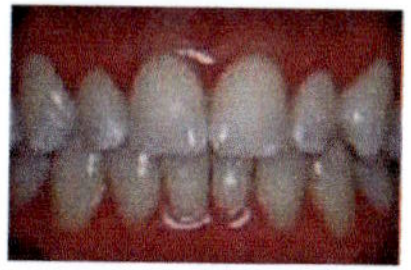 Moderate 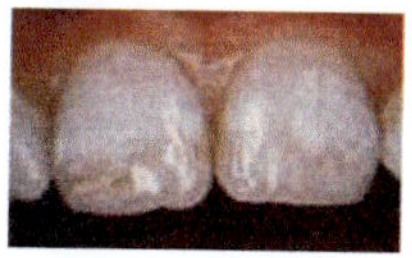 Severe 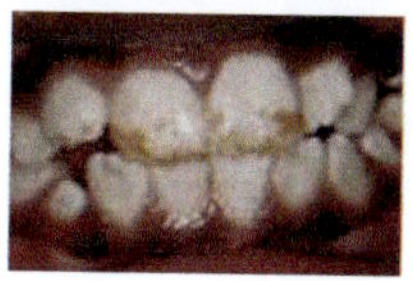	Enamel hypomineralisation with subsurface porosities due to excessive fluoride on ameloblasts during enamel formation, resulting in white opacities presenting as striations affecting homologous teeth In severe cases, possible enamel pitting of the brittle surface may occur as well as post-eruption enamel breakdown.	Qualitative	Calcification	Bracket bond strength may be negatively impacted. Adhesion promoters (Baherimoghadam et al. 2016) Deproteinisation (Sharma et al. 2017)

smooth, indicating a developmental, pre-eruptive lack of enamel matrix formation (Ghanim et al. 2017). For teeth with enamel hypoplasia, defects should be restored to ensure a smooth surface prior to bracket placement. There are currently no clinical reports on bracket bonding and enamel hypoplasia.

Molar incisor hypomineralisation (MIH) is a quantitative defect of the enamel, a type of chronological enamel hypoplasia. Clinically, permanent molars and incisors show demarcated areas of hypomineralisation or opacities, which may be coloured yellow or brownish (Table 3.2). They microscopically correspond to a less dense prism structure with loosely arranged apatite crystals and larger prism sheaths, with significantly reduced mineral density compared to sound enamel, possibly due to retention of proteins during enamel maturation. The irregular apatite and porous enamel structure lead to disruption of bonded margins, post-eruptive enamel breakdown or even restoration loss. In severe cases of MIH, the dentin may also be affected, leading to additional tooth destruction and hypersensitivity. MIH prevalence has been reported (mostly in Europe) to range from 3.6 to 37.5% (Lagarde et al. 2020; Seow 2014).

Regarding adhesion of restorative material to MIH teeth, findings from laboratory and clinical studies highlight the decreased bond strength to affected enamel, attributed to an uneven etching pattern, reduced micro tags within the prism rod, prism capacity to retain moisture and increased protein content (Lagarde et al. 2020).

Deproteinisation of the enamel with NaOCl has been introduced to improve bond strength and adhesion. Results of a clinical study over a two-year period revealed a significantly higher survival rate of resin composites (Sönmez and Saat 2017). However, the results of *in vitro* studies are not in line with the use of NaOCl (Lagarde et al. 2020). Reinforcing the porous enamel with an infiltrant application such as Icon before bonding to increase bond strength and further diminish enamel cracks upon debonding could also be a consideration; however, Icon exhibits inconsistent penetration in MIH-affected enamel (Marouane and Manton 2021). Evidence has revealed erratic or poor penetration of Icon in MIH-affected enamel, regardless of whether etching was performed with phosphoric or hydrochloric acid. The combined use of infiltrants and additional NaOCl application on affected MIH enamel did not significantly enhance bonding agents (Krämer et al. 2018).

Applying a weekly fluoride varnish for a four-week period has also been proposed prior to sealant placement to enhance retention of the material. The fluoride acts through remineralisation of the enamel surface, thus increasing sealant adherence (de Souza et al. 2017).

No clinical studies have been published on orthodontic bonding for MIH-affected teeth and related survival outcomes, possibly because this does not present a significant clinical challenge. The enamel defect is often localised more occlusally and thus does not affect or partially affects the bracket placement position. In severe cases of MIH in anterior teeth, however, when enamel breakdown has occurred, restoration of the defect is essential prior to fixed appliance orthodontic treatment. Furthermore, as with restorative material adhesion, deproteinisation may be considered to enhance the bond strength in severely affected teeth with extended defects covering the entirety of the buccal tooth surface. The latest evidence from a survey on clinical decision-making regarding managing MIH-affected molar teeth reveals that such cases should be managed under a multidisciplinary clinic structure. Meticulous treatment planning and considerations for repeated restorations or even removal of severely affected teeth and orthodontic space closure are appropriate alternatives (Alkadhimi et al. 2022).

3.3.3 Fluorosis

Dental fluorosis refers to developmental defects of enamel induced by fluoride. Dental fluorosis presents as enamel hypomineralisation induced by excessive ingestion of fluoride, i.e. >0.05 mg/kg, which is deposited in the developing tooth during the enamel formation stage and specifically during the secretory and maturation phases of amelogenesis (DenBesten 1999). In fluorosis, the presence and effect of excessive fluoride on ameloblasts during enamel formation result in surface and subsurface porosities. The prevalence of children and adolescents with dental fluorosis ranges between 4 and 70%, with the mildest forms being the most common. Mildly fluorosed teeth are characterised by narrow, diffuse, poorly demarcated enamel, bilateral white lines and increased subsurface porosity. The more severe forms may include a yellow/brownish colouration, and the enamel may present pre-eruptive or post-eruptive breakdown, which may subsequently lead to a greater susceptibility to dental caries.

The order of macroscopic changes is closely linked to a progressive increase in the extent and degree of subsurface porosity or hypomineralisation. A pore volume surpassing a threshold level (10–15%) may favour mechanical damage of the brittle enamel surface during mastication, resulting in pit formation. The severity and distribution of fluorosis depend on the fluoride concentration, the duration of exposure to fluoride, the stage of ameloblast activity and individual variation in susceptibility. Clinically, it is characterised by a pattern of white opacities affecting homologous teeth. The opacities may vary from minor white striations to small or extensive areas of lustreless, opaque enamel and post-eruptive brown staining or enamel pitting (Cutress and Suckling 1990). Several indices have been used in epidemiologic studies, and the most commonly referred to is the classical Dean index (scoring system: 1 = very mild, 2 = mild, 3 = moderate, 4 = severe) (Thylstrup and Fejerskov 1978) (Table 3.2).

Orthodontists may be particularly challenged in geographic areas where fluorosis is endemic. Bracket failure occurs in fluorosed teeth as it is difficult to etch the outer enamel surface during bonding because it is hypermineralised and acid resistant. The reduction in acid solubility of the enamel has been attributed to the incorporation of fluoride in the enamel crystals during the developmental stages of the teeth, resulting in more insoluble fluorapatite crystals. Thus, the tensile bond strength of fluorosed teeth may be negatively impacted (Trakinienė et al. 2019).

A further challenge and consideration for fluorosed teeth may appear during the removal of the fixed appliances: additional and longer enamel microcracks may occur due to the fragile nature of the enamel compared to healthy teeth. This is mainly attributed to the subsurface of fluorotic enamel being extensively hypomineralised, contributing to a greater risk of enamel damage during bracket removal when debonding force is applied (Trakinienė et al. 2019). Applying adhesion protocols that involve promoters has been suggested as an alternative method to improve shear bond strength in orthodontically treated fluorosed cases with fixed appliances. Results of a recent ex vivo study in extracted premolars demonstrated that although adhesion promoters may significantly improve bond strength, their use resulted in excess enamel cracks upon debonding compared to the conventional bonding method (Baherimoghadam et al. 2016).

Deproteinisation of the enamel before bonding on fluorosed enamel has also been suggested as a pretreatment method to increase the bond strength of bracket bonding, based on the rationale of the higher protein content of fluorosed enamel. Evidence from an ex vivo study revealed that applying NaOCl in a 5.25% concentration to the fluorosed enamel surface before acid etching with 37% phosphoric acid and using conventional composite as an adhesive material eliminates organic elements, achieving significantly greater bonding capacity. Deproteinisation allows the acid etchant to penetrate more effectively into the enamel, resulting in better adhesion to the fluorosed enamel (Espinosa et al. 2008; Sharma et al. 2017).

In fluorosed teeth, preserving tooth structure and preventing irreversible damage following debonding should be considered equally with the protocols for improving bracket bond strength. Increasing bond strength may compromise the safety of debonding and increase enamel damage (Bishara et al. 1993). The extent of fluorosis should be taken into consideration collectively. For very mild and mild cases where the fluorotic enamel is in less than half of the tooth surface, conventional bonding techniques aided by adhesion promoters may work effectively (Baherimoghadam et al. 2016), as the enamel is minimally affected and thus no considerations upon debonding are likely to occur. For moderate cases where the entire enamel surface is affected, deproteinisation may be attempted (Sharma et al. 2017); and for more severe cases, orthodontic debonding may be destructive and options other than fixed appliances for orthodontic tooth movement should be considered.

3.4 Concluding Remarks

Orthodontic treatment involving bonding and debonding procedures in patients presenting developmental enamel defects is highly challenging and may incur inevitable additional substrate fractures or loss of the affected enamel. Long-term fixed appliance therapies, including rounds of rebonding procedures should be avoided, and cases should be carefully monitored with frequent clinical documentation throughout the course of the treatment. Personalised treatment planning is highly recommended, involving (i) identification of the extent of the defect and (ii) thorough projection of the patient's objective treatment needs. Severely affected patients should refrain from fixed appliance treatment and search for other alternatives, if any.

References

Ahmed, A.M., Nagy, D., and Elkateb, M.A. (2019). Etching patterns of sodium hypochlorite Pretreated hypocalcified amelogenesis imperfecta primary molars: SEM study. *J. Clin. Pediatr. Dent.* 43 (4): 257–262. Epub 2019 May 16.

Alachioti, X.S., Dimopoulou, E., Vlasakidou, A., and Athanasiou, A.E. (2014). Amelogenesis imperfecta and anterior open bite: etiological, classification, clinical and management interrelationships. *J. Orthod. Sci.* 3 (1): 1–6.

Alkadhimi, A., Cunningham, S.J., Parekh, S. et al. (2022). Decision making regarding management of compromised first permanent molars in patients with molar incisor hypomineralisation: a comparison of orthodontists and paediatric dentists. *J. Orthod.* 49 (1): 7–16.

Arkutu, N., Gadhia, K., McDonald, S. et al. (2012). Amelogenesis imperfecta: the orthodontic perspective. *Br. Dent. J.* 212 (10): 485–489.

Baherimoghadam, T., Akbarian, S., Rasouli, R., and Naseri, N. (2016). Evaluation of enamel damages following orthodontic bracket debonding in fluorosed teeth bonded with adhesion promoter. *Eur. J. Dent.* 10: 193–198.

Bishara, S.E., Fehr, D.E., and Jakobsen, J.R. (1993). A comparative study of the debonding strengths of different ceramic brackets, enamel conditioners, and adhesives. *Am. J. Orthod. Dentofacial. Orthop.* 104: 170–179.

Buonocore, M.G. (1981). Retrospections on bonding. *Dent. Clin. North Am.* 25 (2): 241–255.

Chen, C.F., Hu, J.C., Bresciani, E. et al. (2013). Treatment considerations for patient with *amelogenesis imperfecta*: a review. *Braz. Dent. Sci.* 16 (4): 7–18.

Cutress, T.W. and Suckling, G.W. (1990). Differential diagnosis of dental fluorosis. *J. Dent. Res.*; 69 Spec No:714–20; discussion 721.

Dashash, M., Yeung, C.A., Jamous, I., and Blinkhorn, A. (2013). Interventions for the restorative care of amelogenesis imperfecta in children and adolescents. *Cochrane Database Syst. Rev.* 6 (6): CD007157.

DenBesten, P.K. (1999). Biological mechanisms of dental fluorosis relevant to the use of fluoride supplements. *Community Dent Oral Epidemiol* 27: 41–47.

van Dorp, C.S., Exterkate, R.A., and ten Cate, J.M. (1990). Mineral loss during etching of enamel lesions. *Caries. Res.* 24 (1): 6–10.

Dumbryte, I., Jonavicius, T., Linkeviciene, L. et al. (2015). Enamel cracks evaluation - a method to predict tooth surface damage during the debonding. *Dent. Mater. J.* 34 (6): 828–834.

Eliades, T. (2006). Orthodontic materials research and applications: part 1. Current status and projected future developments in bonding and adhesives. *Am. J. Orthod. Dentofacial. Orthop.* 130 (4): 445–451.

Eliades, T. (2007). Orthodontic materials research and applications: part 2. Current status and projected future developments in materials and biocompatibility. *Am. J. Orthod. Dentofacial. Orthop.* 131 (2): 253–262.

Eliades, T. and Koletsi, D. (2020). Minimizing the aerosol-generating procedures in orthodontics in the era of a pandemic: current evidence on the reduction of hazardous effects for the treatment team and patients. *Am. J. Orthod. Dentofacial. Orthop.* 158 (3): 330–342.

Eliades, T., Gioka, C., Eliades, G., and Makou, M. (2004). Enamel surface roughness following debonding using two resin grinding methods. *Eur. J. Orthod.* 26 (3): 333–338.

Espinosa, R., Valencia, R., Uribe, M. et al. (2008 Fall;). Enamel deproteinization and its effect on acid etching: an in vitro study. *J. Clin. Pediatr. Dent.* 33 (1): 13–19.

Faria-e-Silva, A.L., De Moraes, R.R., Menezes Mde, S. et al. (2011). Hardness and microshear bond strength to enamel and dentin of permanent teeth with hypocalcified amelogenesis imperfecta. *Int. J. Paediatr. Dent.* 21 (4): 314–320.

Ghanim, A., Silva, M.J., Elfrink, M.E.C. et al. (2017). Molar incisor hypomineralisation (MIH) training manual for clinical field surveys and practice. *Eur. Arch. Paediatr. Dent.* 18 (4): 225–242. Epub 2017 Jul 18.

Ioannidis, A., Papageorgiou, S.N., Sifakakis, I. et al. (2018). Orthodontic bonding and debonding induces structural changes but does not alter the mechanical properties of enamel. *Prog Orthod.* 19 (1): 12. https://doi.org/10.1186/s40510-018-0211-7.

Kanemura, N., Sano, H., and Tagami, J. (1999). Tensile bond strength to and SEM evaluation of ground and intact enamel surfaces. *J. Dent.* 27 (7): 523–530.

Koruyucu, M., Bayram, M., Tuna, E.B. et al. (2014). Clinical findings and long-term managements of patients with amelogenesis imperfecta. *Eur. J. Dent.* 8: 546–552.

Krämer, N., Bui Khac, N.N., Lücker, S. et al. (2018). Bonding strategies for MIH-affected enamel and dentin. *Dent. Mater.* 34 (2): 331–340. Epub 2017 Dec 6.

Lagarde, M., Vennat, E., Attal, J.P., and Dursun, E. (2020). Strategies to optimize bonding of adhesive materials to molar-incisor hypomineralization-affected enamel: a systematic review. *Int. J. Paediatr. Dent.* 30 (4): 405–420. Epub 2020 Feb 12.

Marouane, O. and Manton, D.J. (2021). The influence of lesion characteristics on application time of an infiltrate applied to MIH lesions on anterior teeth: an exploratory in vivo pilot study. *J. Dent.* 115: 103814.

Øgaard, B., Bishara, S.E., and Duschner, H. (2004). Enamel effects during bonding-debonding and treatment with fixed appliances. In: *Risk Management in Orthodontics: experts' Guide to Malpractice* (ed. T.M. Graber, T. Eliades, and A.E. Athanasiou), 19–47. Chicago: Quintessence.

Pires Dos Santos, A.P., Cabral, C.M., Moliterno, L.F., and Oliveira, B.H. (2008). Amelogenesis imperfecta: report of a successful transitional treatment in the mixed dentition. *J. Dent. Child (Chic).* 75 (2): 201–206.

Pugach, M.K., Ozer, F., Mulmadgi, R. et al. (2014). Shear bond strength of dentin and deproteinized enamel of amelogenesis imperfecta mouse incisors. *Pediatr. Dent.* 36 (5): 130–136.

Saroğlu, I., Aras, S., and Oztaş, D. (2006). Effect of deproteinization on composite bond strength in hypocalcified amelogenesis imperfecta. *Oral Dis.* 12 (3): 305–308.

Seow, W.K. (2014). Developmental defects of enamel and dentine: challenges for basic science research and clinical management. *Aust. Dent. J.* 59 (Suppl 1): 143–154. Epub 2013 Oct 27.

Shah, P., Sharma, P., Goje, S.K. et al. (2019). Comparative evaluation of enamel surface roughness after debonding using four finishing and polishing systems for residual resin removal-an in vitro study. *Prog. Orthod.* 20 (1): 18.

Shahabi, M., Ahrari, F., Mohamadipour, H., and Moosavi, H. (2014). Microleakage and shear bond strength of orthodontc brackets bonded to hypomineralized enamel following different surface preparations. *J. Clin. Exp. Dent.* 6 (2): e110–e115. https://doi.org/10.4317/jced.51254.

Sharma, R., Kumar, D., and Verma, M. (2017). Deproteinization of fluorosed enamel with sodium hypochlorite enhances the shear bond strength of orthodontic brackets: an in vitro study. *Contemp. Clinic. Dent.* 8 (1): 20–25.

Siegel, S.C. and von Fraunhofer, J.A. (1999a). Comparison of sectioning rates among carbide and diamond burs using three casting alloys. *J. Prosthodont.* 8 (4): 240–244.

Siegel, S.C. and von Fraunhofer, J.A. (1999b). Dental burs--what bur for which application? A survey of dental schools. *J. Prosthodont.* 8 (4): 258–263.

Silverstone, L.M., Saxton, C.A., Dogon, I.L., and Fejerskov, O. (1975). Variation in the pattern of acid etching of human dental enamel examined by scanning electron microscopy. *Caries. Res.* 9 (5): 373–387.

Sönmez, H. and Saat, S. (2017). A clinical evaluation of deproteinization and different cavity designs on resin restoration performance in MIH-affected molars: two-year results. *J. Clin. Pediatr. Dent.* 41: 336–342.

de Souza, J.F., Fragelli, C.B., Jeremias, F. et al. (2017). Eighteen-month clinical performance of composite resin restorations with two different adhesive systems for molars affected by molar incisor hypomineralization. *Clin. Oral Investig.* 21 (5): 1725–1733. Epub 2016 Oct 15.

Thylstrup, A. and Fejerskov, O. (1978). Clinical appearance of dental fluorosis in permanent teeth in relation to histologic changes. *Community Dent Oral Epidemiol* 6: 315–328.

Trakinienė, G., Petravičiūtė, G., Smailienė, D. et al. (2019). Impact of fluorosis on the tensile bond strength of metal brackets and the prevalence of enamel microcracks. *Sci. Rep.* 9 (1): 5957.

Venezie, R.D., Vadiakas, G., Christensen, J.R., and Wright, J.T. (1994). Enamel pretreatment with sodium hypochlorite to enhance bonding in hypocalcified amelogenesis imperfecta: case report and SEM analysis. *Pediatr. Dent.* 16 (6): 433–436.

Witkop, C.J. (1989). Amelogenesis imperfecta, dentinogenesis imperfecta and dentin dysplasia revisited: problems in classification. *J. Oral. Pathol. Med.* 17: 547–553.

Yaman, B.C., Ozer, F., Cabukusta, C.S. et al. (2014). Microtensile bond strength to enamel affected by hypoplastic amelogenesis imperfecta. *J. Adhes. Dent.* 16 (1): 7–14.

Zachrisson, B.U., Skogan, O., and Höymyhr, S. (1980). Enamel cracks in debonded, debanded, and orthodontically untreated teeth. *Am. J. Orthod.* 77 (3): 307–319.

4

Enamel Colour, Roughness and Gloss Changes after Debonding

Andreas Karamouzos, Effimia Koumpia, and Anastasios A. Zafeiriadis

Department of Orthodontics, Faculty of Dentistry, School of Health Sciences, Aristotle University of Thessaloniki, Thessaloniki, Greece

4.1 Introduction

Facial attractiveness is an important social aspect and plays a key role in daily interactions (Cunningham 1986; Shaw 1981). People are sensitive to facial attractiveness because it is an important biological and social signal. Our perceptual and attentional system seems biased towards attractive faces (Nakamura et al. 2017). Related studies suggest that attractiveness influences mating success, personality evaluations, performance, employment prospects and perceived leadership ability (Dion et al. 1972; Flanary 1992; Re and Perrett 2014; Rhodes 2006). This was demonstrated in studies where higher intellectual and social abilities were attributed to individuals with more aesthetic smiles (Eli et al. 2001; Newton et al. 2003; Talamas et al. 2016). In the literature, facial and smile attractiveness are strongly related (Johnson et al. 2017). In social interactions, one's attention is mainly directed towards the eyes and mouth of the speaker (Baker et al. 2018; Van der Geld et al. 2007).

In modern dentistry, the patients' needs are considered regarding function and dental appearance. The oral region is essential in social interactions, and poor oral hygiene or unattractive teeth can lead to

Debonding and Fixed Retention in Orthodontics: An Evidence-Based Clinical Guide, First Edition. Edited by Theodore Eliades and Christos Katsaros.

negative attention. Dental appearance is linked to both cultural factors and individual preferences (Vallittu et al. 1996). An aesthetically pleasing smile depends on tooth size, shape, position, inclination, colour, smile arc, gingival display and the framing of the lips (Akyalcin et al. 2014; Giron de Velasco et al. 2017; Van der Geld et al. 2007). Tooth colour is one of the most important factors in satisfaction with oral appearance and the smile (Cunningham et al. 1990; Kershaw et al. 2008; Montero et al. 2014; Neumann et al. 1989; Van der Geld et al. 2007). Relatively minor changes in the lightness of tooth colour may influence an individual's perceived social appeal (social, intellectual, psychological and relational abilities) (Montero et al. 2014). Moreover, the patients' perception of tooth whiteness, health and attractiveness is significantly affected by the colour of the adjacent lips and gums (Reno et al. 2000).

Dental professionals can deliver high-quality oral care by improving patients' perceived quality of life and offering a functional occlusion combining balanced dentofacial aesthetics. Likewise, current dental patients are more demanding, appearance-conscious individuals seeking care that offers a functional occlusion and an appealing smile (Alkhatib et al. 2005). In several relevant studies of different populations, tooth colour has been shown to be a major concern that involves significant dental care for improvement (Isiekwe and Aikins 2019; Odioso et al. 2000; Xiao et al. 2007).

Optical stability of the teeth is important after orthodontic treatment, regarding enamel colour, translucency and gloss. Generally, the unfavourable effects on enamel caused by bracket bonding and debonding involve a wide array of procedures during acid etching, fixed orthodontic treatment and debonding (Sandison 1981; Sarafopoulou et al. 2018). The subsequent changes include enamel loss caused by enamel etching, inhibition of remineralisation by saliva in the tooth area bonded during treatment, fractures, and scratches caused on the surface during resin removal (Eliades et al. 2004a) (Figure 4.1). As discussed in previous chapters, rotary instruments lead to changes on the enamel surface that may be irreversible. It is also not uncommon to detect composite resin residues even after 30 seconds of polishing the debonded tooth surface (Vieira et al. 1993), while the quantity of residual resin may be product-dependent (Irinoda et al. 2000). Moreover, although not directly caused by orthodontic bonding/debonding procedures, a common complication during orthodontic treatment is the demineralisation and discolouration of enamel due to the accumulation of plaque on the fixed orthodontic

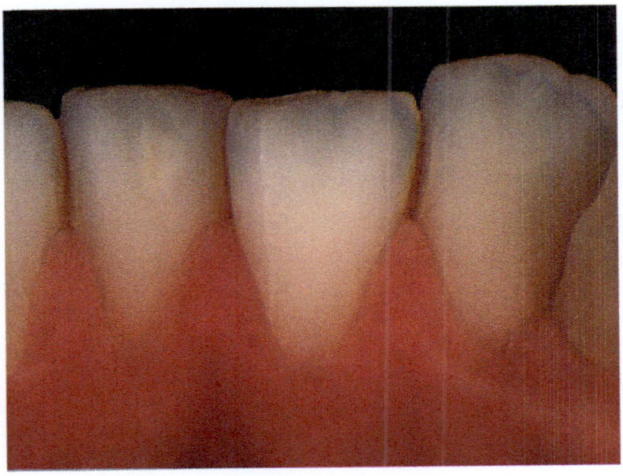

Figure 4.1 Spectrophotometric recording of an enamel colour defect and an enamel fracture on two lower incisors (SpectroShade Micro; MHT, Zurich, Switzerland).

appliances and the impeding of easy access to the tooth surfaces for cleaning (Øgaard 2008). The debonding effects on enamel may affect the tooth's optical attributes to a varying degree since the uppermost tooth layer can be modified on the order of 10 μm by acid etching, debonding, cleaning and polishing (Boncuk et al. 2014; Zhu et al. 2014).

Polishing resin composites has been shown to influence surface roughness (SR) and gloss, and limited significant correlations between colour and both SR and gloss parameters were also found. The effect differs by composite and shade (Hosoya et al. 2011). Orthodontic debonding procedures have also been shown *in vitro* to alter the surface characteristics of two types of porcelain systems commonly used in prosthetic dentistry. While bonding and debonding increased all roughness parameters, they also significantly altered gloss and colour indexes. Post-debond polishing did not restore the surface to the prebond state, regardless of the polishing method (12-fluted carbide bur/Sof-Lex discs in addition to the bur). It is proposed that patients should be informed that restorations may be damaged at the time of bracket debonding (Jarvis et al. 2006).

It has also been indicated that the perception of the appearance of teeth within the oral environment is too complicated to be strictly defined only by colour parameters since it is influenced by many factors, including the concepts of colour, translucency, surface gloss, opacity, iridescence and fluorescence (Johnston and Kao 1989; Terry et al. 2002). Directly measuring three colour parameters obtained from an instrument for a given illumination and observation geometry is inadequate to determine a translucent material's appearance (Johnston and Kao 1989). So, the clinical efficacy of instrumental measurement techniques has been questioned (Okubo et al. 1998), although there are always ongoing developments to improve colour measurement techniques (Joiner 2004). Regardless of the instrumental method used for tooth colour evaluation, the evaluations are ultimately visual (Hindle and Harrison 2000).

This chapter focuses on changes in enamel colour, gloss and roughness resulting from bonding and debonding procedures.

4.2 Tooth Colour Changes Associated with Orthodontic Treatment

4.2.1 Colour Definitions – Vision and Specification

The phenomenon of colour is a psychophysical response to the physical interaction of light energy with an object and the subjective experience of an individual observer (Bridgeman 1987). The eye is sensitive to a spectrum of wavelengths, which, when combined, determine the property known as *colour* (Lynch and Livingston 1995). Three factors can influence the perception of colour: the light source, the object being viewed and the observer viewing the object. The observer's visual system in the eye and brain affects the overall perception of colour (Hill 1987).

Colour vision starts with light absorption by the retinal cone photoreceptors, which transduce electromagnetic energy into electrical voltages. These voltages are transformed into action potentials by a complicated network of cells in the retina. The information is sent to the visual cortex via the lateral geniculate nucleus (LGN) in three separate colour-opponent channels characterised psychophysically, physiologically and computationally. Although some brain areas are more sensitive to colour than others, colour vision emerges through the combined activity of neurons in many different areas (Gegenfurtner and Kiper 2003).

Today, colour science principles are still based on Munsell's basic three-dimensional notation theory from the twentieth century (Nickerson 1969). Colour can be described according to the Munsell colour space in terms of hue, value and chroma. *Hue* is the attribute of colour; it refers to the dominant wavelengths present in its spectral distribution (Billmeyer and Saltzman 1981) and enables one to distinguish between different families of colour – for example, reds, blues and greens. *Value* indicates the lightness of a colour ranging from pure black to pure white. *Chroma* is the degree of colour saturation and describes a colour's strength, intensity or vividness (McLaren 1987).

The Commission Internationale de l' Éclairage (CIE) (1971), an organisation devoted to standardisation in areas such as colour and appearance, developed a system based on a standard light source and standard observer curves that enabled the calculation of tristimulus values, which represent how the human visual system responds to a given colour (McLaren 1987). The CIELAB colour space represents a uniform colour space, with equal distances corresponding to equal perceived colour differences (Figure 4.2). In this three-dimensional colour space, the three axes are L*, a* and b*. The L* value is a measure of the lightness of an object and is quantified on a scale such that perfect black has an L* value of zero and a perfect reflecting diffuser has an L* value of 100. The a* value is a measure of redness (positive a*) or greenness (negative a*). The b* value is a measure of yellowness (positive b*) or blueness (negative b*). The a* and b* co-ordinates approach zero for

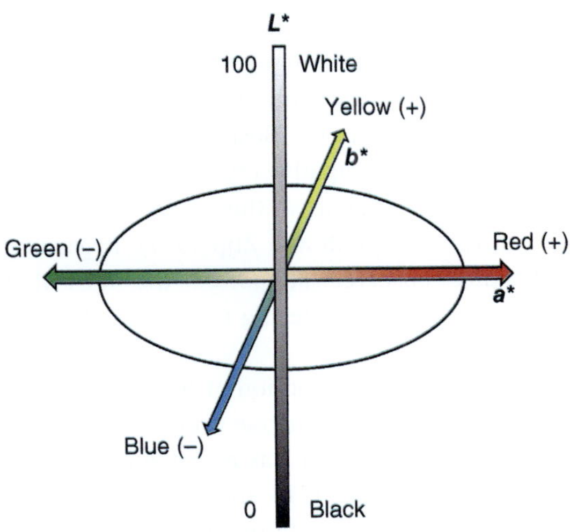

Figure 4.2 The CIELAB colour space. *Source:* Adapted from Paravina and Powers (2004).

neutral colours (white, greys) and increase in magnitude for more saturated or intense colours. The advantage of the CIELAB system is that colour differences can be expressed and calculated in ΔE units that can be related to visual perception and clinical significance (O'Brien et al. 1997) according to the following equation

$$\Delta E = \left[\left(L^*_{i} - L^*_{ii} \right)^2 + \left(a^*_{i} - a^*_{ii} \right)^2 + \left(b^*_{i} - b^*_{ii} \right)^2 \right]^{1/2}$$

where i and ii represent the colour measurements made at two different time intervals.

4.2.2 Tooth Optical Properties

The colour of a tooth is determined by a combination of its optical properties. When light encounters a tooth, four phenomena associated with the interactions of the tooth with the light flux can be described: (i) specular transmission of the light through the tooth, (ii) specular reflection at the surface, (iii) diffuse light reflection at the surface, and (iv) absorption and scattering of light within the dental tissues (Jahangiri et al. 2002). Numerous studies agree that tooth colour is determined mainly by the colour of the dentin and the type of tooth (Pop-Ciutrila et al. 2015). Since the enamel scattering is stronger for shorter (blue range) than for larger (red range) wavelengths and its absorption is small, the enamel plays only a minor role in tooth colour and appearance (Joiner 2004; Spitzer and ten Bosch 1975). Regarding enamel, it was found that the hydroxyapatite crystals contribute to light scattering. Demineralisation increases the scattering coefficient by a factor of about three (ten Bosch and Zijp 1987). Regarding dentin, the optical imbalance observed supported the idea that tubules are the predominant cause of scattering (Hariri et al. 2012; Vaarkamp et al. 1995).

A few studies have reported on the contribution of luminescence in determining tooth colour, with mixed results. In one study, the combination of fluorescence from dentin and enamel was reported as a whiteness or value enhancer (Terry et al. 2002). In another study, it was concluded that under everyday lighting conditions fluorescence does not contribute measurably to visually observed tooth colour (ten Bosch and Coops 1995).

4.2.3 Tooth Colour Measurement and Quantification Thresholds

There are two common methods of analysing *in vivo* the apparent tooth colour: visual determination and instrumental measurement (Billmeyer and Saltzman 1981). Visual determination by comparing teeth and shade guides is considered highly subjective but remains the most frequently applied method in dentistry for colour communication (van der Burgt et al. 1990). However, several factors such as external light conditions, experience, age and fatigue of the human eye and inherent limitations of the contemporary shade guides can influence the consistency of visual colour selection and specification (Billmeyer and Saltzman 1981; Preston 1985; Rubino et al. 1994). The demand for objective colour matching in dentistry, coupled with rapid advances in optical electronic sensors and computer technology, has made instrumental measurement devices a supplementary adjunct to visual tooth colour evaluation (Paravina and Powers 2004). Nowadays, commercial systems, including tristimulus colourimeters, spectroradiometers, spectrophotometers and digital colour analysers, are used in clinical and research settings for objective colour specification (Joiner 2004) (Figure 4.3).

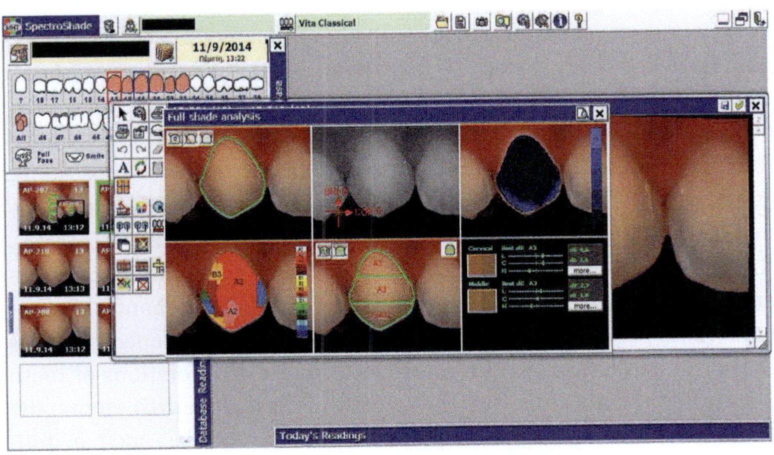

Figure 4.3 Full shade analysis of an upper-right canine with reflectance spectrophotometer software (SpecroShade Micro; MHT, Zurich, Switzerland). The patient's name is masked for anonymity.

Evaluating colour in dental research involves incorporating perceptibility and/or acceptability thresholds to compare the results. The quantitative assessment of a colour difference identifies the difference that is perceivable and the colour difference that is clinically acceptable (Douglas 1997; Paravina et al. 2015). Tooth colour measurement devices can detect and quantify minor colour differences as their limit of detection during *in vitro* quantification of monochromatic samples is considered to be 0.1 ΔE units (Seghi et al. 1989). It has been proposed that ΔE values greater than one unit obtained under ideal viewing conditions are agreed to be visually significant, correlating with 50–50% perceptibility (Kuehni and Marcus 1979; Seghi et al. 1989). In clinical conditions, ΔE values greater than 2.7 (Ragain and Johnston 2000) and 3.3 (Ruyter et al. 1987) and 3.7 (Johnston and Kao 1989) were found to have 50 : 50% acceptability thresholds. In the oral cavity, where the standardisation of light conditions is difficult, the most frequently proposed acceptance limit for tooth colour matching was set to 3.7 ΔE units, beyond which the differences were considered clinically perceivable (Johnston and Kao 1989).

4.2.4 Tooth Colour Changes Related to Orthodontic Treatment

Despite the extensive evidence available on enamel effects associated with fixed appliance therapy (Øgaard et al. 2004), the incidence of tooth colour alterations related to orthodontic treatment has not been thoroughly documented. A search of the relevant literature revealed a small number of well-designed, randomised controlled trials or prospective cohort studies and two systematic reviews assessing the effect of any orthodontic appliance on tooth colour. According to Chen et al. (2015), there is no strong evidence that orthodontic treatment with fixed appliances alters the original enamel colour. On the other hand, Kamber et al. (2018) concluded that the existing low-quality evidence indicates that orthodontic treatment may be associated with alterations of tooth colour that are not consistently clinically discernible. Furthermore, the available evidence seems to support that many variables, such as individual characteristics, patient oral hygiene and dietary preferences, etching pattern, bonding materials, debonding procedures, remnant adhesive protocols, treatment duration, etc., influence tooth colour alterations related to orthodontic treatment. Therefore, this section outlines the results of contemporary research studies concerning the effect of orthodontic treatment on tooth colour.

4.2.5 Aetiology of Colour Changes

Several etiological factors that adversely affect the colour variables of natural teeth by altering their surface and structural characteristics are probably associated with tooth colour alterations related to orthodontic treatment. Dissolution of apatite crystallites during the *acid etching technique* increases the microscopic roughness of the exposed enamel (Retief et al. 1986) and, therefore, the light-scattering characteristics of the tooth surface (ten Bosch and Coops 1995). *White spot lesions*, frequently encountered during orthodontic treatment (Årtun and Thylstrup 1986; Øgaard et al. 1988), can heal or remineralise if they are kept plaque-free (Al-Khateeb et al. 1998), but it is doubtful whether the minerals in these lesions are deposited in the same manner as in sound enamel (Øgaard et al. 2004). Moreover, current methods of *bracket debonding* and *adhesive removal* protocols typically result in alterations in enamel morphology and texture modifications (Zachrisson 2000; Zarrinnia et al. 1995), which cannot be restored with the use of polishing media at the post-finishing stages (Eliades et al. 2004a; Piacentini and Sfondrini 1996). These irreversible changes can affect the optical properties of enamel surfaces such as gloss and lustre, consequently influencing the colour parameters of natural teeth. Occasionally, fractures in the enamel surface following removal of orthodontic brackets (Dumbryte et al. 2013) may provide stagnation areas for development of caries or discolouration (Zachrisson et al. 1980).

Enamel colour alterations after debonding may also derive from the long-term irreversible penetration of *resin tags* into the enamel surface (Eliades et al. 2001). This phenomenon affects the specularly reflected light component, thus influencing the L* values of the tooth substrate (Chung 1994; Leibrock et al. 1997). Furthermore, discolouration of the resin-infiltrated enamel may arise as a result of the colour instability of resin composites, attributed to endogenous changes from physicochemical reactions within the material (Ferracane 1985), exogenous changes from superficial absorption of food colourants (Inokoshi et al. 1996), prolonged exposure to staining materials (Erdemir et al. 2012; Faltermeier et al. 2008) or products arising from corrosion of the orthodontic appliance (Maijer and Smith 1982).

Previous *in vitro* studies have indicated that most of the conventional orthodontic adhesives tested revealed unsatisfactory colour stability (mean $\Delta E > 3.7$ units) after exposure to food colourants and/or artificial photo-ageing (Eliades et al. 2004b; Faltermeier et al. 2008). The discolouration of adhesives has also been linked with changes in b* values towards the yellow (Leibrock et al. 1997). Chemical differences among the resin components as well as differences in filler content and polymerisation conversion affect the colour stability of the various composites (Davis et al. 1995; Eldiwany et al. 1995). Nevertheless, the results of an *in vitro* study have attributed the uptake of tea and coffee stains to the components of the enamel, not the resin tags, with responsibility for the colour changes, as the type of adhesive and the methods of application did not affect the enamel colour change (Jahanbin et al. 2009). However, it is possible that *in vivo* oral conditions can cause colour changes in bonding materials.

Orthodontic forces are known to affect gingival and pulp tissue vascularity and blood flow and to produce significant changes in the number and density of periodontal ligament (PDL) blood vessels (Murrell et al. 1996). Despite the conflicting evidence in the contemporary literature concerning the temporary or long-lasting effects of orthodontic forces on these tissues (Krishnan and Davidovitch 2006), it is assumed that *in vivo* tooth colour measurements may be influenced by *intrinsic parameters* that cannot be reliably simulated by *in vitro* tests. Therefore, *in vivo* tooth colour alterations may result either from the variation of blood flow within the dental pulp and the adjacent gingival tissue (Goodkind and Schwabacher 1987) or from resting salivary flow rates that affect the degree of tooth hydration and thus tooth colour (Dawes 1974).

4.2.6 *In Vitro* vs. *In Vivo* Studies

Enamel discolouration and stain susceptibility after bonding, debonding and clean-up procedures have been evaluated *in vitro* during the last two decades (Boncuk et al. 2014; Eliades et al. 2001; Kim et al. 2006; Shayan et al. 2021; Trakyali et al. 2009; Tuncer et al. 2018; Wriedt et al. 2008; Zaher et al. 2012). Some *in vitro* studies have concluded that bonding/debonding procedures alone do not seem to significantly influence the tooth colour of bovine or human enamel (Trakyali et al. 2009; Wriedt et al. 2008). Conversely, other studies have shown that these procedures significantly affected enamel colour variables (Boncuk et al. 2014; Zaher et al. 2012). Although these studies showed that some alterations in tooth colour are inevitable, regardless of whether these changes are visually perceptible, it must be emphasised that *in vitro* tests may not be a reliable reflection of the clinical situation (Eliades et al. 2004b). Long-term resin discolouration due to the absorption of colourants from the oral environment cannot be estimated *in vitro*. Additionally, the lack of saliva, food colouring and the inability to simulate the mechanical abrasion caused by brushing are limitations of experimental studies (Chen et al. 2015). To gain more reliable results, randomised clinical trials are essential to provide evidence-based information regarding this issue.

In vivo colour determination of natural teeth is affected by many factors presenting in the oral cavity, such as the lighting conditions of the surrounding environment, light scattered from the adjacent perioral and gingival tissues (Goodkind and Schwabacher 1987) and resting salivary flow rates influencing the degree of tooth hydration (Dawes 1974) and, consequently, the reflective index of the underlying surface. Recent longitudinal randomised and non-randomised clinical trials using commercial instrumental devices evaluated *in vivo* the tooth colour alterations associated with orthodontic treatment, concluding that the CIELAB colour parameters of natural teeth present significant differences after the removal of *fixed orthodontic appliances* (Table 4.1) (Al Maaitah et al. 2013; Al-Laban 2015; Çörekçi et al. 2015; Gorucu-Coskuner et al. 2018; Karamouzos et al. 2010; Karamouzos et al. 2019; Kaya et al. 2018; Malekpour et al. 2022; Pinzan-Vercelino et al. 2021; Ratzmann et al. 2018; Tunca and Kaya 2023).

Although there is no data on this issue concerning *aligner orthodontic treatment*, it is assumed that irreversible alterations made to the enamel structure while bonding and debonding composite resin attachments may affect the colour of the enamel surface. Such composite attachments, bonded routinely on the labial surface of multiple teeth, have dimensions ranging from 2 to 5 mm (Dasy et al. 2015), thus involving a considerable enamel area and potentially damaging its outermost layer (Eliades et al. 2020).

Table 4.1 *In vivo* tooth colour evaluation studies related to orthodontic treatment.

Authors, year	Journal	Study design	Patients, teeth	Intervention (source of variation)	Post-debonding cleaning	Outcome timing	ΔE differences measured	Authors' conclusions
Karamouzos et al. (2010)	*AJODO*	pNRS	26 patients Max./ Mand. 4–4	CC and LC adhesives	Carbide bur (low-speed)	Prebonding Post-debonding	2.12–3.61 ΔE units	Chemically cured resin was associated with greater colour changes than light-cured composite. The colour of natural teeth is changed in various ways after fixed orthodontic treatment.
Al Maaitah et al. (2013)	*AJODO*	RCT	34 patients Max./ Mand. 3–3	Self-etching primer and conventional acid etching Male/female Adolescents/adults	Spiral 12-fluted tungsten carbide bur (low-speed)	Prebonding 1 wk post-debonding	The average tooth colour difference after orthodontic treatment was 2.85 ΔE units.	Fixed orthodontic appliances caused tooth colour changes; self-etching primer and conventional acid etching had similar effects on tooth colour; men and adolescents had greater colour changes than girls and adults.

Çörekçi et al. (2015)	*Turk. J. Med. Sci.*	pNRS	28 patients 42, 41, 31, 32	Four LC adhesives: 42/Grengloo, 41/Light Bond, 31/Kurasper F, 32/Transbond XT	Carbide bur (high- and low-speed); Sof-Lex polishing discs	Prebonding 4.3–8.5 mo after bonding	Teeth demonstrated clinically visible colour changes ranging from 1.12 to 3.34 ΔE units.	Teeth may be discoloured with fixed appliances during treatment. Contemporary orthodontic composites have similar effects of enamel discolouration.
Al-Laban (2015)	*J. Bagh. Coll. Dent.*	pNRS	34 patients Max. 3–3	Gingival, middle and incisal thirds of upper anterior teeth Males/females	12-fluted tungsten carbide bur (low-speed); extra-fine Sof-Lex polishing discs	Prebonding Post-debonding	Gingival 4.05 ΔE units Middle 4.95 ΔE units Incisal 3.64 ΔE units	The discolouration of teeth due to orthodontic treatment occurs in the middle third more than the incisal and gingival thirds, and there is no difference between the two sex groups.
Kaya et al. (2018)	*AJODO*	pNRS	20 patients 3–3 max.	3, 6, 12 mo follow-ups during the retention	12-bladed tungsten carbide bur (low-speed)	Post-debonding 3, 6 and 12 mo after debonding	Mean ΔE values were 1.52–3.57 units.	In the first three mo, there was a significant increase in the lightness of the tooth colour.

(*Continued*)

Table 4.1 (Continued)

Authors, year	Journal	Study design	Patients, teeth	Intervention (source of variation)	Post-debonding cleaning	Outcome timing	ΔE differences measured	Authors' conclusions
Gorucu-Coskuner et al. (2018)	*Angle Orthod.*	pNRS	59 patients 3–3 max.	Self-etching primer and conventional acid etching 12-, 24-bladed tungsten carbide burs Sof-Lex XT discs	12-, 24-bladed tungsten carbide burs Sof-Lex polishing discs	Prebonding Post-debonding After polishing	Mean ΔE values were 4.2-4.8 units.	Orthodontic treatment resulted in visible and clinically unacceptable tooth colour alterations regardless of the enamel preparation and clean-up techniques. Polishing reduced the effect of tungsten carbide burs but did not affect the total influence of orthodontic treatment on the tooth colour.
Ratzmann et al. (2018)	*Head Face Med.*	pNRS	15 patients 14, 24	Body and gingival tooth segments	NA	Prebonding Post-debonding 3 mo after debonding	Mean ΔE values were up to 2.3 units.	Within the limitations of this study, the fixed appliance treatment can be seen as a safe method concerning tooth colour.

Karamouzos et al. (2019)	*Orthod. Craniofac. Res.*	pNRS	48 patients Max./ Mand. 4–4	Low-/high-speed carbide bur Prior to and after polishing with Sof-Lex discs 3 and 12 mo follow-up during retention	Carbide burs (low- or high-speed)	After debonding 3 mo later, prior to and following finishing with Sof-Lex discs After 1 yr	Total ΔE differences ranged from 1.4 to 2.1 units.	The greatest changes were exhibited during the first 3 mo in teeth on which high-speed rotary instruments were used (1.6 units). The clinical relevance of this study shows that the colour of natural teeth following the removal of fixed orthodontic appliances changes in the long term.
Pinzan-Vercelino et al. (2021)	*AJODO*	RCT	6 patients Teeth 4, 5, 6 Max./ Mand.	Sof-Lex discs/ Sof-Lex Spiral Wheels	12-blade tungsten carbide bur (low-speed)	Before bonding After tooth polishing 30 d after polishing	Total ΔE differences ranged from 10.88 to 14.1 units.	The fixed orthodontic appliance altered the enamel colour. Sof-Lex discs and Sof-Lex Spiral Wheels resulted in similar enamel colour changes after bracket debonding using two polishing systems.

(*Continued*)

Table 4.1 (Continued)

Authors, year	Journal	Study design	Patients, teeth	Intervention (source of variation)	Post-debonding cleaning	Outcome timing	ΔE differences measured	Authors' conclusions
Tunca and Kaya (2021)	*J. Orofac. Orthop.*	pNRS	25 patients 3–3 max./mand.	Four different LC adhesives	NA	Prebonding Post-debonding	The ΔE values were 1.83–2.18 and 1.41–1.95 for incisors and canines, respectively.	Although statistically fewer enamel colour changes occurred in the Kurasper F group compared with the Grengloo and Light Bond groups, the observed changes were not clinically relevant.
Malekpour et al. (2022)	*J. Orofac. Orthop.*	pNRS	20 patients	Carbide bur/carbide bur and Sof-Lex disc 10 d application of nanohydroxyapatite serum after debonding	Carbide bur/carbide bur and Sof-Lex disc	Immediately 2 and 4 mo after debonding	The mean total colour change was clinically perceptible ($\Delta E > 3.3$).	The applied concentrations of nanohydroxyapatite did not significantly reduce tooth colour changes after debonding in orthodontic treatment. Sof-Lex discs can significantly reduce tooth colour changes in a short time.

CC, chemically cured adhesive; LC, light-cured adhesive; NA, non-applicable; pNRS, prospective non-randomised study; RCT, randomised clinical trial.

4.2.7 ΔE and CIELAB Colour Parameter Changes

Several *in vivo* studies have been conducted to prospectively assess colour alterations of natural teeth associated with fixed orthodontic treatment (Table 4.1). The results of these studies indicated that orthodontic treatment led to an average colour change ranging from 1.12 to 4.95 ΔE units, except for one study (Pinzan-Vercelino et al. 2021) where the ΔE differences ranged from 10.88 to 14.1 units. Most of the studies concluded that orthodontic treatment resulted in visible and clinically acceptable and/or unacceptable tooth colour alterations regardless of the enamel preparation and the bonding/debonding and clean-up techniques. Long-term follow-up studies found that the greatest changes were exhibited during the first three months after the removal of orthodontic appliances (Karamouzos et al. 2019; Kaya et al. 2018). Differences in ΔE values among the *in vivo* studies were explained by the study characteristics, such as study design, setting, colour measurement device, patient number, age, appliances, treatment duration, clinical procedures during bonding and debonding, outcome measured, measurement unit and timing.

Furthermore, pretreatment and post-treatment comparison results showed significant changes in L* (lightness) and b* (yellow/blue axis) values, whereas a* (red/green) values were more stable. Tunca and Kaya (2023) found significant decreases in L* and b* values and insignificant changes in a* values, concluding that the tooth colour becomes darker and shifts towards the colour blue. Other studies found that the mean L* value decreased, whereas the mean a* and b* values increased, implying that the average tooth colour becomes darker and shifts into more red and especially yellow colour ranges (Gorucu-Coskuner et al. 2018; Karamouzos et al. 2010). However, after polishing with discs, L* values showed statistically significant increases (Gorucu-Coskuner et al. 2018; Karamouzos et al. 2019).

In most of the studies, the clinical relevance of the colour changes was addressed by comparing the colour differences with a standard value of clinical detection set to 3.7 ΔE units, beyond which the changes were considered clinically unacceptable (Johnston and Kao 1989). It was found that approximately 13% of the bonded teeth presented visible, clinically significant colour changes at the end of active treatment, whereas the distribution of these teeth among the subjects revealed that 45.44–80% of patients presented at least one tooth with unacceptable colour changes (Çörekçi et al. 2015; Karamouzos et al. 2010).

Although these findings emphasise the potential risk of clinically unacceptable tooth colour changes, only a small percentage of patients complain of tooth colour alterations after orthodontic treatment (Gorucu-Coskuner et al. 2018). This may be explained by the fact that tooth-colour perception and appearance are related to individual facial characteristics such as age, the attractiveness of the entire oral region, skin tone and the colour and volume of adjacent lips and gums (Alkhatib et al. 2005). This variety of factors contributes to the perception of the overall dental appearance and thus may diminish the issue of tooth-colour alterations caused by orthodontic treatment (Karamouzos et al. 2010).

4.2.8 Long-Term Enamel Colour Changes

Long-term enamel colour changes following fixed appliance therapy were recently investigated *in vivo* (Karamouzos et al. 2019; Kaya et al. 2018). Colour changes one year after debonding ranged from 1.4 to 3.57 ΔE units. Both studies indicated that most colour changes occur within the first three months following debonding. The most significant increase was in lightness (L*) (Kaya et al. 2018). Orthodontic debonding and cleaning procedures were also found to have statistically significant long-term effects on the CIELAB colour parameters of treated teeth. Finishing temporarily decreased the enamel colour differences (Karamouzos et al. 2019). It was found that 4.6% of the teeth measured showed visible and clinically significant alterations in colour. The way these teeth were distributed among the patients indicated that almost 30% of cases exhibited at least one tooth showing noticeable colour changes (Karamouzos et al. 2019). The clinical relevance of these studies demonstrates that the colour of natural teeth following the removal of fixed orthodontic appliances changes in the long term.

4.2.9 Types of Teeth

Some differences were found regarding the types of teeth, with canines being the least affected, followed by central incisors, first premolars and ultimately lateral incisors, which were the most affected (Karamouzos et al. 2010). Although canines presented lower ΔE values *in vivo* (1.41–1.95) than incisors (1.83–2.18), the comparison between them was not significant following treatment with fixed appliances (Tunca and Kaya 2023). Another study reported no effect of tooth type on treatment-induced colour change (Al Maaitah et al. 2013).

Regarding the labial surface of upper anterior teeth, the middle third presented significantly higher ΔE values than the incisal and gingival thirds. A possible explanation is that the middle third of the tooth remains unexposed to oral fluids and tooth brushing since it is covered by the bracket (Al-Laban 2015). However, in another clinical study, body and gingival tooth segments presented slight colour differences (Ratzmann et al. 2018).

4.2.10 Gender and Age

Two studies comparing tooth colour changes in relation to gender reveal inconsistent results: one study found no significant difference between male and female groups (Al-Laban 2015), while the other showed that males presented greater tooth colour changes than females as a result of fixed orthodontic treatment. According to the authors, this difference may be related to different dietary habits or the quality of oral hygiene between male and female patients (Al Maaitah et al. 2013). In the same study, adolescents recorded more colour changes than adults, and these were explained by the fact that the teeth of younger patients have increased enamel porosity and are more prone to acid attacks, increasing their susceptibility to staining adsorption.

4.2.11 Etching Pattern

There are conflicting results regarding the effects of different etching procedures on tooth colour. It was found *in vitro* that self-etching created less resin penetration and these systems may produce less iatrogenic colour change in enamel following orthodontic treatment (Boncuk et al. 2014; Zaher et al. 2012). Other *in vitro* studies found no significant differences between teeth treated with conventional etching or self-etching after polishing with regard to colour alteration (Eliades et al. 2001; Joo et al. 2011). Additionally, the type of phosphoric acid (solution or gel) had no significant effect on the colour change of enamel (Shayan et al. 2021).

In vivo tooth colour measurements before and after orthodontic treatment revealed that neither conventional nor self-etching techniques caused statistically different tooth colour alterations (Al Maaitah et al. 2013; Gorucu-Coskuner et al. 2018). As the depth of the resin tags did not influence short-term superficial discolouration, the use of self-etching or conventional etching may not lead to a significant difference in the short term. This was attributed to the similarity between the two protocols of the etching pattern at the uppermost enamel layer, which discolours first, independently of penetration depth (Cinader 2001).

4.2.12 Adhesives

In vitro investigations of the effects of different orthodontic bonding materials on enamel colour alteration indicated that the adhesives tested were associated with changes in the CIELAB colour parameters of bonded teeth (Boncuk et al. 2014; Haghighi et al. 2020; Trakyali et al. 2009). Resin-modified glass ionomer cement showed the fewest colour differences, and chemically cured resin groups showed the highest ΔE values among all orthodontic adhesives tested *in vitro* (Wu et al. 2018; Ye et al. 2013).

Repeated bracket bonding has been shown to influence *in vitro* enamel colour changes similarly to single bonding. However, this does not necessarily mean repeated bonding procedures do not affect the colour parameters. In other words, some steps may result in an increase in the ΔE value, while others result in a decrease, working antagonistically and neutralising the colour change (Tuncer et al. 2018).

Limited *in vivo* evidence indicated that chemically cured composite resins used to bond orthodontic appliances lead to significantly more discolouration to a clinically relevant point than light-cured composite resins (Karamouzos et al. 2010). This may be attributed to chemical differences between the two resins, such as filler content and polymerisation conversion, which may affect their colour stability (Eldiwany et al. 1995; Eliades et al. 2004b; Gioka et al. 2005). Furthermore, the type of filler and monomer, the connection capacity of monomer to filler and the oxidation of the polymer matrix must be considered concerning discolouration of composites. Additionally, most orthodontic resins are flowable and not highly filled polymers, and they may easily absorb staining substances from the oral environment (Chung 1994; Dietschi et al. 1994).

Colour alterations of natural teeth associated with different light-cured orthodontic composites were evaluated *in vivo* in a short-term orthodontic treatment (5.9–8.8 months), and it was found that colour changes in terms of L*, a* and b* values were not significantly different between resins (Çörekçi et al. 2015). Consistent results were found in another clinical trial, where the ΔE value comparisons for the Transbond XT, Kurasper F, Grengloo and Light Bond groups were insignificant (ΔE values of 2.05, 1.83, 2.09 and 2.18, respectively) (Tunca and Kaya 2021).

Moreover, mouthwash use during orthodontic treatment may result in different levels of enamel discolouration (Korkmaz and Bulut 2020). Although these compounds are effective in oral hygiene, it seems that lower concentrations of chlorhexidine should be prescribed to orthodontic patients (Soheilifar et al. 2021).

4.2.13 Resin Removal Techniques

Although the effects of resin removal techniques after debonding on enamel colour have been extensively studied *in vitro* (Boncuk et al. 2014; Eliades et al. 2001; Kim et al. 2006), there is still no agreement on which method is more efficient. Different polishing systems are available, such as diamond and carbide burs, polishing discs, diamond-impregnated rubber wheels, cups, discs and pastes. However, due to their shorter cleaning times, tungsten carbide burs are the most popular adhesive removal tools (Janiszewska-Olszowska et al. 2014). The main purposes of finishing and polishing are to remove scratches, maintain the enamel resistance, avoid decalcification and provide a good aesthetic appearance and surface brightness, avoiding staining and providing a smooth, shiny surface. Thus, a flat, smooth tooth surface allows more specular reflection, precise colour measurement and improved light reflection (Çörekçi et al. 2015; Trakyali et al. 2009). Debonding and adhesive remnant removal have been shown to be more invasive than acid etching regarding enamel colour alterations (Eliades et al. 2001). Removing residual adhesive using a low-speed handpiece and tungsten-carbide bur has shown demonstrably less damage to surface enamel (Hosein et al. 2004). Another study found that a tungsten carbide bur with 12 cutting edges produced less colour alteration than the equivalent with 24 edges (Gorucu-Coskuner et al. 2018).

Debonding and cleaning procedures after orthodontic treatment were also evaluated *in vivo* using two different carbide burs attached to a low- or high-speed handpiece, respectively, in a non-blinded cohort study with a split-mouth design (Karamouzos et al. 2019). A comparison of cleaning procedures and time points regarding ΔE demonstrated greater changes at three months using a high-speed handpiece. Although polishing has been shown to reduce the effects of tungsten carbide burs, there was no overall impact on the effect of orthodontic treatment on tooth colour.

The effect on tooth colour changes after adhesive remnant removal using different etching techniques – 12- and 24-bladed tungsten carbide burs and polishing discs – was evaluated in a recent clinical study (Gorucu-Coskuner et al. 2018). It was found that in the self-etch bonding groups, a 12-bladed tungsten carbide bur caused less colour change than the 24-bladed tungsten carbide bur. According to the authors, as the 24-bladed tungsten carbide bur results in less adhesive removal than the 12-bladed bur, the greater colour change may be due to a remaining undetectable adhesive layer. After polishing with Sof-Lex XT discs, the effect of tungsten carbide burs on tooth colour became insignificant. In another clinical trial, it was found that Sof-Lex discs and Sof-Lex Spiral Wheel polishing systems used after the removal of excess adhesive using a 12-blade tungsten carbide bur on a low-speed handpiece did not appear to significantly damage the enamel surface, and the colour change was similar for each of them (Pinzan-Vercelino et al. 2021).

4.2.14 Quality Assessment of Studies

The quality of evidence from previous colour studies has been analysed in two systematic reviews (Table 4.2). According to Chen et al. (2015), the methodological limitations of the five studies were extensive, influencing the quality of the evidence. Four of the five trials were assessed as being associated with an unclear risk of bias; the remaining trial was deemed to be associated with a high risk of bias. Since most of the included studies were *in vitro,* the conclusions should be interpreted with caution. Thus, the evidence to support the relationship between orthodontic treatment and enamel colour alteration was moderate.

Kamber et al. (2018) identified four clinical studies as eligible for inclusion in their systematic review. Three of them were non-randomised, which means their conclusions may be biased (Papageorgiou et al. 2015), and all

Table 4.2 Systematic reviews of the effect of orthodontic treatment on tooth colour.

Authors, year	Journal	Study design	Inclusion criteria	Study selection and characteristics	Quality of evidence of selected studies	Authors' conclusions
Chen et al. (2015)	*BMC Oral Health*	Systematic review	Randomised controlled trials and prospective controlled clinical studies	Five studies: three randomised controlled trials and two prospective studies (four *in vitro* and one *in vivo*)	Four trials were assessed as being unclear regarding the risk of bias. One was assessed as being at high risk of bias.	There is no strong evidence from this review that orthodontic treatment with fixed appliances alters the original colour of enamel. Further well-designed and -conducted randomised controlled trials are required to facilitate comparisons of results.
Kamber et al. (2018)	*J. Orofac. Orthop.*	Systematic review and meta-analysis	Randomised clinical trials and prospective non-randomised controlled or uncontrolled cohort studies	Four *in vivo* studies: three non-randomised and one randomised	Very low due to the inclusion of non-randomised studies, bias and imprecision	Existing low-quality evidence indicates that orthodontic treatment may be associated with tooth colour alterations that are not consistently clinically discernible. Treatment-induced colour alterations may depend on the bonding material and tooth type, but evidence supporting this is weak.

of the studies were found to be at high or serious risk of bias. The most problematic issues were small sample sizes that may impact the determination of a statistically significant difference between interventions, unclear randomisation, confounding due to uncontrolled variables, lack of blinding and selective reporting or missing data.

Finally, although colour assessments with the CIELAB protocol are more objective and consistent than subjective visual inspections of colour, they are still prone to systematic and random errors (Douglas 1997; Russell et al. 2000). Systematic errors are inherent in all instruments and result from calibration techniques, fluorescence, instrument metamerism and variations in measurement geometry (Seghi et al. 1989). These errors are difficult to manage and can be expected to adversely affect instrument accuracy regardless of the degree of precision or control of the environment (Berns 2000). Uncertainty during the measuring process is associated primarily with random errors.

Several methods have been suggested to reduce the detrimental effect of variability of colour measurements, including the use of multiple measurements and averaging or better control of methodological and environmental factors (Seghi et al. 1989).

4.2.15 Conclusions

Existing evidence from contemporary research studies indicates that orthodontic treatment with fixed appliances seems to be associated with colour alterations of natural teeth. Although the evidence to support this relationship was moderate, most clinical studies demonstrated visually perceptible and clinically acceptable or unacceptable colour alterations following the completion of comprehensive treatment with fixed appliances. This outcome may be caused by the iatrogenic effects on the enamel surface associated with bonding, debonding and cleaning procedures that affect the colour parameters of natural teeth and the long-term intrinsic and extrinsic discolouration of the residual adhesive material after orthodontic treatment.

The clinical relevance of these findings suggests that the clinician should take all necessary precautions to minimise the enamel effects associated with various stages of orthodontic treatment by using appropriate bonding/debonding and polishing procedures and motivating patients to use proper oral hygiene and follow healthy diet habits. Further randomised clinical studies are required to improve the quality of research in this area, allowing additional systematic reviews and meta analyses to strengthen the evidence concerning longitudinal tooth colour changes related to orthodontic treatment and develop clinical approaches to minimise them.

4.3 Tooth Bleaching Considerations After Debonding

In the last two decades, patients and orthodontists have begun to place more emphasis on aesthetics as a reason for treatment, and orthodontics have become part of a much larger explosion in 'cosmetic dentistry' procedures that include tooth whitening and veneers (Micu and Carstairs 2018). A high percentage of private-practice orthodontists in the US (88.8%) had patients who requested tooth whitening and had recommended whitening procedures (76.2%) (Slack et al. 2013), reflecting a constantly increasing trend within the specialty (Micu and Carstairs 2018).

So far, four *in vitro* studies and two *in vivo* studies have tested the effect of bleaching post-orthodontic treatment (Gomes Lde et al. 2013; Hintz et al. 2001; Jadad et al. 2011; Koumpia et al. 2022; Lunardi et al. 2014; Wriedt et al. 2008). In a study of bovine incisors, the response to the bleaching process was found to be independent of enamel alterations caused by bonding/debonding procedures. But the effects of photo-ageing and general discolouration were not considered, and final spectrophotometric measurements were recorded two weeks after debonding (Wriedt et al. 2008).

In an *in vitro* study on human premolars, both experimental and control groups were subjected to whitening, while the experimental group also underwent orthodontic bonding/debonding. Colorimetric readings were taken before and after whitening for 30 days. Control sites responded initially to a greater extent, whereas experimental sites did not respond until after two weeks of continuous whitening. Differences became insignificant at the end of the 30 days of monitoring (Hintz et al. 2001). These findings are in accordance with results from a study with bovine incisors where the influence of bonding/debonding on bleaching was evaluated using three different adhesive systems. Experimental groups showed significantly less teeth whitening than the control group, but there were no statistically significant colour differences between groups after 14 days (Gomes et al. 2013). Bovine incisors were also evaluated to assess the effectiveness of dental bleaching under orthodontic brackets. The presence of bracket bonds negatively affected the effectiveness of bleaching treatments. The bleaching agents were unable to penetrate evenly throughout the specimen, resulting in a poorly lightened area under the bracket (Lunardi et al. 2014).

In one *in vivo* study, the effectiveness of a bleaching agent was assessed in the six anterior maxillary teeth of patients wearing fixed orthodontic appliances. Groups were divided according to the timeline application of the bleaching agent during or after orthodontic treatment. Tooth colour was recorded before and after the application of the bleaching agent, and it was observed that significant tooth bleaching occurred in both groups with and without brackets (Jadad et al. 2011). In another *in vivo* study, the efficacy of bleaching post-debonding was evaluated in three groups of subjects: orthodontically treated patients immediately after debonding, patients in the retention phase and untreated controls. Each group received either a 38% hydrogen peroxide bleaching treatment or a placebo agent. Tooth colour changes were assessed at seven time points for CIELAB colour parameters in all upper incisors and canines (Figure 4.4). Statistically significant differences were observed between the Bleaching-Untreated and Bleaching-Retention subgroups and between different groups of teeth. Based on the results from this study, previous exposure to fixed orthodontic appliances influenced the efficacy of tooth bleaching.

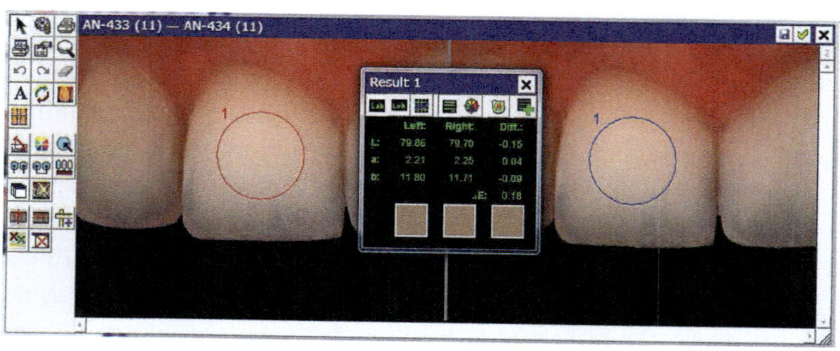

Figure 4.4 Consecutive spectrophotometric recordings of an upper-right central incisor (SpecroShade Micro; MHT, Zurich, Switzerland).

The bleaching effect was greater after orthodontic treatment and with a longer retention period. Canines changed in colour more than incisors (Koumpia et al. 2022).

It has been suggested that different variables in the bonding/debonding procedure may affect the initial response to whitening. Changes in enamel morphology caused by debonding procedures may affect the degree of light reflected from the test surface (Eliades et al. 2004c), and the amount of enamel loss can differ for each surface (van Waes et al. 1997). Most studies agree that the bonding/debonding processes of orthodontic treatment influence the bleaching effect. It seems that with the onset of orthodontic debonding, and as time elapses, the enamel is more susceptible to resin tags that discolour the post-debonded surface, thus increasing the post-bleaching colour difference.

4.4 Enamel Roughness Changes After Debonding

Since the advent of the acid-etch technique (Buonocore 1955) and its use for bracket bonding, a primary concern at the completion of orthodontic treatment has been to restore the enamel surface to its pretreatment state. Removal of orthodontic fixed appliances involves the mechanical removal of adhesive residuals with various abrasive rotary tools or hand instruments. These have been shown to cause enamel loss (Banerjee et al. 2008; Fitzpatrick and Way 1977; Ireland et al. 2005), irreversible enamel damage (Eliades et al. 2004c; Zachrisson and Arthun 1979) and increased enamel roughness, leading to colour alterations (Eliades et al. 2001).

Surface roughness (SR) is defined as a complex of irregularities or small projections and indentations that characterise a surface and influence wetting, quality of adhesion and brightness. Usually, SR is expressed as a measurement representing an averaged and macroscopic measurement of the overall surface topography: average roughness (Ra). Although Ra is considered a poor indicator of surface texture, it is the most frequently recorded value to verify surface topography in dental materials (Abu-Bakr et al. 2001; Kakaboura et al. 2007; Marigo et al. 2001).

Enamel SR can be visualised by profilometry (Mhatre et al. 2015), rugosimetry (Cardoso et al. 2014), scanning electron microscopy (SEM)

(Shah et al. 2019) and atomic force microscopy (AFM) (Kubínek et al. 2007). Profilometry, rugosimetry and AFM provide three-dimensional (3D) numerical data of the SR for subsequent evaluation. SEM gives two-dimensional (2D) information; therefore, visual enamel evaluation indices are required to conduct statistical analysis (Sugsompian et al. 2020). Indices including the enamel surface index (ESI) (Pont et al. 2010), enamel damage index (EDI) (Alessandri Bonetti et al. 2011; Baumann et al. 2011) and enamel surface rating system (ESRS) (Schiefelbein and Rowland 2011) have been employed in SEM studies. Even though SEM is widely applied, it is considered a subjective method (Winchester 1991).

Profile analysis, contact diamond and non-contact laser modes, in addition to laser reflectivity measuring systems, are frequently applied for surface profile measurements (Joniot et al. 2000; Whitehead et al. 1999). Limitations of surface profilometry with respect to the sensitivity of the method have been described (Whitehead et al. 1995, 1996). AFM uses high resolution, at the level of a nanometre, and multiple mechanical 3D scans to analyse surface irregularities (Binnig et al. 1986) and offers several advantages (Kakaboura et al. 2007; Karan et al. 2010; Tholt de Vasconcellos et al. 2006).

At the completion of active orthodontic treatment, bracket debonding and adhesive removal contribute to the formation of prominent areas or grooves on the tooth surface, leading to enamel staining (Joo et al. 2011). Surface roughening may be associated with plaque accumulation and bacterial retention (Bollen et al. 1997; Joo et al. 2011), leading to aesthetic concerns. Although post-orthodontic scarring of the enamel surface seems inevitable, several techniques have been introduced that aim to minimally affect the enamel microstructure. These include hand instruments (pliers, scalers), ultrasonic devices, various burs, aluminium oxide discs, air abrasion units and erbium family diode lasers.

Enamel SR has been extensively evaluated qualitatively (Brauchli et al. 2011; Campbell 1995; Caspersen 1977; Faria-Júnior et al. 2015; Fitzpatrick and Way 1977; Radlanski 2001; Retief and Denys 1979; Shah et al. 2019; Smith et al. 1999; Vieira et al. 1993; Zachrisson 1977) and quantitatively (Eichenberger et al. 2019; Eliades et al. 2004a; Hong and Lew 1995; Hosein et al. 2004; Ireland et al. 2005; Pinzan-Vercelino et al. 2021; Pont et al. 2010; Roush et al. 1997; Shah et al. 2019; Tüfekçi et al. 2004). In an early SEM study, the authors concluded that a green rubber wheel was more effective and less destructive to enamel than a tungsten carbide bur

(Gwinnett and Gorelick 1977). The results of this study contradict those of Zachrisson and Arthun (1979), where tungsten carbide burs scored better than green rubber wheels, but the two studies employed different methods of enamel surface assessment.

Zarrinnia et al. (1995) compared seven different adhesive removal procedures. Diamond burs were found to be extremely destructive, while tungsten carbide burs were more efficient in adhesive removal, followed by Sof-Lex discs and a rubber cup with Zircate paste. In SEM studies using subjective visual assessment, a tungsten carbide bur proved to be the quickest (Eminkahyagil et al. 2006) but fairly aggressive method of adhesive removal. The roughest surface was observed following adhesive removal with Arkansas stone (Osorio et al. 1998) and the smoothest with Sof-Lex aluminium oxide discs (Eminkahyagil et al. 2006) and PoGo micropolishers (Ulusoy 2009), although both techniques were time-consuming (Eminkahyagil et al. 2006; Ulusoy 2009; Zarrinnia et al. 1995). Hong and Lew (1995), using the surface roughness index (SRI), concluded that ultrafine diamond produced the roughest surface and tungsten carbide burs gave the best surface smoothness. EDI following the use of a tungsten carbide bur scored as grade 0 in 8 teeth, grade 1 (acceptable surface, fine scattered scratches) in 13 teeth and grade 2 (rough surface, numerous coarse scratches or slight grooves) in 3 teeth (Alessandri Bonetti et al. 2011). Another SEM study compared the effectiveness of tungsten carbide, fibreglass and polymer burs and a polymer bur with 75% ethanol pretreatment. Polymer burs were less effective and more time-consuming in removing the remaining resin than carbide and fibreglass burs (Soares Tenório et al. 2020).

In quantitative studies of enamel SR, most authors used tungsten carbide burs but stressed the necessity of finishing and polishing procedures. Eliades et al. (2004a) assessed the enamel surface following debonding using two resin removal methods. The enamel surface of 30 premolars was subjected to profilometry, registering four roughness parameters. An eight-bladed carbide bur was used in half the specimens and an ultra-fine diamond bur in the other half, both attached to a high-speed hand piece. In both groups, finishing was achieved with Sof-Lex discs. Resin removal with a diamond bur was twice as fast but more destructive than with a carbide bur. Roughness variables presented elevated values at the resin removal interval that could not be reversed with Sof-Lex discs. Even after polishing, enamel grooves remained, although they had reduced height (Eliades et al. 2004a). This finding is in accordance with other research indicating irreversible changes in enamel post-debonding (Ahrari et al. 2013; Al Shamsi et al. 2007; Banerjee et al. 2008; Karan et al. 2010; Piacentini and Sfondrini 1996; Ryf et al. 2012).

Karan et al. (2010) compared the effects of a tungsten carbide bur and a composite bur on the SR of enamel after debonding. The composite bur provided a smoother enamel surface, but the time required for resin removal was greater than with the carbide bur (Karan et al. 2010). In a study where Sof-Lex discs and fibreglass burs were tested, it was concluded that no clean-up procedure restored enamel to its original roughness, but Sof-Lex discs proved to be the most successful technique (Ozer et al. 2010).

It has been suggested that a one-step polisher and finisher and adhesive residue remover can achieve a smoother enamel surface than a tungsten carbide bur (Janiszewska-Olszowska et al. 2016). Based on the results of Fan et al. (2017), evaluating three resin removal techniques, a OneGloss polisher left enamel surfaces closest to the intact enamel; Super-Snap discs provided acceptable surfaces, although several deep scratches were left; and a diamond bur was not suitable for removing adhesive remnants (Fan et al. 2017).

It has been proposed that the use of a dental loupe by the practitioner may affect the quality of the debonding procedure, causing less enamel damage and better resin removal (Baumann et al. 2011). In an AFM study, enamel SR values were compared after resin removal with a white stone bur, a tungsten carbide bur and a tungsten carbide bur under loupe magnification. The white stone bur was the most time-consuming technique for adhesive removal. The mean times required for resin removal with the carbide bur alone and the carbide bur with a dental loupe were similar (Mohebi et al. 2017).

Enamel surface morphology has also been assessed after lingual bracket debonding using 3D optical interferometric profilometry (Eichenberger et al. 2019). Measurements were made before and after debonding of lingual brackets, following enamel finishing with fine diamond and polishing with 12- and 20-fluted carbide burs. Four roughness parameters were tested, and parameter differences were calculated. Debonding lingual brackets from enamel resulted in an increase in all roughness parameters. The most-affected parameter was the hybrid parameter Sdr, which measures the developed interfacial area ratio, expressed as the percentage of the developed area due to surface texture compared to an ideal plane of the same size. The authors concluded that in lingual debonding, increased roughness may involve a significant area of the enamel surface with the potential to enhance the plaque-retaining capacity of teeth (Eichenberger et al. 2019). In a study using both SEM and AFM, enamel roughness was evaluated using four polishing methods: Sof-Lex disc, sandblaster, tungsten carbide bur and white stone bur. All methods resulted in a clinically acceptable enamel SR below 200 nm, and post-debonded enamel smoothness was similar in the sandblaster and Sof-Lex groups (Sugsompian et al. 2020).

A novel technology that can be used for composite removal is a laser. Although different laser wavelengths have been used for enamel clean-up (Alexander et al. 2002; Smith et al. 1999; Thomas et al. 1996), primarily erbium family lasers have been used for this purpose (Ahrari et al. 2013; Ferreira et al. 2020). Almeida et al. (2009) found that the Er:YAG laser performed significantly better than the conventional technique in removing composite remnants, although it produced a significantly greater amount of enamel loss than the tungsten-carbide bur group. Ahrari et al. (2013) found increased SR and irreversible enamel damage on the tooth surface after clean-up with the diamond bur and the Er:YAG laser compared to the tungsten carbide bur. Similarly, the Er:YAG laser was found to cause more surface irregularity compared to three types of multibladed diamond burs (6-, 12- and 30-bladed) and aluminium oxide sandblasting. The 30-bladed bur created the least-irregular enamel surface, while aluminium oxide sandblasting caused greater enamel wear (Ferreira et al. 2014). Results from laser studies indicate that this method is not recommended for composite removal post-debonding.

Although a threshold for unacceptable SR has not yet been established, an often-cited critical threshold of 0.2 μm of SR has been proposed. Values greater than that can result in increased bacterial adhesion, plaque accumulation and a higher risk of caries (Bollen et al. 1997; Quirynen et al. 1990). Other reports have found no substantial differences in plaque accumulation on surfaces with Ra values from 0.7 to 1.4 μm (Kakaboura et al. 2007; Shintani et al. 1985; Weitman and Eames 1975).

The literature suggests that enamel roughening during adhesive removal depends on the tool used, bur rotation speed and pressure applied to the handpiece. There is much controversy between studies on a universally approved protocol of enamel clean-up after bracket

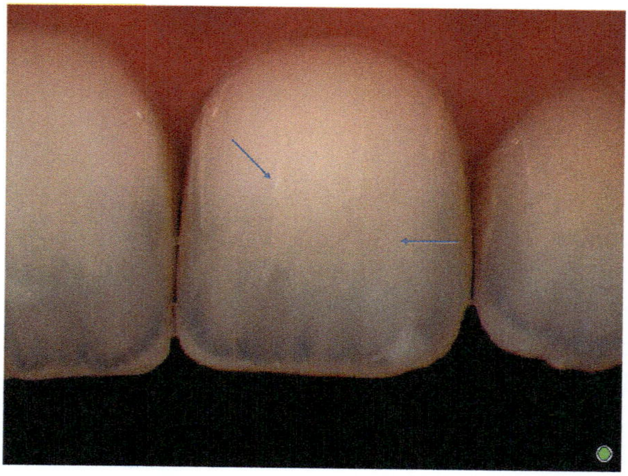

Figure 4.5 Spectrophotometric recordings of an orthodontically treated upper-left central incisor. Note the enamel microfractures and discolouration of adhesive remnants on the tooth surface (SpecroShade Micro; MHT, Zurich, Switzerland).

debonding. Most studies agree that removing residual resin using a tungsten carbide bur on a low- or high-speed handpiece followed by finishing and polishing with aluminium oxide discs appears to restore enamel SR close to its pretreatment conditions. Roughness changes after debonding correspond to irreversible structural and colorimetric alterations caused by orthodontic bonding and debonding (Eliades et al. 2001) (Figure 4.5). The human eye may not be able to clinically perceive these colour alterations (Trakyali et al. 2009), but a roughened enamel surface may facilitate bacterial retention and promote dental caries. Therefore, a smooth enamel surface post-debonding is important for aesthetic reasons and for resisting demineralisation.

4.5 Tooth Gloss Changes After Debonding

Separately from the colour and roughness variables, the perception of the texture and colour of a surface is influenced by the variance of its gloss. Enamel gloss/reflectivity/shine is an optical property that suggests how well the enamel reflects light in a specular (mirror-like) direction

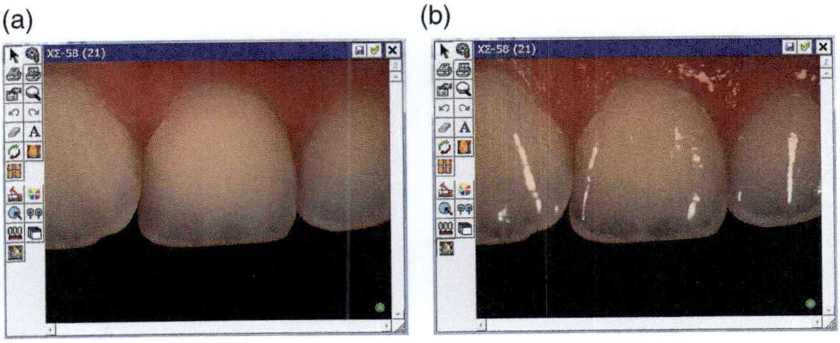

Figure 4.6 Spectrophotometric recordings of an upper-left central incisor. (a) The recorded image is polarised by default. (b) Using the gloss icon tool on the spectrophotometer, the tooth appears with reflections of the incident light (SpecroShade Micro; MHT, Zurich, Switzerland).

(Figure 4.6). *Gloss* is represented by the degree of shine of a surface and is essentially a measure of the difference in the angles formed between the incident and reflected light. The ratio of the angle of specular reflection over that of incidence, defined as *reflectance*, has been shown to be dependent on SR. Increased roughness causes the development of multiple reflecting sites within the same area, with different directions of prism orientation, leading to random or diffuse reflections. Polishing can eliminate enamel SR, which may improve light reflection (Trakyali et al. 2009).

Tooth surface gloss affects the look and vitality of teeth (Terry et al. 2002). On the labial surface of anterior teeth, light reflected from tertiary anatomy adds to vitality, while when this anatomy is worn with age, less vitality is apparent (Figure 4.7). The enamel surface morphology affects the amount and type of reflection. A rough surface permits more diffuse reflection, whereas a flat and smoother surface allows more specular reflection: e.g. the amount of light reflection at enamel surfaces *in vivo* following toothbrushing can be enhanced significantly (Redmalm et al. 1985).

Etching, cleaning and polishing procedures may affect the compositional pattern of enamel surfaces subjected to debonding. Acid etching creates microporosities and increases the surface area of enamel accessible for bonding. This facilitates the infiltration of enamel with bonding resin (tags). Even if there is no subsequent bonding, alterations are found

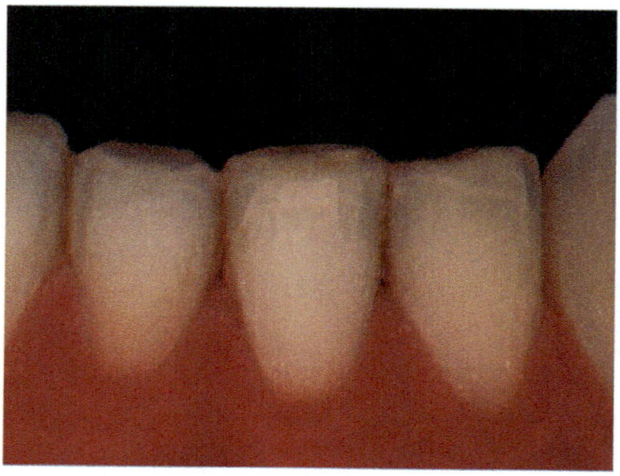

Figure 4.7 Enamel wear of lower incisors (SpecroShade Micro; MHT, Zurich, Switzerland).

in etched enamel after exposure to an oral environment such as higher values in amplitude and hybrid ΣP parameters (Patcas et al. 2015). A hyper-reflexible zone can also be seen, extending as a 10–15 μm wide band below the etched tooth surface that presents differential light reflections (Zentner and Duschner 1996).

The tooth surface following bonding and debonding is mostly composed of cut enamel infiltrated by resin tags, occupying the sites of enamel rods dissolved from acid etching. Consequently, the refractive index of the area may be modified, altering the component of diffusely reflected light. Experiments on bovine enamel have shown that the gloss values measured are different from those of specimens made from resin-based composites (Lefever et al. 2014; Silva et al. 2018).

After acid etching and bonding with conventional composite resins, the enamel surface exhibits changes to a depth of 10–20 μm. Due to the reduced width of the tag (usually no more than 3–5 μm), as well as the increased penetration of the unfilled, liquid resin with low viscosity, no filler particles are usually found in the resin tags. However, composites with nano-particles have been found to penetrate the tag, altering the properties of the resin-enamel adhesive interface (Irinoda et al. 2000; Jogrensen and Shimokobe 1975; Silverstone et al. 1975). It is not easy to safely synthesise evidence relating to the enamel morphology after debonding because of variations in enamel structural properties and standardisation of the debonding technique. Different study findings can be specific to the bonding/debonding protocols used, potentially leading to different results for various debonding protocols.

Effects on the enamel surface can also be found when bonding with a resin-reinforced glass ionomer without prior acid etching. With this method, after debonding and cleaning, the predominating tooth surface features are those of altered enamel. This can be attributed to the fact that mechanical retention with these materials is limited to the flow characteristics of the cement, which allow for adequate enamel moistening and the formation of a reversible hydrolytic molecular bond mechanism between enamel calcium and ionised glass ionomer carboxyl groups (Eliades et al. 2001). SEM has also shown that enamel conditioning with 10% polyacrylic acid before bonding with a light-cured resin-reinforced glass ionomer cement does not alter the fundamental configuration of the enamel surface (Shinya et al. 2008). After bracket bonding with this technique and debonding, no resin tags can be found (Fjeld and Øgaard 2006).

Establishing the relationship between gloss perception, highlighting disparities and roughness is difficult (Methven and Chantler 2012). Increased roughness is correlated with reduced gloss and enhanced diffuse reflectance, which leads to greater lightness (L*) in the Munsell system; however, there is no clear data on the connection between roughness and gloss. It has been shown that surfaces with nominal SR half the wavelength of blue light (approximately 0.2 μm) appear very glossy. Additionally, tooth SR facilitates the buildup of oral pigments, such as coffee, tea and tobacco, which may affect the optical appearance of enamel (Chung 1994; Davis et al. 1995; Eliades et al. 2001).

It is also known that the presence of moisture can influence gloss measurements. The thin layer of water that forms on the tooth surface has a lower refraction index relative to enamel or other adhesive materials due to the development of surface tension at the water–air interface. Under these conditions, surface reflectance can increase as diffuse reflectance is decreased, an effect known as 'wet roughness', which has been shown to increase the smoothness of surfaces in the oral environment. This can also be clinically useful in removing remaining bonding material since the air drying of the adhesive surface can facilitate the differentiation from enamel of adhesive remnants that appear to be relatively whitish (Sifakakis et al. 2018).

Human perceptibility and acceptability of surface gloss on composite resin and tooth specimens can be influenced by gloss variations (Rocha et al. 2020) and can vary under different illuminants (Rocha et al. 2021). Additionally, measurements by gloss meters approximate the perceived gloss since the angular resolution of these instruments is greater than that of the human visual system. Consequently, human eye perception of gloss-meter differences can vary (Sifakakis et al. 2018).

While bleaching treatment with 38% hydrogen peroxide has not been found to change enamel surface gloss (Pedreira De Freitas et al. 2011), different dentifrices have been shown to influence tooth gloss. Teeth that had been left unbrushed for 24 hours exhibited statistically significant lower light reflection values than those recorded immediately after the teeth had been brushed with toothpaste (Redmalm et al. 1985). Fluoride dentifrice containing calcium, phosphate and sodium bicarbonate can effectively improve tooth-surface gloss with regular use (Muñoz et al. 2004), while significantly increased tooth gloss was exhibited after polishing with toothpaste containing nanohydroxyapatite particles (Pedreira De Freitas et al. 2011). Moreover, a low-abrasivity dentifrice containing sodium tripolyphosphate (STP) and aluminium trioxide caused enamel gloss compared to a non-alumina ultra-low-abrasivity STP-containing dentifrice and moderate- and high-abrasivity dentifrices over eight weeks (Milleman et al. 2017).

Research regarding tooth gloss changes after bonding/debonding procedures and the relationship between perceived and physical gloss is limited. Sifakakis et al. (2018) assessed *in vitro* enamel gloss changes caused by orthodontic bracket bonding with a light-cured composite or a light-cured resin-reinforced glass ionomer cement. The buccal surfaces of 20 extracted human upper first premolars were subjected to 60°-angle gloss measurement with a standardised repeated analysis of the same site. Subsequently, a bracket was bonded in half of the specimens with acid-etching and a light-cured composite and in the other half with a light-cured resin-reinforced glass ionomer cement without prior enamel conditioning. Gloss measurements were repeated post-debonding after the removal of the composite/glass ionomer cement with an 18-fluted carbide bur on wet specimens. The authors concluded that the two common bracket bonding protocols examined (acid-etching with a light-cured composite vs. no etching with light-cured resin-reinforced glass ionomer cement) and subsequent debonding and adhesive removal with the same protocol did lead to enamel gloss changes. Teeth bonded with composite/acid-etching exhibited greater enamel gloss changes than resin-reinforced glass ionomer cement/no etching. Since a statistically significant difference was demonstrated although the same adhesive grinding protocol was used, the authors suggest that the bur may have removed the surface layer (already affected by the bonding technique) or may have similarly affected the optical properties of the remaining enamel surface. Less enamel loss occurs after bonding with a resin-modified glass ionomer cement, especially if a slow-speed tungsten carbide bur is used, compared to a high-speed tungsten carbide bur or an ultrasonic scaler (Hosein et al. 2004), a fact that can explain the difference in gloss measurements. The use of ultraviolet light associated with a fluorescent adhesive is proposed for effective adhesive removal compared with conventional lighting without causing further enamel loss (Ribeiro et al. 2017).

Patil et al. (2016) used a custom-made reflectometer to study *in vitro* the effect of various procedures during orthodontic treatment on enamel gloss. The reflectivity of teeth was measured before and after bonding, debonding and polishing with three methods (tungsten carbide burs, Astropol and Sof-Lex discs). None of the methods tested restored the original enamel reflectivity. Tungsten carbide burs provided the least reflectivity of all the systems evaluated, while the closest reproduction of the enamel reflectivity was achieved using Sof-Lex discs.

The limited available literature suggests that common debonding protocols lead to enamel gloss changes, and their effects are possibly minimised by polishing with Sof-Lex discs. However, further research is needed to investigate the effect of several factors, such as bonding adhesives, debonding and polishing modalities and their clinical significance, and/or examine possible ways to minimise the detrimental effects of debonding on tooth gloss using various types of dentifrice.

References

Abu-Bakr, N., Han, L., Okamoto, A., and Iwaku, M. (2001). Evaluation of the surface roughness of compomer by laser scanning microscopy. *Dent. Mater. J.* 20: 172–180.

Ahrari, F., Akbari, M., Akbari, J., and Dabiri, G. (2013). Enamel surface roughness after debonding of orthodontic brackets and various clean-up techniques. *J. Dent. (Tehran)* 10: 82–93.

Akyalcin, S., Frels, L.K., English, J.D., and Laman, S. (2014). Analysis of smile esthetics in American Board of Orthodontic patients. *Angle Orthod.* 84: 486–491.

Al Maaitah, E.F., Abu Omar, A.A., and Al-Khateeb, S.N. (2013). Effect of fixed orthodontic appliances bonded with different etching techniques on tooth color: a prospective clinical study. *Am. J. Orthod. Dentofacial Orthop.* 144: 43–49.

Al Shamsi, A.H., Cunningham, J.L., Lamey, P.J., and Lynch, E. (2007). Three-dimensional measurement of residual adhesive and enamel loss on teeth after debonding of orthodontic brackets: an in-vitro study. *Am. J. Orthod. Dentofacial Orthop.* 131: 301.e9–301.e15.

Alessandri Bonetti, G., Zanarini, M., Incerti Parenti, S. et al. (2011). Evaluation of enamel surfaces after bracket debonding: an in-vivo study with scanning electron microscopy. *Am. J. Orthod. Dentofacial Orthop.* 140: 696–702.

Alexander, R., Xie, J., and Fried, D. (2002). Selective removal of residual composite from dental enamel surfaces using the third harmonic of a Q-switched Nd:YAG laser. *Lasers Surg. Med.* 30: 240–245.

Al-Khateeb, S., Forsberg, C.M., de Josselin de Jong, E., and Angmar-Månsson, B. (1998). A longitudinal laser fluorescence study of white spot lesions in orthodontic patients. *Am. J. Orthod. Dentofacial Orthop.* 113: 595–602.

Alkhatib, M.N., Holt, R., and Bedi, R. (2005). Age and perception of dental appearance and tooth colour. *Gerodontology* 22: 32–36.

Al-Laban, Y.R.A. (2015). Comparison of enamel color alteration between bonded and free unbonded surfaces of maxillary anterior teeth after fixed orthodontic therapy: a prospective clinical study. *J. Baghdad Coll. Dent.* 27: 174–178.

Almeida, H.C., Vedovello Filho, M., Vedovello, S.A. et al. (2009). ER: YAG laser for composite removal after bracket debonding: a qualitative SEM analysis. *Int. J. Orthod. Milwaukee* 20: 9–13.

Årtun, J. and Thylstrup, A. (1986). Clinical and scanning electron microscopic study of surface changes of incipient caries lesions after debonding. *Scand. J. Dent. Res.* 94: 193–201.

Baker, R.S., Fields, H.W. Jr., Beck, F.M. et al. (2018). Objective assessment of the contribution of dental esthetics and facial attractiveness in men via eye tracking. *Am. J. Orthod. Dentofacial Orthop.* 153: 523–533.

Banerjee, A., Paolinelis, G., Socker, M. et al. (2008). An in vitro investigation of the effectiveness of bioactive glass air-abrasion in the 'selective' removal of orthodontic resin adhesive. *Eur. J. Oral Sci.* 116: 488–492.

Baumann, D.F., Brauchli, L., and van Waes, H. (2011). The influence of dental loupes on the quality of adhesive removal in orthodontic debonding. *J. Orofac. Orthop.* 72: 125–132.

Berns, R.S. (2000). *Billmeyer and Saltzman's Principles of Colour Technology*, 3e. New York: Wiley.

Billmeyer, F.W. and Saltzman, M. (1981). *Principles of Colour Technology*, 2e, 1–110. New York: Wiley.

Binnig, G., Quate, C.F., and Gerber, C. (1986). Atomic force microscope. *Phys. Rev. Lett.* 56: 930–933.

Bollen, C.M., Lambrechts, P., and Quirynen, M. (1997). Comparison of surface roughness of oral hard materials to the threshold surface roughness for bacterial plaque retention: a review of the literature. *Dent. Mater.* 13: 258–269.

Boncuk, Y., Cehreli, Z.C., and Polat-Özsoy, Ö. (2014). Effects of different orthodontic adhesives and resin removal techniques on enamel colour alteration. *Angle Orthod.* 84: 634–641.

ten Bosch, J.J. and Coops, J.C. (1995). Tooth color and reflectance as related to light scattering and enamel hardness. *J. Dent. Res.* 74: 374–380.

ten Bosch, J.J. and Zijp, J.R. (1987). Optical properties of dentin. In: *Dentine and Dentine Reactions in the Oral Cavity* (ed. A. Thylstrup, S.A. Leach, and V. Qvist), 59–65. Oxford: IRL Press.

Brauchli, L.M., Baumgartner, E.M., Ball, J., and Wichelhaus, A. (2011). Roughness of enamel surfaces after different bonding and debonding procedures: an in vitro study. *J. Orofac. Orthop.* 72: 61–67.

Bridgeman, I. (1987). The nature of light and its interaction with matter. In: *Colour Physics for Industry* (ed. R. McDonald), 1–34. Huddersfield: H. Charlesworth & Co Ltd.

Buonocore, M.G. (1955). A simple method of increasing the adhesion of acrylic filling materials to enamel surfaces. *J. Dent. Res.* 34: 849–853.

van der Burgt, T.P., ten Bosch, J.J., Borsboom, P.C., and Kortsmit, W.J. (1990). A comparison of new and conventional methods for quantification of tooth colour. *J. Prosthet. Dent.* 63: 155–162.

Campbell, P.M. (1995). Enamel surfaces after orthodontic bracket debonding. *Angle Orthod.* 65: 103–110.

Cardoso, L.A., Valdrighi, H.C., Vedovello Filho, M., and Correr, A.B. (2014). Effect of adhesive remnant removal on enamel topography after bracket debonding. *Dent. Press. J. Orthod.* 19: 105–112.

Caspersen, I.V.A.R. (1977). Residual acrylic adhesive after removal of plastic orthodontic brackets: a scanning electron microscopic study. *Am. J. Orthod.* 71: 637–650.

Chen, Q., Zheng, X., Chen, W. et al. (2015). Influence of orthodontic treatment with fixed appliances on enamel color: a systematic review. *BMC Oral Health* 15: 13.

Chung, K.H. (1994). Effects of finishing and polishing procedures on the surface texture of resin composites. *Dent. Mater.* 10: 325–330.

Cinader, D. (2001). Chemical processes and performance comparisons of Transbond Plus self-etching primer. *Orthod. Perspect.* 8: 5–6.

Commission Internationale de l' Enclairage. (1971). Colourimetry, official recommendations of the International Commission on Illumination. Publication CIE No. 15 (E.1.3.1).

Çörekçi, B., Toy, E., Öztürk, F. et al. (2015). Effects of contemporary orthodontic composites on tooth color following short term fixed orthodontic treatment: a controlled clinical study. *Turk. J. Med. Sci.* 45: 1421–1428.

Cunningham, M.R. (1986). Measuring the physical in physical attractiveness: quasi-experiments on the sociobiology of female facial beauty. *J. Pers. Soc. Psychol.* 50: 925–935.

Cunningham, M.R., Barbee, A.P., and Pike, C.L. (1990). What do women want? Facialmetric assessment of multiple motives in the perception of male facial physical attractiveness. *J. Pers. Soc. Psychol.* 59: 61–72.

Dasy, H., Dasy, A., Asatrian, G. et al. (2015). Effects of variable attachment shapes and aligner material on aligner retention. *Angle Orthod.* 85: 934–940.

Davis, B.A., Friedl, K.H., and Powers, J.M. (1995). Colour stability of hybrid ionomers after accelerated aging. *J. Prosthodont.* 4: 111–115.

Dawes, C. (1974). Rythms in salivary flow rate and composition. *Int. J. Chronobiol.* 2: 253–279.

Dietschi, D., Campanile, G., Holz, J., and Meyer, J.M. (1994). Comparison of the color stability of ten new-generation composites: an in vitro study. *Dent. Mater.* 10: 353–362.

Dion, K., Berscheid, E., and Walster, E. (1972). What is beautiful is good. *J. Pers. Soc. Psychol.* 24: 285–290.

Douglas, R.D. (1997). Precision of in vivo colourimetric assessments of teeth. *J. Prosthet. Dent.* 77: 464–470.

Dumbryte, I., Linkeviciene, L., Malinauskas, M. et al. (2013). Evaluation of enamel micro-cracks characteristics after removal of metal brackets in adult patients. *Eur. J. Orthod.* 35: 317–322.

Eichenberger, M., Iliadi, A., Koletsi, D. et al. (2019). Enamel surface roughness after lingual bracket debonding: an in vitro study. *Materials (Basel)* 13 (12): 4196.

Eldiwany, M., Friedl, K.H., and Powers, J.M. (1995). Color stability of light-cured and post-cured composites. *Am. J. Dent.* 8: 179–181.

Eli, I., Bar-Tal, Y., and Kostovetzki, I. (2001). At first glance: social meanings of dental appearance. *J. Public Health Dent.* 61: 150–154.

Eliades, T., Kakaboura, A., Eliades, G., and Bradley, T.G. (2001). Comparison of enamel colour changes associated with orthodontic bonding using two different adhesives. *Eur. J. Orthod.* 23: 85–90.

Eliades, T., Gioka, C., Eliades, G., and Makou, M. (2004a). Enamel surface roughness following debonding using two resin grinding methods. *Eur. J. Orthod.* 26: 333–338.

Eliades, T., Gioka, C., Heim, M. et al. (2004b). Color stability of orthodontic adhesive resins. *Angle Orthod.* 74: 391–393.

Eliades, T., Kakaboura, A., Eliades, G., and Bradley, T.G. (2004c). Enamel colour alterations associated with orthodontics. In: *Risk Management in Orthodontics: Experts' Guide to Malpractice* (ed. T.M. Graber, T. Eliades, and A.E. Athanasiou), 11–18. Chicago: Quintessence Publishing.

Eliades, T., Papageorgiou, S.N., and Ireland, A.J. (2020). The use of attachments in aligner treatment: analyzing the "innovation" of expanding the use of acid etching-mediated bonding of composites to enamel and its consequences. *Am. J. Orthod. Dentofacial Orthop.* 158: 166–174.

Eminkahyagil, N., Arman, A., Cetinşahin, A., and Karabulut, E. (2006). Effect of resin-removal methods on enamel and shear bond strength of rebonded brackets. *Angle Orthod.* 76: 314–321.

Erdemir, U., Yildiz, E., and Eren, M.M. (2012). Effects of sports drinks on color stability of nanofilled and microhybrid composites after long-term immersion. *J. Dent.* 40: e55–e63.

Faltermeier, A., Rosentritt, M., Reicheneder, C., and Behr, M. (2008). Discolouration of orthodontic adhesives caused by food dyes and ultraviolet light. *Eur. J. Orthod.* 30: 89–93.

Fan, X.C., Chen, L., and Huang, X.F. (2017). Effects of various debonding and adhesive clearance methods on enamel surface: an in vitro study. *BMC Oral Health* 27 (17): 58.

Faria-Júnior, É.M., Guiraldo, R.D., Berger, S.B. et al. (2015). In-vivo evaluation of the surface roughness and morphology of enamel after bracket removal and polishing by different techniques. *Am. J. Orthod. Dentofacial Orthop.* 147: 324–329.

Ferracane, J.L. (1985). Correlation between hardness and degree of conversion during the setting reaction of unfilled dental restorative resins. *Dent. Mater.* 1: 11–14.

Ferreira, F.G., Nouer, D.F., Silva, N.P. et al. (2014). Qualitative and quantitative evaluation of human dental enamel after bracket debonding: a noncontact three-dimensional optical profilometry analysis. *Clin. Oral Investig.* 18: 1853–1864.

Ferreira, F.G., da Silva, E.M., and Vilella, O.V. (2020). A novel method using confocal laser scanning microscopy for three-dimensional analysis of human dental enamel subjected to ceramic bracket debonding. *Microsc. Microanal.* 26: 1053–1060.

Fitzpatrick, D.A. and Way, D.C. (1977). The effects of wear, acid etching, and bond removal on human enamel. *Am. J. Orthod.* 72: 671–681.

Fjeld, M. and Øgaard, B. (2006). Scanning electron microscopic evaluation of enamel surfaces exposed to 3 orthodontic bonding systems. *Am. J. Orthod. Dentofacial Orthop.* 130: 575–581.

Flanary, C. (1992). The psychology of appearance and psychological impact of surgical alteration of the face. In: *Modern Practice in Orthognathic and Reconstructive Surgery* (ed. W.H. Bell), 3–21. Philadelphia, PA: Saunders.

Gegenfurtner, K.R. and Kiper, D.C. (2003). Color vision. *Ann. Rev. Neurosci.* 26: 181–206.

Gioka, C., Bourauel, C., Hiskia, A. et al. (2005). Light-cured or chemically cured orthodontic adhesive resins? A selection based on the degree of cure, monomer leaching, and cytotoxicity. *Am. J. Orthod. Dentofacial Orthop.* 127: 413–419.

Giron de Velasco, J., de la Cuadra, P., and Urizar, G. (2017). The influence of maxillary incisor torque on the esthetic perception of the smile. *Int. J. Esthet. Dent.* 12: 378–395.

Gomes Lde, O., Mathias, P., Rizzo, P. et al. (2013). Effect of dental bleaching after bracket bonding and debonding using three different adhesive systems. *Dent. Press. J. Orthod.* 18: 61–68.

Goodkind, R.J. and Schwabacher, W.B. (1987). Use of a fiber-optic colourimeter for in vivo colour measurements of 2830 anterior teeth. *J. Prosthet. Dent.* 58: 535–542.

Gorucu-Coskuner, H., Atik, E., and Taner, T. (2018). Tooth color change due to different etching and debonding procedures. *Angle Orthod.* 88: 779–784.

Gwinnett, A.J. and Gorelick, L. (1977). Microscopic evaluation of enamel after debonding: clinical application. *Am. J. Orthod.* 71: 651–665.

Haghighi, A.H.S., Emami, M., Fakhri, E., and Rezaei, Y. (2020). Effects of orthodontic adhesives on dental enamel color alteration using chemically cured and light-cured composites. *Front. Dent.* 17: 1–9.

Hariri, I., Sadr, A., Shimada, Y. et al. (2012). Effects of structural orientation of enamel and dentine on light attenuation and local refractive index: an optical coherence tomography study. *J. Dent.* 40: 387–396.

Hill, A.R. (1987). How we see colour. In: *Colour Physics for Industry* (ed. R. McDonald), 211–281. Huddersfield: H. Charlesworth & Co Ltd.

Hindle, J.P. and Harrison, A. (2000). Tooth colour analysis by a new optoelectronic system. *Eur. J. Prosthodont. Restor. Dent.* 8: 57–61.

Hintz, J.K., Bradley, T.G., and Eliades, T. (2001). Enamel colour changes following whitening with 10 per cent carbamide peroxide: a comparison of orthodontically-bonded/debonded and untreated teeth. *Eur. J. Orthod.* 23: 411–415.

Hong, Y.H. and Lew, K.K. (1995). Quantitative and qualitative assessment of enamel surface following five composite removal methods after bracket debonding. *Eur. J. Orthod.* 17: 121–128.

Hosein, I., Sherriff, M., and Ireland, A.J. (2004). Enamel loss during bonding, debonding, and cleanup with use of a self-etching primer. *Am. J. Orthod. Dentofacial Orthop.* 126: 717–724.

Hosoya, Y., Shiraishi, T., Odatșu, T. et al. (2011). Effects of polishing on surface roughness, gloss, and color of resin composites. *J. Oral Sci.* 53: 283–291.

Inokoshi, S., Burrow, M.F., Kataumi, M. et al. (1996). Opacity and color changes of tooth-colored restorative materials. *Oper. Dent.* 21: 73–80.

Ireland, A.J., Hosein, I., and Sherriff, M. (2005). Enamel loss at bond-up, debond and clean-up following the use of a conventional light-cured composite and a resin-modified glass polyalkenoate cement. *Eur. J. Orthod.* 27: 413–419.

Irinoda, Y., Matsumura, Y., Kito, H. et al. (2000). Effect of sealant viscosity on the penetration of resin into etched human enamel. *Oper. Dent.* 25: 274–282.

Isiekwe, G.I. and Aikins, E.A. (2019). Self-perception of dental appearance and aesthetics in a student population. *Int. Orthod.* 17: 506–512.

Jadad, E., Montoya, J., Arana, G. et al. (2011). Spectrophotometric evaluation of color alterations with a new dental bleaching product in patients wearing orthodontic appliances. *Am. J. Orthod. Dentofacial Orthop.* 140: e43–e47.

Jahanbin, A., Ameri, H., and Khaleghimoghaddam, R. (2009). Effect of adhesive types on enamel discolouration around orthodontic brackets. *Aust. Orthod. J.* 25: 19–23.

Jahangiri, L., Reinhardt, S.B., Mehra, R.V., and Matheson, P.B. (2002). Relationship between tooth shade value and skin color: an observational study. *J. Prosthet. Dent.* 87: 149–152.

Janiszewska-Olszowska, J., Szatkiewicz, T., Tomkowski, R. et al. (2014). Effect of orthodontic debonding and adhesive removal on the enamel - current knowledge and future perspectives - a systematic review. *Med. Sci. Monit.* 20: 1991–2001.

Janiszewska-Olszowska, J., Tomkowski, R., Tandecka, K. et al. (2016). Effect of orthodontic debonding and residual adhesive removal on 3D enamel microroughness. *PeerJ* 4: e2558.

Jarvis, J., Zinelis, S., Eliades, T., and Bradley, T.G. (2006). Porcelain surface roughness, color and gloss changes after orthodontic bonding. *Angle Orthod.* 76: 274–277.

Jogrensen, K.D. and Shimokobe, H. (1975). Adaptation of resinous restorative materials to acid etched enamel surfaces. *Scand. J. Dent. Res.* 83: 31–36.

Johnson, E.K., Fields, H.W. Jr., Beck, F.M. et al. (2017). Role of facial attractiveness in patients with slight-to-borderline treatment need according to the Aesthetic Component of the Index of Orthodontic Treatment Need as judged by eye tracking. *Am. J. Orthod. Dentofacial Orthop.* 151: 297–310.

Johnston, W.M. and Kao, E.C. (1989). Assessment of appearance match by visual observation and clinical colorimetry. *J. Dent. Res.* 68: 819–822.

Joiner, A. (2004). Tooth colour: a review of the literature. *J. Dent.* 32 (Suppl 1): 3–12.

Joniot, S.B., Grégoire, G.L., Auther, A.M., and Roques, Y.M. (2000). Three-dimensional optical profilometry analysis of surface states obtained after finishing sequences for three composite resins. *Oper. Dent.* 25: 311–315.

Joo, H.J., Lee, Y.K., Lee, D.Y. et al. (2011). Influence of orthodontic adhesives and clean-up procedures on the stain susceptibility of enamel after debonding. *Angle Orthod.* 81: 334–340.

Kakaboura, A., Fragouli, M., Rahiotis, C., and Silikas, N. (2007). Evaluation of surface characteristics of dental composites using profilometry, scanning electron, atomic force microscopy and gloss-meter. *J. Mater. Sci. Mater. Med.* 18: 155–163.

Kamber, R., Papageorgiou, S.N., and Eliades, T. (2018). Does orthodontic treatment have a permanent effect on tooth color? *J. Orofac. Orthop.* 79: 73–82.

Karamouzos, A., Athanasiou, A.E., Papadopoulos, M.A., and Kolokithas, G. (2010). Tooth-color assessment after orthodontic treatment: a prospective clinical trial. *Am. J. Orthod. Dentofacial Orthop.* 138: 537.e1–537.e8.

Karamouzos, A., Zafeiriadis, A.A., Kolokithas, G. et al. (2019). In vivo evaluation of tooth colour alterations during orthodontic retention: a split-mouth cohort study. *Orthod. Craniofac. Res.* 22: 124–130.

Karan, S., Kircelli, B.H., and Tasdelen, B. (2010). Enamel surface roughness after debonding. *Angle Orthod.* 80: 1081–1088.

Kaya, Y., Alkan, Ö., Değirmenci, A., and Keskin, S. (2018). Long-term follow-up of enamel color changes after treatment with fixed orthodontic appliances. *Am. J. Orthod. Dentofacial Orthop.* 154: 213–220.

Kershaw, S., Newton, J.T., and Williams, D.M. (2008). The influence of tooth colour on the perceptions of personal characteristics among female dental patients: comparisons of unmodified, decayed and 'whitened' teeth. *Br. Dent. J.* 204: E9.

Kim, S.P., Hwang, I.N., Cho, J.H., and Hwang, H.S. (2006). Tooth color changes associated with the bracket bonding and debonding. *Korean J. Orthod.* 36: 114–124.

Korkmaz, Y.N. and Bulut, M. (2020). Effect of mouthwashes on the discoloration of bracket-bonded tooth surfaces: an in vitro study. *Clin. Oral Investig.* 24: 3855–3861.

Koumpia, E., Eliades, T., Knösel, M., and Athanasiou, A.E. (2022). Colour assessment of bleaching effect on orthodontically treated teeth. *Eur. J. Orthod.* 44: 537–547.

Krishnan, V. and Davidovitch, Z. (2006). Cellular, molecular, and tissue-level reactions to orthodontic force. *Am. J. Orthod. Dentofacial Orthop.* 129: 469.e1–469.e32.

Kubínek, R., Zapletalová, Z., Vůjtek, M. et al. (2007). Sealing of open dentinal tubules by laser irradiation: AFM and SEM observations of dentine surfaces. *J. Mol. Recognit.* 20: 476–482.

Kuehni, R.G. and Marcus, R.T. (1979). An experiment in visual scaling of small colour differences. *Colour Res. Appl.* 4: 83–91.

Lefever, D., Krejci, I., and Ardu, S. (2014). Laboratory evaluation of the effect of toothbrushing on surface gloss of resin composites. *Am. J. Dent.* 27: 42–46.

Leibrock, A., Rosentritt, M., Lang, R. et al. (1997). Colour stability of visible light-curing hybrid composites. *Eur. J. Prosthodont. Restor. Dent.* 5: 125–130.

Lunardi, N., Correr, A.B., Rastelli, A.N. et al. (2014). Spectrophotometric evaluation of dental bleaching under orthodontic bracket in enamel and dentin. *J. Clin. Exp. Dent.* 6: e321–e326.

Lynch, D. and Livingston, W. (1995). *Color and Light in Nature* (ed. D. Lynch and W. Livingston), 31–47. Cambridge: Cambridge University Press.

Maijer, R. and Smith, D.C. (1982). Corrosion of orthodontic bracket bases. *Am. J. Orthod.* 81: 43–48.

Malekpour, B., Ajami, S., Salehi, P., and Hamedan, S. (2022). Use of nano-hydroxyapatite serum and different finishing/polishing techniques to reduce enamel staining of debonding after orthodontic treatment: a randomized clinical trial. *J. Orofac. Orthop.* 83: 205–214.

Marigo, L., Rizzi, M., La Torre, G., and Rumi, G. (2001). 3-D surface profile analysis: different finishing methods for resin composites. *Oper. Dent.* 26: 562–568.

McLaren, K. (1987). Colour space, colour scales and colour difference. In: *Colour Physics for Industry* (ed. R. McDonald), 97–115. Huddersfield: H. Charlesworth & Co Ltd.

Methven, T.S. and Chantler, M.J. (2012). Problems of perceiving gloss on complex surfaces. In: *Predicting Perceptions: Proceedings of the 3rd International Conference on Appearance* (ed. S. Padilla, M.J. Chantler, J. Harris, and M.R. Pointer), 43–47. Edinburgh: Lulu Press.

Mhatre, A.C., Tandur, A.P., Reddy, S.S. et al. (2015). Enamel surface evaluation after removal of orthodontic composite remnants by intraoral sandblasting technique and carbide bur technique: a three-dimensional surface profilometry and scanning electron microscopic study. *J. Int. Oral Health* 7: 34–39.

Micu, M. and Carstairs, C. (2018). From improving egos to perfecting smiles: orthodontics and psychology, 1945–2000. *Can. Bull. Med. Hist.* 35: 309–336.

Milleman, K.R., Milleman, J.L., Young, S., and Parkinson, C. (2017). Randomized controlled trial to explore the effect of experimental low abrasivity dentifrices on enamel gloss and smoothness, and the build-up of extrinsic tooth stain. *J. Clin. Dent.* 28: 1–8.

Mohebi, S., Shafiee, H.A., and Ameli, N. (2017). Evaluation of enamel surface roughness after orthodontic bracket debonding with atomic force microscopy. *Am. J. Orthod. Dentofacial Orthop.* 151: 521–527.

Montero, J., Gómez-Polo, C., Santos, J.A. et al. (2014). Contributions of dental colour to the physical attractiveness stereotype. *J. Oral Rehabil.* 41: 768–782.

Muñoz, C.A., Stephens, J.A., Proskin, H.M., and Ghassemi, A. (2004). Clinical efficacy evaluation of calcium, phosphate, and sodium bicarbonate on surface-enamel smoothness and gloss. *Compend. Contin. Educ. Dent.* 25: 32–39.

Murrell, E.F., Yen, E.H., and Johnson, R.B. (1996). Vascular changes in the periodontal ligament after removal of orthodontic forces. *Am. J. Orthod. Dentofacial Orthop.* 110: 280–286.

Nakamura, K., Arai, S., and Kawabata, H. (2017). Prioritized identification of attractive and romantic partner faces in rapid serial visual presentation. *Arch. Sex. Behav.* 46: 2327–2338.

Neumann, L.M., Christensen, C., and Cavanaugh, C. (1989). Dental esthetic satisfaction in adults. *J. Am. Dent. Assoc.* 118: 565–570.

Newton, J.T., Prabhu, N., and Robinson, P.G. (2003). The impact of dental appearance on the appraisal of personal characteristics. *Int. J. Prosthodont.* 16: 429–434.

Nickerson, D. (1969). History of the Munsell color system. *Color Eng.* 7: 42–51.

O'Brien, W.J., Hemmendinger, H., Boenke, K.M. et al. (1997). Colour distribution of three regions of extracted human teeth. *Dent. Mater.* 13: 179–185.

Odioso, L.L., Gibb, R.D., and Gerlach, R.W. (2000). Impact of demographic, behavioral, and dental care utilization parameters on tooth color and personal satisfaction. *Compend. Contin. Educ. Dent. Suppl.* 29: S35–S41; quiz S43.

Øgaard, B. (2008). White spot lesions during orthodontic treatment: mechanisms and fluoride preventive aspects. *Semin. Orthod.* 14: 183–193.

Øgaard, B., Rolla, G., and Arends, J. (1988). Orthodontic appliances and enamel emineralization. Part 1. Lesion development. *Am. J. Orthod. Dentofacial Orthop.* 94: 68–73.

Øgaard, B., Bishara, S.E., and Duschner, H. (2004). Enamel effects during bonding-debonding and treatment with fixed appliances. In: *Risk Management in Orthodontics: Experts' Guide to Malpractice* (ed. T.M. Graber, T. Eliades, and A.E. Athanasiou), 19–46. Chicago: Quintessence.

Okubo, S.R., Kanawati, A., Richards, M.W., and Childress, S. (1998). Evaluation of visual and instrument shade matching. *J. Prosthet. Dent.* 80: 642–648.

Osorio, R., Toledano, M., and García-Godoy, F. (1998). Enamel surface morphology after bracket debonding. *ASDC J. Dent. Child.* 65: 313–317.

Ozer, T., Başaran, G., and Kama, J.D. (2010). Surface roughness of the restored enamel after orthodontic treatment. *Am. J. Orthod. Dentofacial Orthop.* 137: 368–374.

Papageorgiou, S.N., Xavier, G.M., and Cobourne, M.T. (2015). Basic study design influences the results of orthodontic clinical investigations. *J. Clin. Epidemiol.* 8: 1512–1522.

Paravina, R.D. and Powers, J.M. (2004). *Esthetic Color Training in Dentistry*, 1e. UK: Elsevier-Mosby Ltd.

Paravina, R.D., Ghinea, R., Herrera, L.J. et al. (2015). Color difference thresholds in dentistry. *J. Esthet. Restor. Dent.* 27: S1–S9.

Patcas, R., Zinelis, S., Eliades, G., and Eliades, T. (2015). Surface and interfacial analysis of sandblasted and acid-etched enamel for bonding orthodontic adhesives. *Am. J. Orthod. Dentofacial Orthop.* 147: S64–S75.

Patil, H.A., Chitko, S.S., Kerudi, V.V. et al. (2016). Effect of various finishing procedures on the reflectivity (shine) of tooth enamel - an in-vitro study. *J. Clin. Diagn. Res.* 10: ZC22-7.

Pedreira De Freitas, A.C., Botta, S.B., Teixeira Fde, S. et al. (2011). Effects of fluoride or nanohydroxiapatite on roughness and gloss of bleached teeth. *Microsc. Res. Tech.* 74: 1069–1075.

Piacentini, C. and Sfondrini, G. (1996). A scanning electron microscopy comparison of enamel polishing methods after air-rotor stripping. *Am. J. Orthod. Dentofacial Orthop.* 109: 57–63.

Pinzan-Vercelino, C.R.M., Souza Costa, A.C., Gurgel, J.A., and Salvatore Freitas, K.M. (2021). Comparison of enamel surface roughness and color alteration after bracket debonding and polishing with 2 systems: a split-mouth clinical trial. *Am. J. Orthod. Dentofacial Orthop.* 160: 686–694.

Pont, H.B., Özcan, M., Bagis, B., and Ren, Y. (2010). Loss of surface enamel after bracket debonding: an in-vivo and ex-vivo evaluation. *Am. J. Orthod. Dentofacial Orthop.* 138: 387.e1–387.e9.

Pop-Ciutrila, I.S., Ghinea, R., Perez Gomez, M.D.M. et al. (2015). Dentine scattering, absorption, transmittance and light reflectivity in human incisors, canines and molars. *J. Dent.* 43: 1116–1124.

Preston, J.D. (1985). Current status of shade selection and colour matching. *Quintessence Int.* 1: 47–58.

Quirynen, M., Marechal, M., Busscher, H.J. et al. (1990). The influence of surface free energy and surface roughness on early plaque formation. An in vivo study in man. *J. Clin. Periodontol.* 17: 138–144.

Radlanski, R.J. (2001). A new carbide finishing bur for bracket debonding. *J. Orofac. Orthop.* 62: 296–304.

Ragain, J.C. and Johnston, W.M. (2000). Color acceptance of direct dental restorative materials by human observers. *Color Res. Appl.* 25: 278–285.

Ratzmann, A., Schwahn, C., Treichel, A. et al. (2018). Assessing the effect of multibracket appliance treatment on tooth color by using electronic measurement. *Head Face Med.* 22: 14–22.

Re, D.E. and Perrett, D.I. (2014). The effects of facial adiposity on attractiveness and perceived leadership ability. *Q. J. Exp. Psychol. (Hove)* 67: 676–686.

Redmalm, G., Johannsen, G., and Ryden, H. (1985). Lustre changes on teeth. The use of laser light for reflexion measurements on the tooth surface–in vivo. *Swed. Dent. J.* 9: 29–35.

Reno, E.A., Sunberg, R.J., Block, R.P., and Bush, R.D. (2000). The influence of lip/gum color on subject perception of tooth color. *J. Dent. Res.* 79: 381.

Retief, D.H. and Denys, F.R. (1979). Finishing of enamel surfaces after debonding of orthodontic attachments. *Angle Orthod.* 49: 1–10.

Retief, D.H., Busscher, H.J., de Boer, P. et al. (1986). A laboratory evaluation of three etching solutions. *Dent. Mater.* 2: 202–206.

Rhodes, G. (2006). The evolutionary psychology of facial beauty. *Annu. Rev. Psychol.* 57: 199–226.

Ribeiro, A.A., Almeida, L.F., Martins, L.P., and Martins, R.P. (2017). Assessing adhesive remnant removal and enamel damage with ultraviolet light: an in-vitro study. *Am. J. Orthod. Dentofacial Orthop.* 151: 292–296.

Rocha, R.S., Fagundes, T.C., Caneppele, T., and Bresciani, E. (2020). Perceptibility and acceptability of surface gloss variations in dentistry. *Oper. Dent.* 45: 134–142.

Rocha, R.S., de Carvalho, V.G., Galvão, M. et al. (2021). Perceptibility and acceptability of surface gloss variation under different illuminants. *Oper. Dent.* 46: E98–E104.

Roush, E.L., Marshall, S.D., Forbes, D.P., and Perry, F.U. (1997). In vitro study assessing enamel surface roughness subsequent to various final finishing procedures after debonding. *Northwest. Dent. Res.* 7: 2–6.

Rubino, M., Barcia, J.A., Jimenez del Barco, L., and Romero, J. (1994). Colour measurement of human teeth and evaluation of a colour guide. *Colour Res. Appl.* 19: 19–22.

Russell, M.D., Gulfraz, M., and Moss, B.W. (2000). In vivo measurement of colour changes in natural teeth. *J. Oral Rehabil.* 27: 786–792.

Ruyter, I.E., Nilner, K., and Moller, B. (1987). Color stability of dental composite resin materials for crown and bridge veneers. *Dent. Mater.* 3: 246–251.

Ryf, S., Flury, S., Palaniappan, S. et al. (2012). Enamel loss and adhesive remnants following bracket removal and various clean-up procedures in vitro. *Eur. J. Orthod.* 34: 25–32.

Sandison, R. (1981). Tooth surface appearance after debonding. *Br. J. Orthod.* 8: 199–201.

Sarafopoulou, S., Zafeiriadis, A.A., and Tsolakis, A.I. (2018). Enamel defects during orthodontic treatment. *Balk. J. Dent. Med.* 22: 64–73.

Schiefelbein, C. and Rowland, K. (2011). A comparative analysis of adhesive resin removal methods. *Int. J. Orthod. Milwaukee* 22: 17–22.

Seghi, R.R., Hewlett, E.R., and Kim, J. (1989). Visual and instrumental colourimetric assessments of small colour differences on translucent dental porcelain. *J. Dent. Res.* 68: 1760–1764.

Shah, P., Sharma, P., Goje, S.K. et al. (2019). Comparative evaluation of enamel surface roughness after debonding using four finishing and polishing systems for residual resin removal-an in vitro study. *Prog. Orthod.* 20: 18.

Shaw, W.C. (1981). The influence of children's dentofacial appearance on their social attractiveness as judged by peers and lay adults. *Am. J. Orthod.* 79: 399–415.

Shayan, A.M., Behroozian, A., Sadrhaghighi, A. et al. (2021). Effect of different types of acid-etching agents and adhesives on enamel discoloration during orthodontic treatment. *J. Dent. Res. Dent. Clin. Dent. Prospects Winter* 15: 7–10.

Shintani, H., Satou, J., Satou, N. et al. (1985). Effects of various finishing methods on staining and accumulation of Streptococcus mutans HS-6 on composite resins. *Dent. Mater.* 1: 225–227.

Shinya, M., Shinya, A., Lassila, L.V. et al. (2008). Treated enamel surface patterns associated with five orthodontic adhesive systems–surface morphology and shear bond strength. *Dent. Mater. J.* 27: 1–6.

Sifakakis, I., Zinelis, S., Eliades, G. et al. (2018). Enamel gloss changes induced by orthodontic bonding. *J. Orthod.* 45: 269–274.

Silva, E.M.D., Maia, J.N.D.S.M.D., Mitraud, C.G. et al. (2018). Can whitening toothpastes maintain the optical stability of enamel over time? *J. Appl. Oral Sci.* 26: e20160460.

Silverstone, L.M., Saxton, C.A., Dogon, I.L., and Fejerskov, O. (1975). Variation in the pattern of acid etching of human dental enamel examined by scanning electron microscopy. *Caries Res.* 9: 373–387.

Slack, M.E., Swift, E.J. Jr., Rossouw, P.E., and Phillips, C. (2013). Tooth whitening in the orthodontic practice: a survey of orthodontists. *Am. J. Orthod. Dentofacial Orthop.* 143: S64–S71.

Smith, S.C., Walsh, L.J., and Taverne, A.A. (1999). Removal of orthodontic bonding resin residues by CO_2 laser radiation: surface effects. *J. Clin. Laser Med. Surg.* 17: 13–18.

Soares Tenório, K.C., Neupmann Feres, M.F., Tanaka, C.J. et al. (2020). In vitro evaluation of enamel surface roughness and morphology after orthodontic debonding: traditional cleanup systems versus polymer bur. *Int. Orthod.* 18: 546–554.

Soheilifar, S., Khodadadi, H., Naghdi, N., and Farhadian, M. (2021). Does a diluted chlorhexidine-based orthodontic mouthwash cause less discoloration compared to chlorhexidine mouthwash in fixed orthodontic patients? A randomized controlled trial. *Int. Orthod.* 19: 406–414.

Spitzer, D. and ten Bosch, J.J. (1975). The absorption and scattering of light in bovine and human enamel. *Calcif. Tissue Res.* 17: 129–137.

Sugsompian, K., Tansalarak, R., and Piyapattamin, T. (2020). Comparison of the enamel surface roughness from different polishing methods: scanning electron microscopy and atomic force microscopy investigation. *Eur. J. Dent.* 14: 299–305.

Talamas, S.N., Mavor, K.I., and Perrett, D.I. (2016). Blinded by beauty: attractiveness bias and accurate perceptions of academic performance. *PLoS One* 11: e0148284.

Terry, D.A., Geller, W., Tric, O. et al. (2002). Anatomical form defines color: function, form and aesthetics. *Pract. Proced. Aesthet. Dent.* 14: 59–67.

Tholt de Vasconcellos, B., Miranda-Júnior, W.G., Prioli, R. et al. (2006). Surface roughness in ceramics with different finishing techniques using atomic force microscope and profilometer. *Oper. Dent.* 31: 442–449.

Thomas, B.W., Hook, C.R., and Draughn, R.A. (1996). Laser-aided degradation of composite resin. *Angle Orthod.* 66: 281–286.

Trakyali, G., Ozdemir, F.I., and Arun, T. (2009). Enamel colour changes at debonding and after finishing procedures using five different adhesives. *Eur. J. Orthod.* 31: 397–401.

Tüfekçi, E., Merrill, T.E., Pintado, M.R. et al. (2004). Enamel loss associated with orthodontic adhesive removal on teeth with white spot lesions: an in vitro study. *Am. J. Orthod. Dentofacial Orthop.* 125: 733–739.

Tunca, M. and Kaya, Y. (2023). Effect of various orthodontic adhesives on enamel colour changes after fixed treatment. *J. Orofac. Orthop.* 84: 125–133.

Tuncer, N.I., Pamukcu, H., and Polat-Ozsoy, O. (2018). Effects of repeated bracket bonding on enamel color changes. *Niger. J. Clin. Pract.* 21: 1093–1097.

Ulusoy, C. (2009). Comparison of finishing and polishing systems for residual resin removal after debonding. *J. Appl. Oral Sci.* 17: 209–215.

Vaarkamp, J., ten Bosch, J.J., and Verdonschot, E.H. (1995). Propagation of light through human dental enamel and dentine. *Caries Res.* 29: 8–13.

Vallittu, P.K., Vallittu, A.S.J., and Lassila, V.P. (1996). Dental aesthetics—a survey of attitudes in different groups of patients. *J. Dent.* 24: 335–338.

Van der Geld, P., Oosterveldb, P., Van Heckc, G., and Kuijpers-Jagtman, A.M. (2007). Smile attractiveness self-perception and influence on personality. *Angle Orthod.* 77: 759–765.

Vieira, A.C., Pinto, R.A., Chevitarese, O., and Almeida, M.A. (1993). Polishing after debracketing: its influence upon enamel surface. *J. Clin. Pediatr. Dent.* 18: 7–11.

van Waes, H., Matter, T., and Krejci, I. (1997). Three-dimensional measurement of enamel loss caused by bonding and debonding of orthodontic brackets. *Am. J. Orthod. Dentofacial Orthop.* 112: 666–669.

Weitman, R.T. and Eames, W.B. (1975). Plaque accumulation on composite surfaces after various finishing procedures. *Oral Health* 65: 29–33.

Whitehead, S.A., Shearer, A.C., Watts, D.C., and Wilson, N.H. (1995). Comparison of methods for measuring surface roughness of ceramic. *J. Oral Rehabil.* 22: 421–427.

Whitehead, S.A., Shearer, A.C., Watts, D.C., and Wilson, N.H. (1996). Surface texture changes of a composite brushed with "tooth whitening" dentifrices. *Dent. Mater.* 12: 315–318.

Whitehead, S.A., Shearer, A.C., Watts, D.C., and Wilson, N.H. (1999). Comparison of two stylus methods for measuring surface texture. *Dent. Mater.* 15: 79–86.

Winchester, L. (1991). Direct orthodontic bonding to porcelain: an in vitro study. *Br. J. Orthod.* 18: 299–308.

Wriedt, S., Keller, S., and Wehrbein, H. (2008). The effect of debonding and/or bleaching on enamel color - an in-vitro study. *J. Orofac. Orthop.* 69: 169–176.

Wu, H.-M., Ye, C., and Chen, D. (2018). Comparative study of enamel discoloration related to bonding with different orthodontic adhesives and cleaning-up with different procedures. *Shanghai Kou Qiang Yi Xue* 27: 257–260.

Xiao, J., Zhou, X.D., Zhu, W.C. et al. (2007). The prevalence of tooth discolouration and the self-satisfaction with tooth colour in a Chinese urban population. *J. Oral Rehabil.* 34: 351–360.

Ye, C., Zhao, Z., Zhao, Q. et al. (2013). Comparison of enamel discoloration associated with bonding with three different orthodontic adhesives and cleaning-up with four different procedures. *J. Dent.* 41: e35–e40.

Zachrisson, B.J. (1977). A posttreatment evaluation of direct bonding in orthodontics. *Am. J. Orthod.* 71: 173–189.

Zachrisson, B.U. (2000). Bonding in orthodontics. In: *Orthodontics, Current Principles and Techniques*, 3e (ed. T.M. Graber and R.L. Vanarsdall), 557–645. St. Louis: Mosby.

Zachrisson, B.U. and Arthun, J. (1979). Enamel surface appearance after various debonding techniques. *Am. J. Orthod.* 75: 121–127.

Zachrisson, B.U., Skogan, O., and Höymyhr, S. (1980). Enamel cracks in debonded, debanded, and orthodontically untreated teeth. *Am. J. Orthod.* 77: 307–319.

Zaher, A.R., Abdalla, E.M., Abdel Motie, M.A. et al. (2012). Enamel colour changes after debonding using various bonding systems. *J. Orthod.* 39: 82–88.

Zarrinnia, K., Eid, N.M., and Kehoe, M.J. (1995). The effect of different debonding techniques on the enamel surface: an in vitro qualitative study. *Am. J. Orthod. Dentofacial Orthop.* 108: 284–293.

Zentner, A. and Duschner, H. (1996). Structural changes of acid etched enamel examined under confocal laser scanning microscope. *J. Orofac. Orthop.* 57: 202–209.

Zhu, J.J., Tang, A.T., Matinlinna, J.P., and Hägg, U. (2014). Acid etching of human enamel in clinical applications: a systematic review. *J. Prosthet. Dent.* 112: 122–135.

5

Aerosol Production during Resin Removal with Rotary Instruments

Anthony J. Ireland, Christian J. Day, and Jonathan R. Sandy

Department of Orthodontics, Bristol Dental School, University of Bristol, Bristol, UK

5.1 Introduction

Following the completion of a course of fixed appliance treatment, it is necessary to remove the brackets, bands and tubes along with any residual adhesive from the teeth. Hopefully the enamel surfaces will be returned as nearly as possible to their original pretreatment condition. However, the process of orthodontic debonding and enamel clean-up is not without risk. One such risk is the production of airborne particulates as a result of the use of rotary instruments at any or all of the following points during the process:

- Flash removal prior to ceramic bracket debonding
- Removal of residual adhesive following fixed appliance bracket and band removal
- Removal of fractured brackets (mainly ceramic brackets)

The particulates produced have the potential to be inhaled by the patient or operator, including the orthodontist, orthodontic therapist and orthodontic assistant.

Debonding and Fixed Retention in Orthodontics: An Evidence-Based Clinical Guide, First Edition. Edited by Theodore Eliades and Christos Katsaros.

5.1.1 What Are Airborne Particulates, and Where Might They End Up?

Airborne particulates can be classified according to how they are produced or, perhaps more importantly in the current context, according to their size and, therefore, inhalation risk. Particles produced and emitted directly into the air are known as *primary particles*, and solid particles produced as the result of a chemical reaction between two or more gases are known as *secondary particles* (Concawe 2017).

In orthodontics, both primary and secondary particulates may be produced during debonding, but classifying particles according to their size is perhaps more relevant in the clinical setting. However, a classification of particulates according to absolute size would be of little benefit in terms of describing the potential inhalation risk. It is how they behave in the air that is important, and this behaviour depends on the combination of three factors: particulate size, mass and shape. The mass median aerodynamic diameter (MMAD) in micrometres (μm) determines how far a particle may penetrate the human respiratory system. The depth of this penetration, along with the chemical composition and concentration of the particulates, determines the potential health risk of their inhalation.

To illustrate, consider the particulates typically produced during orthodontic debonding and enamel clean-up, shown in Figure 5.1. They are many different sizes, and once generated, they can be expected to behave differently in the air surrounding a patient's mouth. The largest particles will probably fall quickly out of the air as a result of gravity and end up on the patient's skin and the operator's gloves, with only the smallest particles perhaps being inhaled by the patient and operator. However, this simplistic approach ignores the importance of mass and shape in determining particulate behaviour in the air. As mentioned, it is more relevant to describe airborne particulates according to their MMAD in micrometres (μm) rather than their geometric diameter. This is important because particles with different diameters may behave similarly in how they move within an air stream and, as a result, may be deposited at similar sites within the respiratory system due to their different shapes and masses. This would be the case with the particles shown in Figure 5.1, which were all collected from the air during orthodontic debonding using an impactor, which collects particulates according to MMAD rather than geometric size.

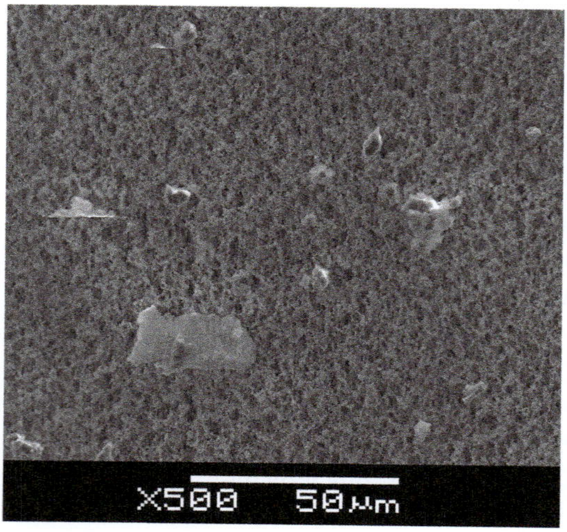

Figure 5.1 A scanning electron microscope image of the various shapes and sizes of particles produced during enamel clean-up following orthodontic debonding.

Various definitions have been applied to particulate size, but useful descriptors include the following (BS EN 481:1993 1993):

The *inhalable fraction* is the mass fraction of particles that can be inhaled through the nose or mouth.

The *thoracic fraction* is the mass fraction of particles that pass the larynx. The median value of particle sizes able to penetrate beyond the larynx is approximately 10 µm.

The *respirable fraction* is the mass fraction of particles that can reach the deeper parts of the lungs to the alveoli. The median value of the distribution of particle sizes in this category is 4.25 µm.

When particles have an MMAD in the range of 50–100 µm, they are sometimes referred to as *splatter*, are readily visible and may end up on the patient's lips and skin or the operator's gloves (Figure 5.2) and protective goggles (Figure 5.3). From a respiratory risk perspective, these particles are of less concern and form the inhalable fraction, which may enter the mouth and nose.

Of more concern in terms of potential respiratory effects are aerosols where the particle MMAD is less than 10 µm, known as PM_{10}

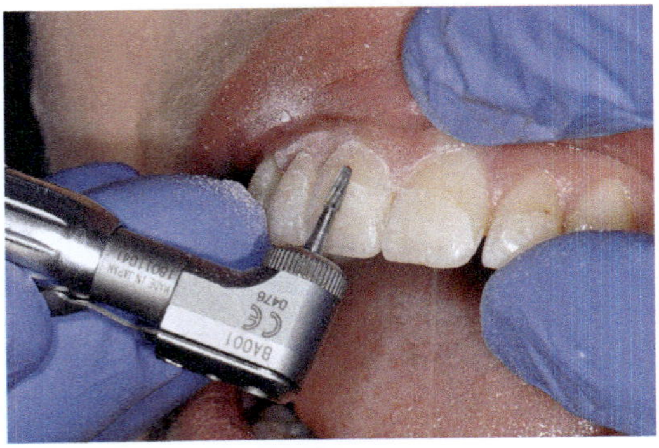

Figure 5.2 Airborne particles produced during enamel clean-up landing on the patient's lips and operator's gloves.

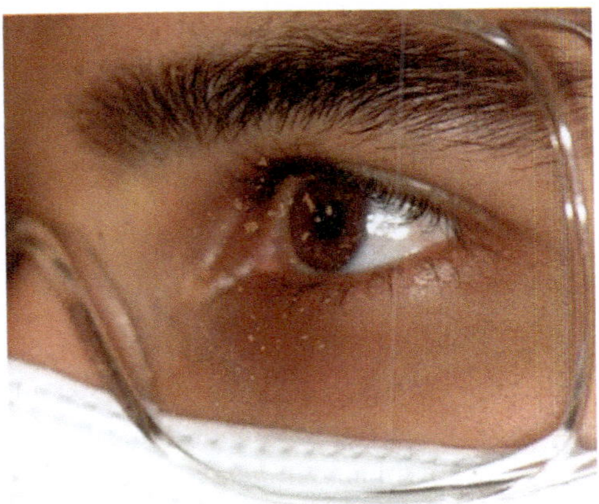

Figure 5.3 Airborne splatter particles visible on the operator's protective goggles.

(PM = particulate matter), as these are most likely to be inhaled and deposited in the human respiratory system. The lungs act as a serial filter such that the larger PM_{10} particles are likely only to reach the pharynx, whereas particles with smaller aerodynamic diameters may be deposited deeper within the respiratory system. Large particles are mostly deposited within the epithelial lining of the upper respiratory tract via inertial impaction, particularly where the airflow changes direction abruptly, e.g. at the bifurcation of the trachea or bronchi, or by gravity.

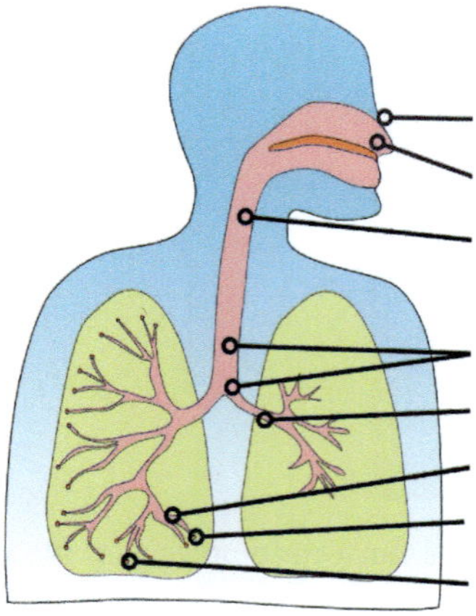

Figure 5.4 A schematic of the human respiratory system and where particulates may be deposited with respect to their mass median aerodynamic diameter (MMAD) and how these relate to the Marple Cascade Impactor stages. Inhalable particulates enter the nose and mouth, the thoracic subfraction of inhalable particulates penetrate beyond the larynx, and the respirable subfraction reach the alveoli of the lungs.

Other key sizes often described are $PM_{2.5}$ (MMAD less than 2.5 μm), which may reach the terminal bronchi, and ultrafines (MMAD less than 0.1 μm), which may reach as deep as the alveoli of the lungs. With decreasing air velocity in the deeper parts of the lungs, these small particles may sediment onto the walls of the bronchioles and alveoli (Möller et al. 2004). Even if they are not inhaled immediately following production, such small particulates can remain airborne almost indefinitely within modest air turbulence and continue to pose an inhalation risk some considerable time after their production (Hext et al. 1999). Figure 5.4 illustrates where particulates with differing MMADs may be deposited in the human respiratory system.

5.1.2 Why Do Airborne Particulates Present a Potential Health Risk?

Airborne particles may pose a potential health risk depending on their aerodynamic diameter (MMAD), chemical composition and solubility and the microbial content of any aerosol (bioaerosol).

5.1.2.1 Aerodynamic Diameter and Lung Clearance

Larger particulates reaching the pharynx, trachea and perhaps the primary bronchi are cleared by the epithelial mucociliary escalator within a few minutes of inhalation or at most one to two days later. This escalator, confined to the conducting zone of the respiratory tree, comprises ciliated cells that move the mucus produced by the goblet cells (Figure 5.5), along with any entrapped particulates, upwards towards the pharynx, where they are either expectorated or swallowed.

The smallest particulates (MMAD less than 1 μm) may reach the respiratory zone and the terminal alveoli of the lungs. This is beyond the mucociliary escalator, so particulate clearance is delayed until the particulates are consumed by the alveolar macrophages. This clearance may take days or even months and, in some cases, may never happen (Hext et al. 1999).

Ultrafine particles (MMAD less than 0.1 μm) penetrate to the depth of the terminal alveoli and may translocate across the alveolar walls and enter the pulmonary interstitium (Ferin et al. 1992) or bloodstream (Seaton 1996; Seaton et al. 1995). Not only do ultrafines penetrate the deeper parts of the lungs, but animal studies have shown them to elicit a greater inflammatory response within the lungs per given mass than larger particles (Oberdörster 2000).

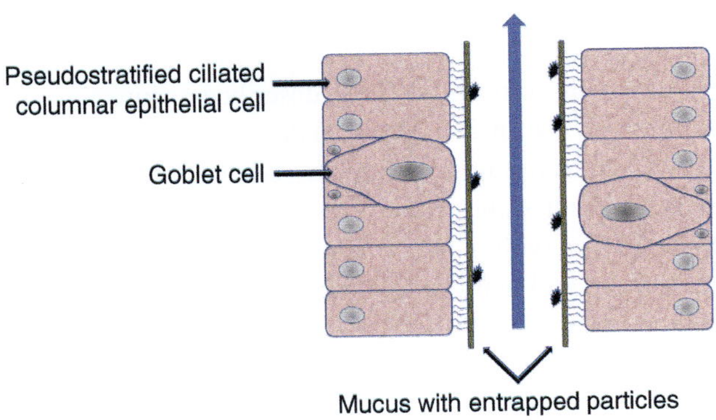

Figure 5.5 Mucociliary escalator lining the conductive airways of the respiratory tree. The large arrow indicates the direction of clearance of the particles towards the pharynx.

5.1.2.2 Chemical Composition and Solubility

In addition to the physical attribute of aerodynamic diameter, the chemical composition and solubility of an aerosol can determine the health risk it poses. For example, it has been suggested that aerosols containing transition metals such as iron, vanadium and nickel have the potential to cause harm as a result of their ability to produce free radicals within biological systems. These free radicals can reduce the built-in antioxidative mechanisms that would otherwise help to protect lung tissues (Donaldson et al. 1997; Gilmour et al. 1997; Li et al. 1997). The damage caused by this mechanism has been linked to increased respiratory and cardiovascular hospital admissions (Bell et al. 2009; Zanobetti et al. 2009).

Other soluble molecules in an aerosol that can dissolve in the pulmonary fluid and enter the systemic circulation include lead, which can cause disease of the central nervous system (Vincent 2005), and cadmium, which can cause kidney damage (Vincent 2005). Organic carbon, elemental carbon and nitrates have also been associated with respiratory and cardiovascular disease (Peng et al. 2009).

5.1.2.3 Bioaerosols

Bioaerosols can consist of nonviable biomolecules (e.g. bacterial endotoxins), nonviable microorganisms or viable microorganisms (Boreson et al. 2004). Respirable bioaerosols may contain viruses with a size range of 0.001–0.025 μm (Božič et al. 2013), bacteria in the range of 0.25–20 μm and fungi in the range of 1–30 μm (Gregory 1973). Therefore, the probability of a particle (or droplet) carrying a microorganism increases with greater aerodynamic diameter.

The effect of inhaling bioaerosols has been described as infectious or allergenic (Griffiths 1994), with infectivity related to the aerodynamic diameter, particulate concentration, organism viability, pathogenicity, airflow, climate and host resistance (Cole and Cook 1998). Examples of health problems associated with bioaerosols include specific respiratory diseases such as asthma and acute respiratory distress syndrome, and less-specific respiratory tract infections, including nasal congestion (Chew et al. 1999; Husman 1996; Skulberg et al. 2004; Teeuw et al. 1994; Wallace 1996; Wyon et al. 2000).

In addition to bacteria, fungi have been implicated in the aetiology of allergic responses and infectious episodes (Gravesen 1979), leading to headaches and eye, nose, sinus and throat symptoms (Kuhn and

Ghannoum 2003). Specific microorganisms may also be responsible for characteristic diseases, e.g. Aspergillus causing aspergillosis (Latge 1999).

Inhalation of viruses may also have significant adverse health effects. The common cold and influenza travel in aerosolised droplets, and the hepatitis B (Toroglu et al. 2003) and human immunodeficiency viruses (Johnson and Robinson 1991) in aerosolised blood.

5.1.2.4 Dental Bioaerosols

The bacterial cell count of human saliva and dental plaque have been reported to be in the region of 10^8 per millilitre and 10^{11} per gram, respectively (Gibbons and Houte 1975), and are thought to contain between 300 and 500 different bacterial species (Moore and Moore 1994; Paster et al. 2001). During routine dental procedures involving the use of a high-speed handpiece, the aerosol produced may contain bacterial concentrations of up to 100 000 per cubic foot in the surrounding ambient air (Bentley et al. 1994). This aerosol may contain microorganisms commonly found in the mouth and pharynx (Greco and Lai 2008; Toroglu et al. 2001). Inhalation of such a bioaerosol may lead to lower respiratory tract disease, with oral bacteria implicated in the aetiology of pneumonia following aspiration of contaminated saliva or plaque (Finegold 1991; Scannapieco et al. 1998). A number of oral bacteria have been isolated from infected lungs, including *S. intermedius*, *Actinomyces* spp., *A. actinomycetemcomitans* and *C. rectus* (Christensen et al. 1993; Kuijper et al. 1992; Rams and Slots 1992; Spiegel and Telford 1984).

5.1.3 What Are the Occupational Health Risks?

Exposure to particulate-containing aerosols can lead to a number of health conditions, with the effect depending on the type of particle inhaled and the site of deposition within the lung. Rhinitis, laryngitis, bronchitis and asthma can all be caused by inhalable dust deposited in the nasopharynx and bronchi. Pneumoconiosis, emphysema, asbestosis and mesothelioma can be due to respirable particles deposited in the terminal bronchioles and alveoli (Vincent 2005).

In occupations other than dentistry, two particulates in particular pose serious health risks: asbestos and silica. With asbestos, the particles produced are not only large in terms of geometric size but also fibrous and flexible. Despite their large size, they have a small MMAD and can penetrate the deeper regions of the lungs. Beyond the mucociliary escalator, their geometric size, shape and inert nature mean they are difficult for the alveolar macrophages and mesothelial cells of the pleura to clear from lung tissues (Feder et al. 2017), and their presence is associated with the long-term development of asbestosis and/or mesothelioma. There are no known safe levels of exposure to asbestos fibres.

Crystalline silica particles reaching the deeper areas of the lungs, beyond the mucociliary escalator, are also ingested by the alveolar macrophages. As a result, these cells secrete inflammatory cytokines, leading to a proliferation of fibroblasts, which in turn produce collagen to surround the silica particles. This results in nodular fibrosis and destruction of the surrounding lung tissue (Leung et al. 2012), which can eventually lead to silicosis (pneumoconiosis), for which there is no known cure. Silicosis is usually associated with workers in industries such as mining, the building industry and stonemasonry, where large amounts of silica dust are produced.

As a result of the health implications of these and other particulates, there are strict workplace exposure limits for many materials, including silica (HSE 2018). The following section discusses how these limits may pertain to orthodontics, based on the evidence that airborne particulates are created during orthodontic appliance removal with rotary instruments.

5.1.4 Are Dental Personnel at Risk from Particulate Inhalation?

Even though particles may reach different levels within the respiratory system and therefore may be rapidly cleared or remain in place indefinitely, is there any evidence within dentistry that this causes any health risks?

Dental laboratory technicians are exposed to a wide variety of potentially harmful substances within the laboratory, including methyl methacrylate (MMA) used in the construction of removable orthodontic appliances; gypsum dust used in the production and trimming of plaster models; silica in sandblasters and porcelain fabrication; and metal alloys used in the manufacture of dentures, crowns and bridges. These metal alloys may include cobalt, chromium, molybdenum, aluminium, nickel and beryllium and may present as particulates or vapours. Cristobalite is a toxic form of respirable crystalline silica found in some casting investment materials. White asbestos (chrysotile) was historically used in dental laboratories and has since been replaced by ceramic-based ring lining materials, although the toxicity of the ceramic fibres in these materials is unknown since the fibres are similar in size to those of asbestos. There have been reports of dentists and dental technicians exposed to either asbestos-containing periodontal dressings or asbestos lining papers used in metal casting succumbing to mesothelioma (Fry 2009; Reid et al. 1991; Taira et al. 2009).

Although the amount of dust produced in a dental laboratory makes it difficult to form an association between reported cases of pneumoconiosis and any specific agent (Radi et al. 2002), the prevalence of pneumoconiosis amongst dental technicians in the literature is sufficiently common – from 4.5 to 16% (Choudat et al. 1993; Froudarakis et al. 1999; Radi et al. 2002; Rom et al. 1984; Selden et al. 1995; Sherson et al. 1988) – for it to be referred to as dental technician pneumoconiosis (DTP). The prevalence of pneumoconiosis in the normal population is around 3.7% (Choudat et al. 1993).

Although dentists and their assistants may be exposed to aerosols when placing and removing restorations and when adjusting crowns and dentures, there are no reported cases of pneumoconiosis in dentists.

5.1.5 What Is the Evidence that Airborne Particulates Are Created during Orthodontic Appliance Removal with Rotary Instruments?

Before describing the available evidence, it is worth revisiting what happens during orthodontic debonding. In the case of metallic brackets, debonding pliers are used to remove the bracket from the tooth surface by promoting crack initiation and propagation (Figures 5.6 and 5.7), usually in the region of the bonding adhesive. However, cohesive failure within the resin is only one of the possible modes of bond failure. The others include

- Cohesive within the enamel
- At the adhesive resin–enamel surface interface
- Cohesive within the adhesive resin
- At the adhesive resin–bracket base interface
- Cohesive within the bracket
- Mixed-mode failure at two or more of these sites

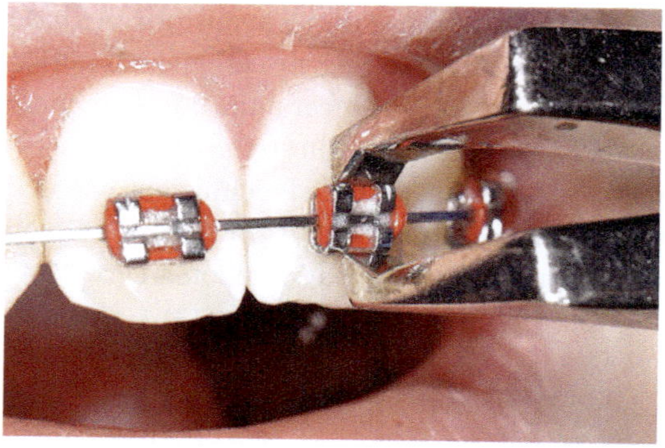

Figure 5.6 Bracket debonding pliers being used to remove a metallic bracket at the completion of treatment.

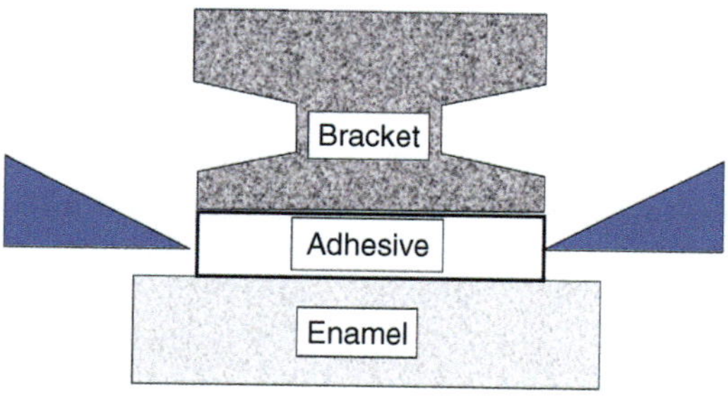

Figure 5.7 Schematic of a bracket bonded to the enamel surface. The blades of the debonding pliers are usually applied at the margins of the adhesive to initiate and promote crack propagation and bracket debonding.

Of these modes of failure, cohesive enamel and bracket failure are, fortunately, the least common. Failure at the enamel–resin interface is much more common and almost inevitably involves some enamel loss, either at debonding or during subsequent enamel clean-up. This is due to the nature of the mechanical bond between the adhesive resin and the enamel (Figure 5.8).

Ceramic brackets can fracture during treatment or at the time of debonding and may involve entirely ceramic cohesive failure or be part of a mixed-mode failure. In both cases, the remainder of the ceramic may need to be removed from the tooth using a diamond bur in a high-speed handpiece under water coolant spray. This has the potential to

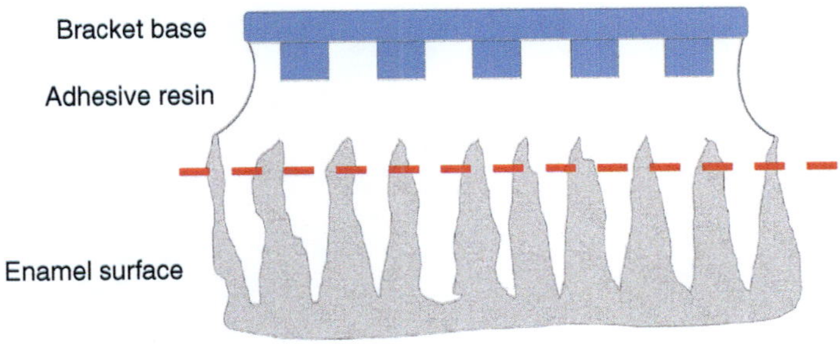

Figure 5.8 Schematic of the bracket base and adhesive resin penetrating the previously etched enamel surface. The dashed line indicates a potential locus of bond failure at the time of bracket debonding, which may macroscopically appear to be at the interface between the enamel and adhesive. Instead, there is likely to be some enamel loss as the bulk of the adhesive is removed at clean-up, and some adhesive resin will remain within the enamel surface.

create an aerosol containing ceramic particulates in addition to adhesive resin and enamel particulates.

A number of studies have been published investigating the particulates produced at the time of orthodontic debonding and enamel clean-up. Following the removal of metallic brackets, bands and residual adhesive, it is known that both PM_{10} and $PM_{2.5}$ particulates are produced. This means both thoracic and respirable fractions are generated in the air within the clinical environment (Ireland et al. 2003).

Typically, the residual adhesive on the enamel surface following bracket debonding is removed using a rotary instrument. This may be a spiral-fluted tungsten carbide bur in a slow- or high-speed handpiece, with or without water coolant spray. A laboratory study by Day et al. (2008) looked at the effect of handpiece speed (high-speed vs. slow-speed) and water coolant spray (no water coolant vs. water coolant) on the particulates produced. In order to determine the MMAD and, therefore, lung-penetration depth, air sampling was carried out during simulated debonding and enamel clean-up using a Marple Personal Cascade Impactor. This impactor simulates the various levels within the respiratory system and offers eight sampling stages, with differing MMAD cut-offs for collecting particulates ranging from approximately 15 to less than 0.5 μm (Figure 5.9). The filter media from each impactor stage collects particles within a small MMAD range. In this study, once collected, the filter from each stage was viewed

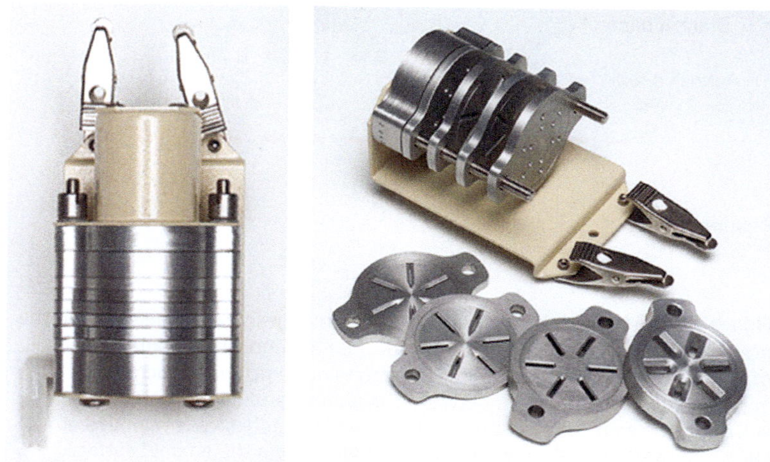

Figure 5.9 Marple Personal Cascade Impactor assembled and disassembled stages.

under scanning electron microscopy (SEM) to assess the presence of particulates at each stage and enable X-ray analysis and thereby help determine the chemical composition of any collected particles. Particles were identified at each impactor stage, where the MMAD cut-off was 8 μm or less for both the slow- and high-speed handpieces and under both water coolant and no water coolant.

All four enamel clean-up methods produced particles with MMADs as small as 0.75 μm or less, which would be respirable and be expected to be deposited in the alveoli of the lungs. These would take months to be cleared following initial early ingestion by alveolar macrophages. However, the greatest number of smaller particles were produced with the high-speed handpiece, particularly in combination with water cooling, whereas the greatest concentration of large particulates was seen when the slow-speed handpiece was used without water coolant, as illustrated in Figure 5.10.

X-ray analysis of the particles from the filters showed a wide variety of materials. The commonest were calcium, phosphorus, silica and aluminium. It was supposed that the calcium and phosphorus were from the tooth enamel and the silica, aluminium and lanthanum were from the bonding resin or the resin-modified glass polyalkenoate band cement.

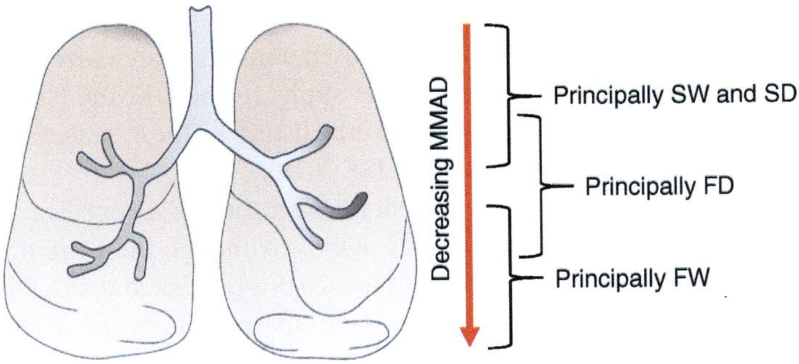

Figure 5.10 Diagram showing the deposition site of the greatest particulate concentrations with each method of clean-up (SW = slow speed and water coolant, SD + slow speed no water coolant, FD = high speed no water coolant, FW = high speed and water coolant).

In the earlier study by Ireland et al. (2003), tungsten was detected and was probably from the debonding bur. In this later study by Day et al. (2008), iron was detected at impactor stages 4 to 8, corresponding to the $PM_{2.5}$ fraction, and was probably from the bearings of the handpiece. Iron is a highly toxic transition metal and, in the $PM_{2.5}$ fraction, is deposited in the deeper regions of the lung, where it is cleared by absorption into the blood or the lymphatic system. The most frequently detected material at all impactor stages was silica. Although there are no reported cases of silicosis among orthodontists, there are strict workplace exposure limits for this material.

5.1.6 What Are Workplace Exposure Limits (WELs), and How Do Particulates Produced During Orthodontic Debonding Compare with Them?

Workplace exposure limits (WELs), previously known as maximum exposure limits (MELs), threshold limit values (TLVs), reference exposure levels (RELs) or occupational exposure limits (OELs), can be defined as the maximum permitted concentration of chemicals, fumes, dust or fibres to which a worker can be exposed over an extended period. They are usually expressed as a time weighted average (TWA) over either 8 hours or a shorter 15-minute period, with the latter primarily used for short-term exposure to materials that may cause fairly rapid irritation, e.g. to the eyes. WELs are the maximum level of inhalable or respirable particles to which a worker should be exposed, and there are currently over 500 substances to which these limits apply. In the UK, the latest Health and Safety Executive (HSE) guidance listing of these materials and their limits was published in 2018 (HSE 2018).

Perhaps of greatest relevance to orthodontics are the WELs for silica, a filler component of many resin bonding agents. Although there are no published short-term exposure limits, there are HSE-published WELs for long-term, 8-hour exposure to silica ranging from 6 mg/m^3 for inhalable particulates to between 2.4 and 0.08 mg/m^3 for respirable particulates. In the USA, Collins et al. (2005) looked at a large number of studies reporting silicosis in mine workers in order to come up with a chronic REL, which is the concentration at or below which no adverse health effects from long-term (lifetime) exposure would be expected in the general population (OEHHA 2000). Chronic RELs are based on the reported adverse health effects occurring at the lowest dose: for respirable silica, this is 3 μg/m^3 (Collins et al. 2005; OEHHA 2000), which is much lower than the UK WEL of 0.1 mg/m^3 advised by the HSE. Finkelstein (2000) suggested that 30 years of exposure to silica at 0.1 mg/m^3 would lead to a lifetime risk of silicosis of 25%, and a lifetime exposure at 0.1 mg/m^3 would lead to an increased risk of lung cancer of 30% or more.

In a recent study by Vig et al. (2019) investigating particulate production during debonding and enamel clean-up following the use of both conventional metal and flash-free ceramic brackets, particulates were identified in all three fractions – inhalable, thoracic and respirable. This was both a laboratory and a clinical investigation, and silica was identified within each fraction using X-ray analysis. In addition to the qualitative part of this study, a quantitative analysis of particulate concentration within the respirable fraction (<5 μm MMAD) was also carried out. Although the WEL for dust was not exceeded, the WEL for silica (0.1 mg/m^3) was exceeded in every experiment. However, it was unlikely that all the particulates were silica, and it was impossible to determine what fraction consisted of silica alone. In this study, each debonding took around 20 minutes to complete, and the WEL for silica is the time-weighted average over 8 hours. Although it is unlikely that any single operator would debond continuously for 8 hours, the effects of the airborne particulates from debonding carried out by other clinicians in multisurgery clinical set-ups could contribute to such an exposure, particularly as it is known that such small particulates can remain airborne for many hours in non-turbulent air (Hext et al. 1999).

5.1.7 What Methods Can Be Used to Reduce the Orthodontist's Exposure to Airborne Particulates Produced During Appliance Debonding and Enamel Clean-Up?

In the study by Vig et al. (2019), the laboratory experiment and clinical trial were performed in the presence of high-volume evacuator (HVE) suction to reduce the level of particulates in the ambient air. This followed a study by Johnston et al. (2009), who looked at two different methods that may be used to reduce the exposure risk of airborne particulates to the orthodontist and any assistants: HVE and a face mask (Figure 5.11). The simulated orthodontic debonding and enamel clean-up methods used were similar to those of Day et al. (2008) and included the use of a tungsten carbide bur in a slow- or high-speed handpiece, with or without the use of a water coolant. In addition, the simulated debonding of polycrystalline ceramic brackets was investigated.

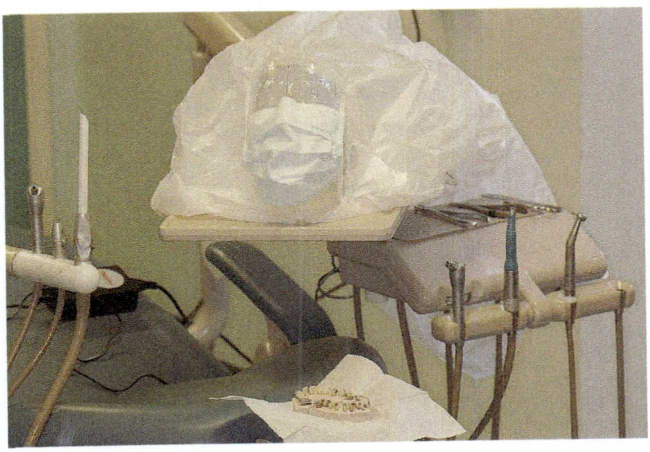

Figure 5.11 The experimental setup used by Johnston et al. (2009) to test the effect of high-volume suction or a facemask on particulate levels. The air sampler in this case is in a sealed bag behind a clear plastic mannequin head with a paper facemask over the nose and mouth.

This entailed flash removal with a tungsten carbide bur in a slow-speed handpiece without water coolant before normal bracket removal and enamel clean-up. It also simulated the removal of fractured ceramic brackets using a diamond bur in a high-speed handpiece with water cooling, followed by conventional enamel clean-up using a slow-speed tungsten carbide bur without water coolant.

A Marple Personal Cascade Impactor was used for qualitative analysis of the particulates produced, which included chemical composition and the possible level they might reach in the lungs. Quantitative analysis was also carried out using a pDr-1200 real-time active air sampler to determine the concentration of particles (mg/m^3) produced with an MMAD of 5 µm or less.

The results showed that using HVE led to a 43.5% reduction in the concentration of respirable particulates produced at debonding of metal brackets and subsequent enamel clean-up using a tungsten carbide bur in a slow-speed handpiece without water cooling. In the case of ceramic brackets and HVE, the concentration of particulates was reduced by 25% when enamel clean-up was carried out using a tungsten carbide bur in a high-speed handpiece with water cooling. Previous work on suction devices has also shown them to be capable of reducing the level of airborne particulates, with HVE being more effective than low-volume evacuator (LVE) suction (Jacks 2002). However, unlike in the study by Johnston et al. (2009), Nimmo et al. (1990) described HVE as more effective in reducing the concentration of particulates for the patient but less effective for the operator, who is still exposed to similar, moderate levels of particulates.

Face masks provide a physical barrier, and many can filter out particles 1 µm or greater in diameter (Lipp and Edwards 2002). In the same study by Johnston et al. (2009), a face mask was much more efficient than HVE, reducing particulate concentration by up to 96%; this was similar to the results reported by Checchi et al. (2005), where the reduction was 85–86% (Checchi et al. 2005). However, it should be remembered that both were laboratory studies, and factors such as breathing, the moisture associated with breathing and the fit of the mask on the moving face cannot easily be replicated; all of these may dramatically reduce efficiency in the clinical setting (Pippin et al. 1987; Weber et al. 1993).

When ceramic brackets fracture during treatment or debonding and require removal with a diamond bur in a high-speed handpiece with water cooling, a large number of airborne particulates are produced. Once again, the face mask in the study by Johnston et al. (2009) reduced the concentration of airborne particulates to levels comparable with those following normal ceramic bracket debonding and enamel clean-up with a slow-speed tungsten carbide bur under dry conditions without water cooling.

5.1.8 What about Bioaerosols Produced During Orthodontic Debond and Enamel Clean-Up?

In addition to the solid particulates created during orthodontic debonding, bioaerosols containing both solid particulates and microbial contaminants can be created. It has been shown that within as little as five minutes of starting debonding and enamel clean-up, there is a significant increase in the concentration of bioaerosols compared to preoperative resting room levels and that these bioaerosols can contain microorganisms derived from the patient's oral cavity (Toroglu et al. 2001).

Orthodontists have traditionally perceived themselves to be at less risk of contracting disease from their patients than general dental practitioners, probably because their patients tend to be mainly children and young adults (Woo et al. 1992). Perhaps because of this perceived lower risk, orthodontists are less likely to adhere to infection control procedures (McCarthy et al. 1997). Certainly the use of rotary instruments would suggest otherwise. The early work on the contamination risk of dental bioaerosols used traditional microbiological culture techniques to directly identify the microbial species present. However, it is now known that approximately 50% of intraoral microbes cannot be cultured in the laboratory. Instead, polymerase chain reaction (PCR) and denaturing gradient gel electrophoresis (DGGE) techniques can be used to identify other microbial species (Muyzer and Smalla 1998).

PCR and DGGE techniques have since been used by Dawson et al. (2016) in a clinical trial to investigate the effect of preprocedural rinsing prior to debonding on the bacterial load and biodiversity of the aerosol produced. The patients included in the trial had all reached the end of a course of upper and lower fixed appliance treatment and were about to be debonded. They were divided into three groups, and each group was allocated a different method of composite removal at appliance debonding:

1) A slow-speed handpiece run dry with a tungsten carbide bur, but no preprocedural mouth rinse
2) A slow-speed handpiece run dry with a tungsten carbide bur following the use of 0.2% chlorhexidine gluconate preprocedural mouth rinse
3) A slow-speed handpiece run dry with a tungsten carbide bur following the use of a sterile water preprocedural mouth rinse

Air sampling was performed using an Andersen 6 Stage Viable Impactor. Within each of the six stages, corresponding to different levels in the human respiratory tree, was a glass petri dish containing culture medium. The six stages, the droplet size and corresponding respiratory levels are shown in Figure 5.12.

This study reported a marked increase in bacterial load during debonding and enamel clean-up compared to the background level of no clinical activity in all three groups, consistent with previous research

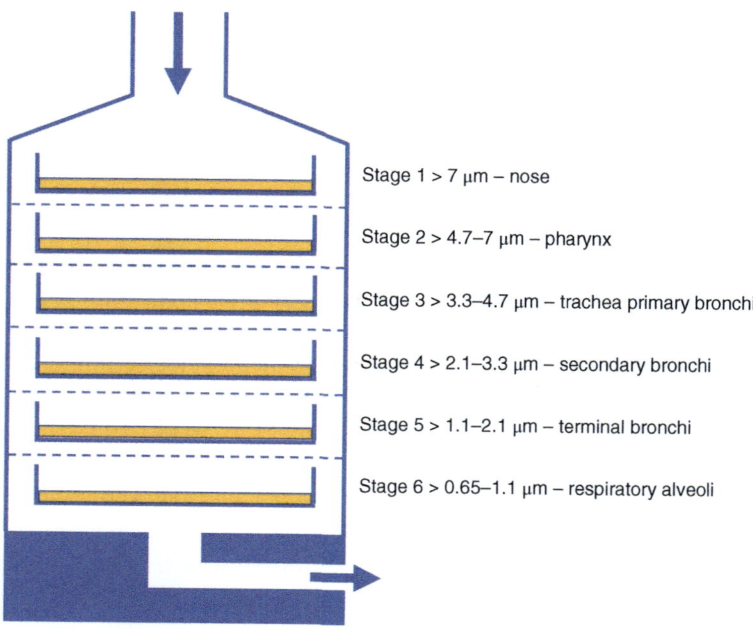

Figure 5.12 Viable impactor with cut-off stages.

(Toroglu et al. 2001). However, unlike previous studies, the bacterial load of the sampled air at debonding appeared to increase following the use of a preprocedural mouth rinse, whether sterile water or chlorhexidine. A likely explanation may lie in chlorhexidine's mode of action, which loosens plaque from tooth surfaces. Also, due to differences in composition, viscosity and surface tension between chlorhexidine and saliva, chlorhexidine droplets may be more easily displaced from the tooth and therefore aerosolised, leading to an increase in the number of bacterial colony-forming units observed. In the absence of any possible pharmacological effect, it is possible that with both the sterile water and chlorhexidine preprocedural rinse, the increased bacterial numbers were due to the simple mechanical cleansing action of the liquid prior to enamel clean-up.

Two different methods were used to assess biodiversity in this study: (i) counting the number of morphologically different colony types present on the culture plates and (ii) counting the number of individual bands produced by DGGE. Counting the cultured colonies suggested that rinsing with either water or chlorhexidine also increased biodiversity compared with nonrinsing, as did the results of the PCR/DGGE. Biodiversity was greatest at the first impactor stage and least at the sixth stage, corresponding to the deepest parts of the lung. When bacterial load and diversity were measured without any clinical procedures being performed, bacteria were still detected. Although previous work has shown that less than 1% of airborne particles are normally contaminated with bacteria (Tham and Zuraimi 2005), this may be expected to be higher in the dental clinic due to the number and diversity of aerosol particulates and because respirable particulates may remain airborne for several days in non-turbulent air.

5.1.9 How Can the Risk of Inhalation of Dental Particulates during Orthodontic Debond and Enamel Clean-Up Be Minimised?

To summarise, from the published evidence on the aerosols produced during enamel clean-up with rotary instruments at the completion of a course of orthodontic appliance therapy:

1) Particulates are produced in the inhalable, thoracic and respirable fractions, meaning they can potentially penetrate as far as the alveoli of the lungs.

2) These particulates may contain various elements, including iron, tungsten, silica, carbon, calcium and phosphorus, and probably arise from the adhesive bonding resin, glass polyalkenoate band cement, debonding bur and dental handpiece.
3) The lowest concentration of particulates is generated by cleaning the residual adhesive from the enamel surface using a spiral-fluted tungsten carbide bur in a slow-speed handpiece without a water coolant spray.
4) The highest concentration of particulates is generated by cleaning the residual adhesive from the enamel surface using a spiral-fluted tungsten carbide bur in a high-speed handpiece with a water coolant spray.
5) The use of a facemask by the operator is the most effective method of reducing the risk of inhalation of particulates produced during orthodontic debonding and enamel clean-up. The concentration of particulates in the ambient air can also be reduced by using high-volume evacuation held close to the patient's mouth during enamel clean-up.
6) Bioaerosols are also produced in the inhalable, thoracic and respirable fractions, meaning they can potentially penetrate as far as the alveoli of the lungs.
7) Using preprocedural water or chlorhexidine increases the number and diversity of airborne bacteria produced during enamel clean-up and is not recommended.

References

Bell, M.L., Ebisu, K., Peng, R.D. et al. (2009). Hospital admissions and chemical composition of fine particle air pollution. *Am. J. Respir. Crit. Care Med.* 12: 1115–1120.

Bentley, C.D., Burkhart, N.W., and Crawford, J.J. (1994). Evaluating spatter and aerosol contamination during dental procedures. *J. Am. Dent. Assoc.* 125: 579–584.

Boreson, J., Dillner, A.M., and Peccia, J. (2004). Correlating bioaerosol load with PM2.5 and PM10cf concentrations: a comparison between natural desert and urban-fringe aerosols. *Atmos. Environ.* 38: 6029–6041.

Božič, A.L., Šiber, A., and Podgornik, R. (2013). Statistical analysis of sizes and shapes of virus capsids and their resulting elastic properties. *J. Biol. Phys.* 39: 215–228.

BS EN 481:1993. (1993). *Workplace atmospheres. Size fraction definitions for measurements of airborne particles*. British Standards Institution.

Checchi, L., Montevecchi, M., Moreschi, A. et al. (2005). Efficacy of three face masks in preventing inhalation of airborne contaminants in dental practice. *J. Am. Dent. Assoc.* 136: 877–882.

Chew, F.T., Goh, D.Y.T., Ooi, B.C. et al. (1999). Association of ambient air-pollution levels with acute asthma exacerbation among children in Singapore. *Allergy* 54: 320–329.

Choudat, D., Triem, S., Weill, B. et al. (1993). Respiratory symptoms, lung function and pneumoconiosis among self-employed dental technicians. *Br. J. Ind. Med.* 50: 443–449.

Christensen, P.J., Kutty, K., Adlam, R.T. et al. (1993). Septic pulmonary embolism due to periodontal disease. *Chest* 104: 1927–1929.

Cole, E.C. and Cook, C.E. (1998). Characterization of infectious aerosols in health care facilities: an aid to effective engineering controls and preventive strategies. *Am. J. Infect. Control.* 26: 453–464.

Collins, J.F., Salmon, A.G., Brown, J.P. et al. (2005). Development of a chronic inhalation reference level for respirable crystalline silica. *Regul. Toxicol. Pharm.* 43: 292–300.

Concawe. (2017). An introduction to air quality.

Dawson, M., Soro, V., Dymock, D. et al. (2016). Ireland AJ a microbiological assessment of aerosol generated during debond of fixed orthodontic appliances. *Am. J. Orthodont. Dentofacial Orthoped.* 150: 831–838.

Day, C.J., Price, R., Sandy, J.R., and Ireland, A.J. (2008). The inhalation of aerosols produced during the removal of fixed orthodontic appliances: a comparison of four enamel clean-up methods. *Am. J. Orthod. Dentofacial Orthop.* 133: 11–17.

Donaldson, K., Brown, D.M., Mitchell, C. et al. (1997). Free radical activity of PM10: iron-mediated generation of hydroxyl radicals. *Environ. Health Perspect.* 105: 1285.

Feder, I.S., Tischoff, I., Theile, A. et al. (2017). The asbestos fibre burden in human lungs: new insights into the chrysotile debate. *Eur. Respir. J.* 49: 1–10.

Ferin, J., Oberdorster, G., and Penney, D. (1992). Pulmonary retention of ultrafine and fine particles in rats. *Am. J. Respir. Cell Mol. Biol.* 6: 535–542.

Finegold, S.M. (1991). Aspiration pneumonia. *Rev. Infect. Dis.* 13: S737–S742.

Finkelstein, M.M. (2000). Silica, silicosis, and lung cancer: a risk assessment. *Am. J. Ind. Med.* 38: 8–18.

Froudarakis, M.E., Voloudaki, A., Bouros, D. et al. (1999). Pneumoconiosis among Cretan dental technicians. *Respiration* 66: 338–342.

Fry, C. (2009). An investigation into asbestos related disease in the dental industry. *Br. Dent. J.* 206: 515–516.

Gibbons, R.J. and Houte, J.V. (1975). Bacterial adherence in oral microbial ecology. *Annu. Rev. Microbiol.* 29: 19–44.

Gilmour, P., Brown, D., Beswick, P. et al. (1997). Surface free radical activity of PM 10 and ultrafine titanium dioxide: a unifying factor in their toxicity? *An. Occupat. Hyg.* 41: 32–38.

Gravesen, S. (1979). Fungi as a cause of allergic disease. *Allergy* 34: 135–154.

Greco, P.M. and Lai, C.H. (2008). A new method of assessing aerosolized bacteria generated during orthodontic debonding procedures. *Am. J. Orthod. Dentofacial. Orthop.* 133 (4 Suppl): S79–S87.

Gregory, P.H. (1973). *The Microbiology of the Atmosphere*, 2nde. Aylesbury, UK: Leonard Hall.

Griffiths, W.D. (1994). The assessment of bioaerosols: a critical review. *J. Aerosol Sci.* 25: 1425–1458.

Hext, P., Rogers, K. and Paddle, G. (1999). The health effects of PM2.5 (including ultrafine particles). Concawe report no. 99/60.

HSE (2018). *EH40/2005 Workplace Exposure Limits*, 3rd ed. Health and Safety Executive.

Husman, T. (1996). Health effects of indoor-air microorganisms. *Scand. J. Work Environ. Health* 22: 5–13.

Ireland, A.J., Moreno, T., and Price, R. (2003). Air particles produced as a result of enamel clean up following the removal of orthodontic fixed appliances. *American Journal of Orthodontics and Dentofacial Orthopedics* 124: 683–686.

Jacks, M.E. (2002). A laboratory comparison of evacuation devices on aerosol reduction. *J. Dent. Hyg.* 76: 202–206.

Johnson, G.K. and Robinson, W.S. (1991). Human immunodeficiency virus-1 (HIV-1) in the vapors of surgical power instruments. *J. Med. Virol.* 33: 47–50.

Johnston, N.J., Price, R., Day, C.J., and Sandy, J.R. (2009). Ireland AJ quantitative and qualitative analysis of particulate production during simulated clinical orthodontic debonds. *Dent. Mater.* 25: 1155–1162.

Kuhn, D.M. and Ghannoum, M.A. (2003). Indoor mold, toxigenic fungi, and Stachybotrys chartarum: infectious disease perspective. *Clin. Microbiol. Rev.* 16: 144–172.

Kuijper, E.J., Wiggerts, H.O., Jonker, G.J. et al. (1992). Disseminated actinomycosis due to Actinomyces meyeri and Actinobacillus actinomycetemcomitans. *Scand. J. Infect. Dis.* 24: 667–672.

Latge, J.P. (1999). Aspergillus fumigatus and aspergillosis. *Clin. Microbiol. Rev.* 12: 310–350.

Leung, C.C., Yu, I.T., and Chen, W. (2012). Silicosis. *The Lancet.* 379: 2008–2018.

Li, X., Gilmour, P., Donaldson, K., and MAcnee, W. (1997). In vivo and in vitro proinflammatory effects of particulate air pollution (PM10). *Environ. Health Perspect.* 105: 1279.

Lipp, A. and Edwards, P. (2002). Disposable surgical face masks for preventing surgical wound infection in clean surgery. *Cochrane Database Syst. Rev.* (1): (Art. No.: CD002929).

McCarthy, G.M., Mamandras, A.H., and MacDonald, J.K. (1997). Infection control in the orthodontic office in Canada. *Am. J. Orthod. Dentofacial. Orthop.* 112: 275–281.

Möller, W., Häußinger, K., Winkler-Heil, R. et al. (2004). Mucociliary and long-term particle clearance in the airways of healthy non-smoker subjects. *J. Appl. Phys.* 97: 2200–2206.

Moore, W.E. and Moore, L.V. (1994). The bacteria of periodontal diseases. *Periodontol 2000* 5: 66–77.

Muyzer, G. and Smalla, K. (1998). Application of denaturing gradient gel electrophoresis (DGGE) and temperature gradient gel electrophoresis (TGGE) in microbial ecology. *Antonie Van Leeuwenhoek* 73: 127–141.

Nimmo, A., Werley, M.S., Martin, J.S., and Tansy, M.F. (1990). Particulate inhalation during the removal of amalgam restorations. *J. Prosthet. Dent.* 63: 228–233.

Oberdörster, G. (2000). Pulmonary effects of inhaled ultrafine particles. *Int. Arch. Occ. Env. Hea.* 74: 1–8.

Office of Environmental Health Hazard Assessment (OEHHA). (2000). Air toxics hot spots program risk assessment guidelines part III: Technical support document for the determination of noncancer chronic reference exposure levels.

Paster, B.J., Boches, S.K., Galvin, J.L. et al. (2001). Bacterial diversity in human subgingival plaque. *J. Bacteriol.* 183: 3770–3783.

Peng, R.D., Bell, M.L., Geyh, A.S. et al. (2009). Emergency admissions for cardiovascular and respiratory diseases and the chemical composition of fine particle air pollution. *Environ. Health Perspect.* 117: 957–963.

Pippin, D.J., Verderame, R.A., and Weber, K.K. (1987). Efficacy of face masks in preventing inhalation of airborne contaminants. *J. Oral Maxillofac. Surg.* 45: 19–23.

Radi, S., Dalphin, J.C., Manzoni, P. et al. (2002). Respiratory morbidity in a population of French dental technicians. *Occup. Environ. Med.* 59: 398–404.

Rams, T.E. and Slots, J. (1992). Systemic manifestations of oral infections. In: *Contemporary Oral Microbiology and Immunology* (ed. J. Slots and M.A. Taubman), 500–523. St. Louis, Mo: Mosby.

Reid, A.S., Causton, B.E., Jones, J.S., and Ellis, I.O. (1991). Malignant mesothelioma after exposure to asbestos in dental practice. *Lancet* 338: 696.

Rom, W.N., Lockey, J.E., Lee, J.S. et al. (1984). Pneumoconiosis and exposures of dental laboratory technicians. *Am. J. Public Health* 74: 1252–1257.

Scannapieco, F.A., Papandonatos, G.D., and Dunford, R.G. (1998). Associations between oral conditions and respiratory disease in a national sample survey population. *Ann. Periodontol.* 3: 251–256.

Seaton, A. (1996). Particles in the air: the enigma of urban air pollution. *J. Roy. Soc. Med.* 89: 604.

Seaton, A., Godden, D., Macnee, W., and Donaldson, K. (1995). Particulate air pollution and acute health effects. *Lancet* 345: 176–178.

Selden, A.I., Persson, B., Bornberger-Dankvardt, S.I. et al. (1995). Exposure to cobalt chromium dust and lung disorders in dental technicians. *Thorax* 50: 769–772.

Sherson, D., Maltbaek, N., and Olsen, O. (1988). Small opacities among dental laboratory technicians in Copenhagen. *Br. J. Ind. Med.* 45: 321–324.

Skulberg, K.R., Skyberg, K., Kruse, K. et al. (2004). The effect of cleaning on dust and the health of office workers: an intervention study. *Epidemiology* 15: 71–78.

Spiegel, C.A. and Telford, G. (1984). Isolation of Wolinella recta and Actinomyces viscosus from an actinomycotic chest wall mass. *J. Clin. Microbiol.* 20: 1187–1189.

Taira, M., Sasaki, M., Kimura, S., and Araki, Y. (2009). Characterization of aerosols and fine particles produced in dentistry and their health risk assessments. *Nano. Biomed.* 1: 9–15.

Teeuw, K.B., Vandenbroucke-Grauls, C.M.J.E., and Verhoef, J. (1994). Airborne gram-negative bacteria and endotoxin in sick building syndrome. A study in Dutch governmental office buildings. *Arch. Intern. Med.* 154: 2339–2345.

Tham, K.W. and Zuraimi, M.S. (2005). Size relationship between airborne viable bacteria and particles in a controlled indoor environment study. *Indoor Air* 15: 48–57.

Toroglu, M.S., Haytac, M.C., and Köksal, F. (2001). Evaluation of aerosol contamination during debonding procedures. *Angle. Orthod.* 71: 299–306.

Toroglu, M.S., Bayramoglu, O., Yarkin, F., and Tuli, A. (2003). Possibility of blood and hepatitis B contamination through aerosols generated during debonding procedures. *Angle. Orthod.* 73: 571–578.

Vig, P., Atack, N.E., Sandy, J.R. et al. (2019). Particulate production during debonding of fixed appliances: laboratory investigation and randomized clinical trial to assess the effect of using flash-free ceramic brackets. *Am. J. Orthod. Dentofacial. Orthop.* 155: 767–778.

Vincent, J.H. (2005). Health-related aerosol measurement: a review of existing sampling criteria and proposals for new ones. *J. Environ. Monit.* 7: 1037–1053.

Wallace, L. (1996). Indoor particles: a review. *J. Air Waste Manag. Assoc.* 46 (2): 98–126.

Weber, A., Willeke, K., Marchioni, R. et al. (1993). Aerosol penetration and leakage characteristics of masks used in the health care industry. *Am. J. Infect. Control.* 21: 167–173.

Woo, J., Anderson, R., Maguire, B., and Gerbert, B. (1992). Compliance with infection control procedures among California orthodontists. *Am. J. Orthod. Dentofacial. Orthop.* 102: 68–75.

Wyon, D.P., Tham, K.W., Croxford, B. et al. (2000). The effects of health and self estimated productivity of 2 experimental interventions which reduced airborne dust levels in office premises. In: *Proceedings of the Healthy Buildings 2000 Conference, Helsinki, Finland*, 641–646.

Zanobetti, A., Franklin, M., Koutrakis, P., and Schwartz, J. (2009). Fine particulate air pollution and its components in association with cause-specific emergency admissions. *Environ. Health.* 8: 58.

6

Evidence on Airborne Pathogen Management from Aerosol-Inducing Practices in Dentistry – How to Handle the Risk

Despina Koletsi[1], *Georgios N. Belibasakis*[2], *and Theodore Eliades*[1]

[1] *Clinic of Orthodontics and Pediatric Dentistry, Center of Dental Medicine, University of Zurich, Zurich, Switzerland*
[2] *Division of Oral Diseases, Department of Dental Medicine, Karolinska Institutet, Huddinge, Sweden*

6.1 Introduction

Everyday clinical practice of dental/orthodontic practitioners is related to a working environment linked to certain potential hazards. For one, airborne material particulates are produced during and/or after practicing on composites/restorations, with high rotary instrumentation (Cokic et al. 2020; Ireland et al. 2003); further, this is also allied to potentially infectious bacteria, viruses or other microorganisms residing in the patients' oral cavity (Dawson et al. 2016). Aerosolized microorganisms, including airborne pathogens may arise upon active performance of high-powered handpiece utilization during routine dental procedures. Resin removal after orthodontic debonding, attachment grinding after aligner treatment (Iliadi et al. 2020), tooth and material grinding for restorations, or routine practice professional oral prophylaxis using high-speed ultrasonic scalers, may substantiate an increased dynamic for

Previously published as Koletsi, D., Belibasakis, G.N., and Eliades, T. (2020). Interventions to reduce aerosolized microbes in dental practice: A systematic review with network meta-analysis of randomized controlled trials. *J. Dent. Res.* 99 (11): 1228–1238.

Debonding and Fixed Retention in Orthodontics: An Evidence-Based Clinical Guide, First Edition. Edited by Theodore Eliades and Christos Katsaros.

spatter related contamination, within the dental practice environment and including the practices' personnel and patients (Laheij et al. 2012).

The potentially pathogenic capacity of aerosols produced in dentistry depends on the combination of in-service compressed air and water spray with tooth and material debris, plaque, blood, calculus and saliva mixture, always allied to patient's dynamic for an airborne disease. In this respect, research has long identified the role of microorganisms being present within the dental unit waterlines' (DUWL) coupled with their potential to mix-up with oral cavity risk factors, namely blood and saliva. As a result, aerosols may set the basis for a risk for disease transmission and cross contamination within the dental clinic environment, however, this in turn is largely dependent on patients' pathogenic potential for induction of an airborne disease (Harrel and Molinari 2004; Laheij et al. 2012).

A range of interventions have been proposed to reduce environmental and/or patient/professional related aerosol induced contamination, mainly directed towards the use of antiseptic agents as pre-procedural mouthwash rinse solutions (Logothetis and Martinez-Welles 1995; Sethi et al. 2019). Use of alternative schemes have also been reported, such as high volume evacuators (Holloman et al. 2015), or in-service instrumentation coolant agents (Jawade et al. 2016) and antiseptic agents directly applied to the DUWLs (Mamajiwala et al. 2018).

The American Dental Association (ADA) council on scientific affairs and dental practice, has issued recommendations for infection control against spatter and droplet forming aerosols, for over 20 years. Protective eyewear, high volume evacuator, appropriate positioning of the patients and rubber dams were recognized as the foremost protection strategies (ADA Council 1996). Latest reports appear to focus on attention to specific occupational practices, identified as most prone to bio-aerosol stimulation. The performance of oral prophylaxis measures in-office, through ultrasonic scaling (Joshi et al. 2017; Sethi et al. 2019), but also enamel clean-up practices after orthodontic fixed appliance debonding with high speed instrumentation (Dawson et al. 2016), have been most frequently discussed.

The present chapter aims to map the available evidence on interventions upheld to minimize aerosol contamination in dental and orthodontic office and provide a conceivable ranking of the effectiveness of the existing approaches. The chapter largely describes data available from the most recent network meta-analysis on the topic (Koletsi et al. 2020).

6.2 Existing Evidence

Existing evidence stems from a variety of interventions, pertaining solely on clinical trials either randomized or not, under typical dental/orthodontic office, university or hospital settings and includes both direct and indirect comparisons of treatment alternatives of a wide range. Ultrasonic scaling, enamel clean-up procedures during orthodontic bracket debonding after fixed appliance treatment, restorative procedures have been identified as the most frequently investigated clinical procedures, while implicated interventions pertain mostly to the investigation of antiseptic agents, acting as pre-procedural solutions. Related outcomes were mostly framed under the microbial count measurement in droplets/aerosol after the respective dental procedures (Koletsi et al. 2020).

More specifically, the body of evidence upon which the conclusions of the present chapter are relied constitutes 29 randomized controlled trials (RCTs) (21) or prospective clinical trials (8), while synthesized data findings come from 11 RCTs (Feres et al. 2010; Gupta et al. 2014; Holloman et al. 2015; Joshi et al. 2017; Kaur et al. 2014; Mohan and Jagannathan 2016; Rani et al. 2014; Reddy et al. 2012; Retamal-Valdes et al. 2017; Saini 2015; Waghmare et al. 2018). A considerable amount of studies was published within the last decade (24/29; 82.8%), with 15 out of 24, since 2015. Parallel trials predominated (23/29; 79.3%), while the number of patients contributing each studies' findings ranged from 18 to 120 across the study samples. Publication period spread across almost 30 years, ranging from 1992 to 2020. Table 6.1 outlines the overall picture of information on the included studies.

Descriptively, the level of the existing source of evidence may be summarized as follows: the most common dental procedure examined was ultrasonic scaling (24/29; 82.8%), while 2 studies reported on outcomes after debonding procedures of orthodontic fixed appliances (Dawson et al. 2016; Toroglu et al. 2001), air-polishing (Logothetis and Martinez-Welles 1995), tooth restoration through with the use of high-speed air turbine (Purohit et al. 2009) and other dental prophylaxis procedures without instrumentation justification (NCT02319668 2017). All studies pertained roughly to the assessment of bacterial load colony forming units (CFUs) after the application of a number of interventions prior or simultaneously to a commonly described dental procedure, namely, as aforementioned, ultrasonic scaling, but also enamel clean-up after debonding procedures, or tooth restoration. In essence, blood agar plates

Table 6.1 Characteristics of the relevant included studies ($n = 29$), in alphabetical order.

Study ID	Participants	Intervention (one or > 1)	Comparator (one or > 1)	Outcome
Dawson et al. 2016 nRS, parallel 3-arm Setting: hospital orthodontic department	18 patients at *orthodontic bracket debonding*; age NR; air sampling for 15 min during debonding (including chairside high volume aspirator)	1) slow-speed handpiece, 0.2% CHX gluconate PMR 2) slow-speed handpiece, sterile water PMR Rinse duration: 1 min	Slow-speed handpiece, no PMR	Bacterial load in CFUs (anaerobic culture), with PCR and DGGE, at 30 cm sampling distance [no mouthrinse performed better]
Devker et al. 2012 nRS, parallel-3 arm (plus within group control)Setting: NR	90 patients; age 18–45; air sampling for 10 min during ultrasonic scaling Split-mouth controls used in each group	1) 0.2% CHX prior to scaling Rinse duration: 2 min 2) HVE attachment used during ultrasonic scaling (140 mmHg)	Combination of 0.2% CHX plus HVE attachment Rinse duration: 2 min	Bacterial load in CFUs (aerobic culture), with blood agar plates and colony counters, at 15, 30, 90 cm sampling distance
dos Santos et al. 2014 nRS, cross-over Setting: university	23 patients during *orthodontic treatment* (at dental prophylaxis procedure with aerosolized sodium bicarbonate); age: 10–40; air sampling for 4 min during prophylaxis procedure	0.2% CHX PMR Rinse duration: 1 min	No PMR	Bacterial load (aerobic culture) in CFUs, with blood agar plates and colony counters, at no measurable sampling distance (reports: clinician's face, 10 cm lower than the mouth, patient's thoracic region)

Feres et al. 2010 RCT, parallel 4-arm Setting: university	60 patients (not advanced periodontitis); age 30–70; air sampling for 10 min during ultrasonic scaling	1) 0.05% CPC prior to scaling 2) 0.12% CHX prior to scaling Rinse duration: 1 min	1) water PMR 2) 2. no PMR	Bacterial load in CFUs (anaerobic culture), at 30 cm sampling distance. Also, samples for 39 oral/periodontal bacterial species were analyzed using the checkerboard DNA–DNA hybridization technique (mean DNA % probe counts)
Fine et al. 1992 RCT, cross-over Setting: university	18 patients (ADA periodontal case type I, II); age: NR (adults); air sampling for 10 min during ultrasonic scaling	Antiseptic mouthwash (not-specified) PMR Rinse duration: 30 s	5% hydroalcochol control rinse	Bacterial load (aerobic culture) in CFUs, at 5 cm sampling distance
Gupta et al. 2014 RCT, parallel 3-arm Setting: university	24 patients (chronic periodontitis); age 25–55; air sampling for 30 min during ultrasonic scaling plus 30 min thereafter	1) 0.2% CHX PMR 2) HRB PMR Rinse duration: 1 min	Water PMR	Bacterial load (aerobic culture) in CFUs, at 30 cm sampling distance
Holloman et al. 2015 RCT, parallel 2-arm Setting: university	52 patients; age mean 45 (intervention group), mean 40 (control); air sampling (duration NR) during ultrasonic scaling, plus 35 min thereafter	Isolite (dental isolation system attached to high-volume suction hose)	Saliva ejector (attached to low-volume suction hose)	Bacterial load (anaerobic culture) in CFUs, at 15 cm sampling distance

(*Continued*)

Table 6.1 (Continued)

Study ID	Participants	Intervention (one or > 1)	Comparator (one or > 1)	Outcome
Jawade et al. 2016 RCT, parallel 3-arm Setting; university	30 patients (chronic periodontitis); age 22–55; air sampling for 20 min during ultrasonic scaling plus 20 min thereafter	1) Ultrasonic liquid coolant: 2% PI plus distilled water 2) Ultrasonic liquid coolant: 0.12% CHX plus distilled water	Distilled water (coolant)	Bacterial load (culture NR) in CFUs, at 40 cm to 2 m
Joshi et al. 2017 RCT, parallel 4-arm Setting: university	40 patients (chronic gingivitis); age mean 32.4; air sampling for 30 min during ultrasonic scaling plus 30 minthereafter	1) 0.05% CPC PMR (47°) 2) 0.2% CHX PMR (47°) Rinse duration: 1 min	1) 0.05% CPC PMR (18°) 2) 0.2% CHX PMR (18°) Rinse duration: 1 min	Bacterial load (aerobic culture) in CFUs, at 30 cm sampling distance
Kaur et al. 2014 RCT, parallel 3-arm Setting: university	60 patients; age 20–50; air sampling for 10 min during ultrasonic scaling plus 30 min thereafter – both prior and after PMR	1) 0.2% CHX PMR 2) 1% PI PMR Rinse duration: NR	OZ irrigation	Bacterial load (aerobic and anaerobic culture) in CFUs, at 22–275 cm sampling distance
King et al. 1997 RCT, split-mouth Setting: university	12 patients; age 21–63 (mean 39); sampling for 5 min during ultrasonic scaling plus 25 min thereafter	Ultrasonic scaler with aerosol reduction device (i.e. high volume suction tube attached to scaler)	Ultrasonic scaler without aerosol reduction device	Bacterial load (aerobic culture) in CFUs, at 15 cm sampling distance

Logothetis and Martinez-Welles 1995 RCT, parallel 3-arm Setting: university	18 patients; age 25–54, mean 38; sampling for 30 min during air polishing plus 30 minutes thereafter	1) 0.12% CHX PMR 2) Antiseptic mouthwash with essential oils PMR Rinse duration: 30 s	Distilled water Rinse duration: 30 s	Bacterial load (aerobic culture) in CFUs, at 60–275 cm sampling distance
Mamajiwala et al. 2018 RCT, parallel 3-arm Setting: university	60 patients (moderate to severe gingivitis); age 15–55; sampling for 20 min during ultrasonic scaling	1) CHX added in DUWL 2) CIN added in DUWL	Distilled water in DUWL	Bacterial load in CFUs (aerobic and anaerobic culture), within the range of 30 cm sampling distance
Mohan and Jagannathan 2016 RCT, parallel 2-arm Setting: university	20 patients; age 25–40; sampling during ultrasonic scaling/duration NR	0.2% CHX PMR Rinse duration: 1 min	Normal saline PMR Rinse duration: 1 min	Bacterial load (culture NR) in CFUs, at 90 cm sampling distance
Narayana et al. 2016 nRS, parallel 3-arm (plus within group control) Setting: NR	45 patients; age NR; air sampling during ultrasonic scaling for 5 min	1) 0.12% CHX PMR 2) HVE Rinse duration: 30 s	Combination of 0.12% CHX and HVE Rinse duration: 30 s	Bacterial load (aerobic culture) in CFUs, with blood agar plates and colony counters; sampling distance NR
Paul et al. 2020 nRS, parallel 3-arm Setting: university	60 patients; age 18–55 (mean 37.4, SD 10.3); air sampling during ultrasonic scaling for 20 min	1) 0.2% CHX PMR 2) 1% PI PMR Rinse duration: 1 min	94.5% AV PMR Rinse duration: 1 min	Bacterial load (aerobic culture) in CFUs, at 30 cm sampling distance

(*Continued*)

Table 6.1 (Continued)

Study ID	Participants	Intervention (one or > 1)	Comparator (one or > 1)	Outcome
Purohit et al. 2009 nRS, parallel 2-arm (plus within group control) Setting: university	20 patients; age NR; air sampling during (a) ultrasonic scaling (oral prophylaxis) and (b) tooth restoration through high-speed air turbine handpiece	1) Ultrasonic scaling with 0.12% CHX PMR 2) High speed air turbine tooth restoration with 0.12% CHX PMR Rinse duration: 30 s	1. Ultrasonic scaling without 0.12% CHX PMR 2. High speed air turbine tooth restoration without 0.12% CHX PMR Rinse duration: 30 seconds	Bacterial load (aerobic culture) in CFUs, at 15–60 cm sampling distance
Rajachandrasekaran et al. 2019 nRS, parallel 2-arm Setting: university	50 patients; age 20–50; air sampling during ultrasonic scaling for 30 min	0.12% CHX PMR Rinse duration: 1 min	HRB PMR Rinse duration: 1 min	Bacterial load (aerobic culture) in CFUs, at 60–275 cm sampling distance (selective isolation of bacteria strains)
Rani et al. 2014 RCT, parallel 3-arm Setting: hospital	36 patients; age 18–35; air sampling during ultrasonic scaling for 10 min	1) 0.2% CHX PMR 2) HRB PMR Rinse duration: 30 s	Water PMR Rinse duration: 30 s	Bacterial load (culture NR) in CFUs, at patient's and operator's chest (30 cm)
Reddy et al. 2012 RCT, parallel 3-arm Setting: hospital	30 patients; age NR; sampling during ultrasonic scaling/duration NR	1) 0.2% tempered CHX (47 °C) PMR 2) 0.2% non-tempered CHX PMR Rinse duration: 1 min	Sterile water PMR Rinse duration: 1 min	Bacterial load (culture NR) in CFUs, at 10 cm sampling distance

Retamal-Valdes et al. 2017 RCT, parallel 4-arm Setting: dental office	60 patients; age 18–70; sampling during ultrasonic scaling for 10 min	1) 0.075% CPC+ 0.28% Zn + 0.05% SF PMR 2) 0.12 CHX PMR Rinse duration: 1 min	1) Water PMR 2) No PMR Rinse duration: 1 min	Bacterial load (anaerobic culture) in CFUs, at patient's chest and operator's forehand (15-30 cm). Also, samples for oral/periodontal bacterial species were analysed using the checkerboard DNA–DNA hybridization technique (mean DNA % probe counts)
Saini 2015 RCT, parallel 3-arm Setting: university	120 patients (chronic periodontitis); age 18–55; sampling during ultrasonic scaling for 10 min-plus 30 pause, plus 10 after assignment to PMR	1) CIO_2 PMR 2) 0.2% CHX PMR Rinse duration: 1 min	Water PMR Rinse duration: 1 min	Bacterial load (culture NR) in CFUs, at 30-245 cm sampling distance (mainly 30 cm)
Swahney et al. 2015 RCT, parallel 3-arm parallel Setting: university	60 patients (mild to moderate gingivitis); age 25–54; sampling during ultrasonic scaling (duration NR)	1) CHX 0.2% PMR 2) Listerine PMR 3) Water PMR (all with suction) Rinse duration: 1 min	1) CHX 0.2% PMR 2) Listerine PMR 3) Water PMR (all without suction) Rinse duration: 1 min	Distribution of microbial growth in percentages, at sampling distance 15 cm
Sethi et al. 2019 RCT, parallel 3-arm Setting: university	60 patients (moderate to severe gingivitis); age 18–55 (mean 29.26; SD, 2.8); sampling during ultrasonic scaling for 20 min	1) CHX as ultrasonic coolant 2) CIN PMR as ultrasonic coolant	Distilled water as ultrasonic coolant	Bacterial load (aerobic culture) in CFUs, at 30 cm sampling distance

(*Continued*)

Table 6.1 (Continued)

Study ID	Participants	Intervention (one or > 1)	Comparator (one or > 1)	Outcome
Shetty et al. 2013 RCT, parallel 3-arm Setting: university	60 patients; age NR; sampling during ultrasonic scaling for 10 min	1) 0.2% CHX PMR 2) Tea tree oil PMR Rinse duration: NR	Distilled water Rinse duration: NR	Bacterial load (aerobic culture) in CFUs, at 15–30 cm
Swaminathan et al. 2014 RCT, parallel 3-arm Setting: university	30 patients; age 18–50; sampling during ultrasonic scaling for 30 min	1) 0.2% CHX PMR 2) HRB PMR Rinse duration: 1 min	Normal Saline PMR Rinse duration: 1 min	Bacterial load (aerobic culture) in CFUs, at 30–90 cm sampling distance
Toroglu et al. 2001 nRS, parallel 2-arm (plus within group control) Setting: NR	26 patients; age intervention group 11–13; age control group 10–15; sampling during orthodontic debonding procedures (5 min working time, plus 25 min thereafter)	Debonding/adhesive removal, through the use of an air turbine handpiece, with water cooling and slow speed evacuation (0.2% CHX as within group control) Rinse duration: 1 minute	Standard orthodontic procedures that did not require turbine handpiece, with slow speed evacuator	Bacterial load (aerobic culture) in CFUs, at or less than 30 cm sampling distance; also specific tests for Staphylococcus, Streptococcus and oxidase activity

Waghmare et al. 2018 RCT, parallel 3-arm Setting: NR	60 patients; age 20–28; sampling during ultrasonic scaling for 30 min	1) 1% ClO_2 PMR 2) 0.2% CHX PMR Rinse duration: 1 min	Normal Saline PMR Rinse duration: 1 min	Bacterial load (aerobic culture) in CFUs, at 30 cm sampling distance
NCT02319668 2017 RCT, parallel 2-arm Setting: NR	38 patients; age 18–64, mean 27.9, SD 10.5; sampling during dental prophylaxis (not-specified procedure)	0.2% CHX PMR Rinse duration: 1 min	No PMR	Bacterial load (anaerobic culture) in CFUs, at certain positions around dental unit

AV, *aloe vera*; CFUs, colony forming units; CHX, chlorhexidine; CIN, cinnamon; CIO2, chlorine dioxide; CPC, cetylpiridinium chloride; DGGE, denaturing gradient gel electrophoresis; DUWL, dental unit waterline; HRB: herbal mouthwash; HVE, high volume evacuator; NR, not reported; nRS, non-randomized prospective studies; OZ, ozone; PCR, polymerase chain reaction; PMR, pre-procedural mouth rinse; PI, povidone iodine; SD, standard deviation; SF, sodium fluoride; Zn, zinc lactate.

Source: According to findings of Koletsi et al. *J. Dent. Res.* 99 (11): 1228–1238.

were used across the studies to collect the aerosolized bacteria, while subsequently aerobically and/or anaerobically incubated and analyzed in colony counters. The sampling distance ranged between 5 and 275 cm, away from patients' oral cavity, with the majority of trials investigating close-up distances, such as patient's thoracic region, clinician's face, or specific targets around the dental unit, where the presence of clinic staff might be at stake. These targets were within the range of 15 to 90 cm. Interestingly, only two studies reported on additional specification of bacterial species, via checkerboard DNA-DNA hybridization techniques, measuring mean percentage DNA probe counts (Feres et al. 2010; Retamal-Valdes et al. 2017). Yet, these included primarily oral/periodontal microbes, rather than species that may cause non-oral opportunistic infections. Air sampling across studies pertained to a duration of 5 minutes during the dental procedure until 35 minutes after its completion. The variety of the reported interventions, irrespective of the dental procedure implemented in practice were as follows: pre-procedural mouthrinse (PMR) with chlorhexidine (CHX) 0.2%, 0.12% or tempered CHX 0.2%, cetylpiridinium chloride PMR (CPC) 0.05%, use of high volume evacuator (HVE) jointly with CHX or alone, ultrasonic scaler with high-volume suction tube attached, herbal PMR (i.e. oil tree, *aloe vera*), ozone (OZ), povidone iodine PMR (PI), CHX 0.12% or PI used as ultrasonic coolants, CHX or cinnamon (CIN) used in dental unit waterlines (DUWLs), chlorine dioxide (CIO_2), as well as control non-active interventions such as water, distilled water, normal saline, simple saliva ejector, or no PMR at all. For the interventions that pertained to PMR solutions, the duration was 30 seconds to 2 minutes (Table 6.1).

6.2.1 Existing Evidence from Synthesized Data Including Direct and Indirect Comparisons of Interventions

The network map of the identified interventions and their contribution and comparisons within the network is presented in Figure 6.1, while interventions were examined under a setting of procedural ultrasonic scaler in-practice, in adult patients; nevertheless, extrapolations may be reasonable for similar dental or orthodontic procedures such as enamel clean-up after fixed appliance debonding practices. A total of 16 direct and 29 indirect comparisons have been ultimately formulated. The results of the synthesized data from both direct and indirect comparisons in terms of the network map, following an augmented

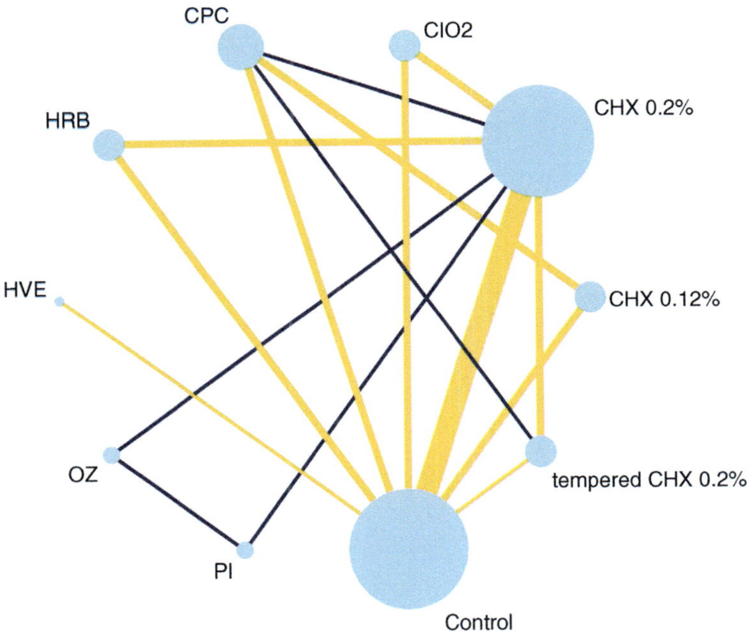

Figure 6.1 Network plot, with all contributing interventions and their comparison matrix. Edge colours indicate risk of bias (RoB) of the contributing studies to the relative comparisons (dark blue: "low RoB"; yellow: "some concerns"). Size of the light blue nodes is analogous to the contribution of the sample size for each intervention overall. *Source:* Adapted from Koletsi et al. 2020 / with permission of SAGE.

format under multivariate meta-analysis of RCTs (White 2015), are collectively presented in Table 6.2 and also in Figure 6.2. As noted, tempered chlorhexidine (CHX) 0.2% compared to control was most effective towards reduced post-procedural bacterial load with a mean difference (MD) of −0.92 (95% CI: −1.54, −0.29) in $\log_{10}$ CFUs. A similar trend was noted for CHX 0.2% compared to control (MD: -0.74; 95 CI%: −1.07, −0.40), as well as for chloride dioxide (ClO_2) versus control (MD: -0.68; 95%CI: −1.01, −0.34).

The overall rank score of the effectiveness of each intervention has been identified, by examining the surface under the curve cumulative ranking (SUCRA) value (Chaimani et al. 2013). Relative rankings for the competing treatments are presented through ranking probabilities for each

Table 6.2 League table, indicating network meta-analysis (NMA) mean differences in log10 CFUs (colony forming units), below the diagonal.

CHX 0.12%		0.50 (−0.66, 1.66)					0.03 (−1.01, 1.08)		
0.31 (−0.83, 1.45)	temp. CHX 0.2%	0.93 (0.01, 1.85)					0.17 (−0.80, 1.14)		0.21 (−0.42, 0.84)
−0.60 (−1.65, 0.44)	−0.92 (−1.54, −0.29)	Control			−0.31 (−0.89, 0.27)	−0.28 (−1.25, 0.68)	−0.47 (−1.66, 0.72)	−0.62 (−1.13, −0.11)	−0.84 (−1.00, −0.68)
−0.11 (−1.72, 1.50)	−0.42 (−1.77, 0.93)	0.50 (−0.76, 1.75)	PI	−0.22 (−1.25, 0.81)					−0.24 (−1.41, 0.93)
0.11 (−1.40, 1.63)	−0.20 (−1.44, 1.03)	0.72 (−0.42, 1.85)	0.22 (−0.85, 1.29)	OZ					−0.02 (−1.06, 1.02)
−0.29 (−1.49, 0.91)	−0.61 (−1.47, 0.25)	0.31 (−0.28, 0.90)	−0.18 (−1.57, 1.20)	−0.40 (−1.68, 0.87)	HVE				
−0.14 (−1.46, 1.19)	−0.45 (−1.46, 0.56)	0.47 (−0.38, 1.31)	−0.03 (−1.50, 1.45)	−0.25 (−1.62, 1.12)	0.16 (−0.87, 1.19)	HRB			−0.13 (−1.04, 0.79)

0.04 (−0.95, 1.03)	−0.27 (−1.09, 0.54)	0.64 (−0.12, 1.40)	0.15 (−1.28, 1.57)	−0.07 (−1.39, 1.25)	0.33 (−0.63, 1.30)	0.18 (−0.93, 1.28)	CPC		−0.01 (−0.98, 0.96)
0.07 (−1.00, 1.15)	−0.24 (−0.88, 0.39)	0.68 (0.34, 1.01)	0.18 (−1.06, 1.42)	−0.04 (−1.16, 1.08)	0.37 (−0.31, 1.04)	0.21 (−0.66, 1.07)	0.03 (−0.75, 0.81)	ClO_2	−0.08 (−0.20, 0.03)
0.13 (−0.93, 1.19)	−0.18 (−0.78, 0.41)	0.74 (0.40, 1.07)	0.24 (−0.97, 1.45)	0.02 (−1.06, 1.10)	0.42 (−0.25, 1.10)	0.27 (−0.57, 1.11)	0.09 (−0.66, 0.84)	0.06 (−0.21, 0.33)	CHX 0.2%

Comparisons are indicated by the column vs the row defining the intervention prior to ultrasonic scaling. Negative (−) mean differences are in favor of the column presented interventions, indicating reduced pathogen load. Direct meta-analysis results are presented above the diagonal in a similar manner. Mean differences for comparisons in the opposite direction may be obtained through conversion of negative to positive values and vice versa.

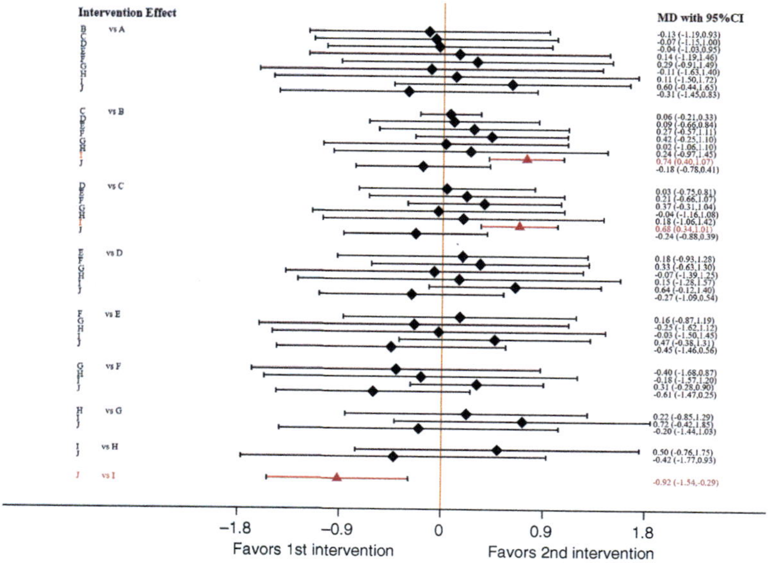

Figure 6.2 Interval plot, allowing for graphical representation of effect sizes (and respective 95% Confidence Intervals), by treatment comparisons across the network. [A, CHX 0.12%; B, CHX 0.2%; C, ClO_2; D, CPC; E, HRB; F, HVE; G, OZ; H, PI; I, Control; J, tempered CHX 0.2%]. *Source:* Adapted from Koletsi et al. 2020 / with permission of SAGE.

identified outcome. The SUCRA values represent the surface under the curve ("surface under cumulative ranking"). A high SUCRA value corresponds to an intervention with high probabilities of being in the first ranks of treatment of choice. Ranking of the interventions of the network in order of effectiveness, towards induction of reduced microbial load, from aerosols produced during ultrasonic in-practice service revealed the following, based on both the cumulative probability of intervention effectiveness, as well as the probability of being ranked as best treatment of choice: the tempered CHX 0.2% at 47 °C was ranked as the most effective in achieving reduced bacterial load after the use of ultrasonic scaling in dental practice both with regard to overall % SUCRA value (78.6%), as well as with respect to being the most likely intervention to be ranked as 1st treatment of choice (31.2%) (Figure 6.3; Table 6.3). In terms of overall SUCRA values for effectiveness, the tempered CHX 0.2% was followed by conventional CHX 0.2% (66.4%), ClO_2, (59.0%) and ozone (OZ) (57.2%)

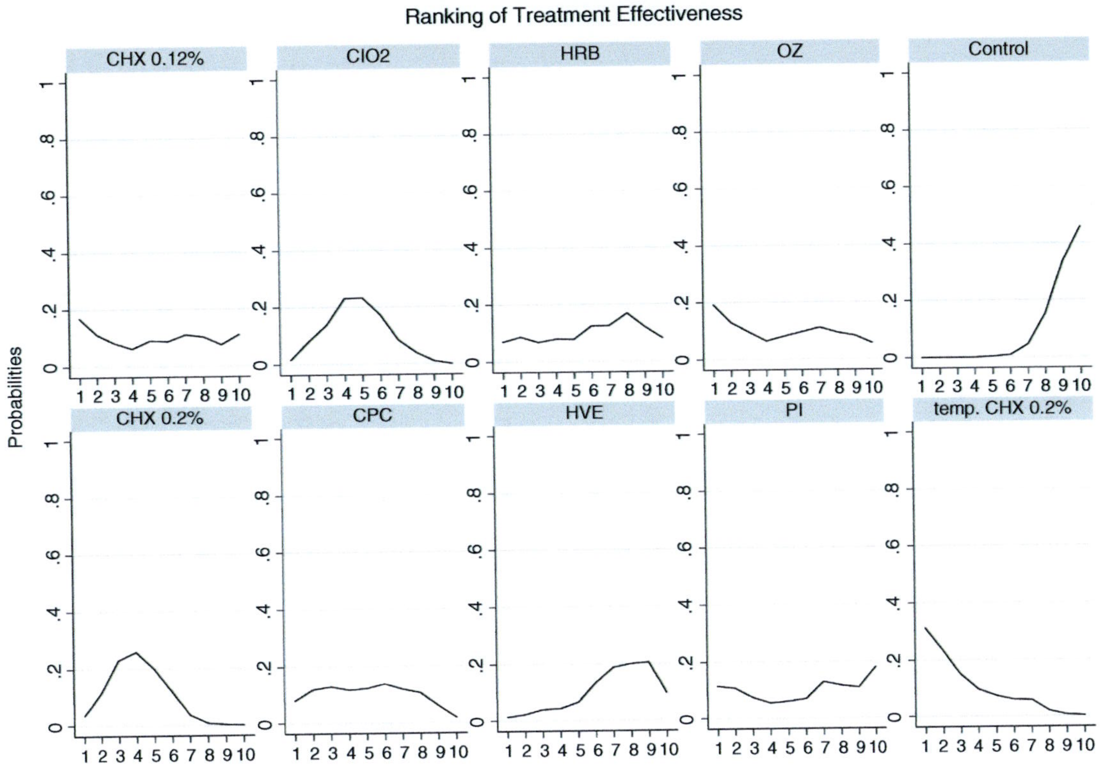

Figure 6.3 Rankograms for the 10 competing interventions. Horizontal axis describes the order of the ranks, while vertical shows the probability (0–1 scale) of each intervention to be ranked 1st, 2nd, ... 10th, in terms of effectiveness for decreased pathogen load after ultrasonic scaler usage. *Source:* Adapted from Koletsi et al. 2020 / with permission of SAGE.

Table 6.3 The ranking probability of each treatment to be considered the 1st choice of interest, the second, the third, the fourth, as well as the overall % SUCRA values for treatment effectiveness.

	Interventions (ranking probabilities in %)									
Ranking	CHX 0.12%	CHX 0.2%	ClO_2	CPC	HRB	HVE	OZ	PI	Control	Temp. CHX 0.2%
Best (1st)	16.9	3.5	1.6	8.0	7.0	1.3	19.2	11.3	0.0	31.2
2nd	11.2	11.3	8.0	11.8	8.7	2.2	12.9	10.6	0.0	23.3
3rd	8.2	23.0	13.7	12.8	6.8	3.9	9.6	7.3	0.0	14.7
4th	6.2	25.9	23.0	11.6	7.9	4.2	6.4	5.3	0.0	9.5
SUCRA values (%)	53.0	66.4	59.0	55.9	44.4	31.5	57.8	44.2	9.1	78.6

CHX, chlorhexidine; ClO_2, chlorine dioxide, CPC, cetylpiridinium chloride; HRB, herbal substance related treatment; HVE, high volume evacuator; OZ, ozone; PI, povidone iodine; Control, any non-active intervention (water, normal saline, no treatment); SUCRA, surface under the cumulative ranking value; temp CHX, tempered (47 °C) chlorhexidine.

(Table 6.3). In terms of being the "1st treatment of choice", it was followed by OZ (19.2%), CHX 0.12% (16.9), and povidone iodine (PI) (11.3%).

6.2.2 Evidence Based on Single Study Estimates

As for single study estimates from both randomized and non-randomized trials, regarding aerosol reducing intervention strategies for alternate dental procedures, use of solutions as ultrasonic scaler coolants, as extracts for the DUWLs, air-polishing practices, or enamel clean-up after fixed appliance orthodontic treatment and debonding procedures have been described. Specifically, CHX in concentration of either 0.12% or 0.2%, CIN, or PI have been reported as significantly effective strategies when used as ultrasonic coolants, compared to control water use ($p<0.001$). Similar findings were confirmed for CHX and CIN, when used as DUWL extracts ($p<0.001$). In addition, CHX 0.12% as PMR was more effective than HRB related solution, when used prior to air-polishing procedures ($p<0.001$). Last, with regard to potentially hazardous diverse dental procedures routinely used, tooth restoration activities with high-speed handpiece were considered more "aerosol pathogen inductive" than ultrasonic scaling ($p<0.001$); however, this effect was eliminated after PMR with CHX 0.12%. Likewise, debonding and enamel clean-up activities in orthodontic practices were more prone to producing contaminated aerosols than routine orthodontic practices ($p = 0.001$) (Table 6.4).

6.2.3 Quality and Confidence of Existing Evidence

The assessment of the quality of the evidence for the comparisons of the identified 4 most effective interventions according to SUCRA values of ranking described above, including the non-active control intervention, revealed a range from very low to moderate level of confidence for the results of the interventions contributing to the network map, and was based on the CINeMA framework originally framed on GRADE, overall and across comparisons (Nikolakopoulou et al. 2020; Papakonstantinou et al. 2020). The most prevalent reason for downgrading confidence levels was within study bias, thus raising "some concerns", with all contributing comparisons being prone to this limitation. Likewise, imprecision was also an issue, mostly from indirect evidence. Major concerns were raised with regard to imprecision, solely in comparisons related to OZ. Moderate confidence levels were framed for comparisons related to tempered CHX 0.2%, conventional CHX 0.2% and CIO_2, all compared to control.

6.3 Findings in Context

Major concerns have been raised with regard to working environment of health care professionals and major efforts are endorsed to minimize the dissemination of microbial and potentially pathogenic load of generated aerosols across medical disciplines, which has been particularly vital in the era of a pandemic (World Health Organization 2020). Dental practice is one of the frontline representatives of high risk population against aerosolized particulates, including bacterial, viral and fungal pathogens (Laheij et al. 2012). Workforce involved are constantly confronted with potentially hazardous compounds as a by-product of standard care delivery to patients; this, might be particularly alarming since small-sized

Table 6.4 Quantitative data from individual single studies for pathogen load (colony counts[a]) after aerosol inductive dental procedure.

#	Study ID	Dental procedure/ Setting	Comparison	MD (95% CIs)[a]	P-value
1	Dawson et al. 2016	Enamel clean-up after orthodontic fixed appliance debonding with slow-speed handpiece and tungsten carbide bur (*simulated pharynx level*)	CHX 0.2% as PMR vs. Sterile water PMR	0 (−2.3, 2.3)	1.0
			CHX 0.2% as PMR vs. No rinse	2.5 (0.5, 4.5)	**0.01**
		Enamel clean-up after orthodontic fixed appliance debonding with slow-speed handpiece and tungsten carbide bur (*simulated respiratory alveoli level*)	CHX 0.2% as PMR vs. Sterile water PMR	0.4 (−1.1, 1.9)	0.60
			CHX 0.2% as PMR vs. No rinse	1.2 (−1.1, 3.5)	0.31
2	Jawade et al. 2016	Use of coolants during ultrasonic scaling	CHX 0.12% vs. PI coolant	−33.3 (−55.3, −11.2)	**0.003**
			CHX 0.12% vs. Water coolant	−97.3 (−117.5, −77.1)	**<0.001**
			PI vs. Water coolant	−64.1 (−91.9, −36.2)	**<0.001**

3	Logothetis and Martinez-Welles 1995	Air-polishing	CHX 0.12% as PMR vs. HRB as PMR	−71.2 (−79.7, −62.7)	**<0.001**
			Water as PMR vs. HRB as PMR	−69.5 (−80.2, −58.8)	**<0.001**
			HRB as PMR vs. Water as PMR	1.7 (−11.2, 14.6)	0.80
4	Mamajiwala et al. 2018	Use of solution extracts in DUWLs during ultrasonic scaling (aerobic counts)	CHX vs. CIN in DUWLs	32.5 (−15.7, 80.7)	0.19
			CHX vs. Water in DUWLs	−814.0 (−872.1, −755.9)	**<0.001**
			CIN vs. Water in DUWLs	−846.5 (−906.1, −786.9)	**<0.001**
		Use of solution extracts in DUWLs during ultrasonic scaling (anaerobic counts)	CHX vs. CIN in DUWLs	−57.1 (−69.1, −45.1)	**<0.001**
			CHX vs. Water in DUWLs	−318.2 (−338.0, −298.4)	**<0.001**
			CIN vs. Water in DUWLs	−261.1 (−282.2, −240.0)	**<0.001**
5	Purohit et al. 2009	Comparison between 2 dental procedures in the presence of CHX 0.12% PMR	Ultrasonic scaling vs. tooth restoration through high-speed handpiece	1.6 (−0.5, 3.7)	0.13
		Comparison between 2 dental procedures without PMR	Ultrasonic scaling vs. tooth restoration through high-speed handpiece	−13.1 (−16.3, −9.9)	**<0.001**

(*Continued*)

Table 6.4 (Continued)

#	Study ID	Dental procedure/ Setting	Comparison	MD (95% CIs)[a]	P-value
6	Sethi et al. 2019	Use of coolants during ultrasonic scaling	CHX 0.2% vs. CIN coolant	51.5 (31.5, 71.5)	**<0.001**
			CHX 0.2% vs. Water coolant	−768.8 (−864.2, −673.4)	**<0.001**
			CIN vs. Water coolant	−820.3 (−915.4, −725.2)	**<0.001**
7	Toroglu et al. 2001	Comparison between 2 orthodontic procedures	Debonding/composite removal (air turbine handpiece, with water cooling and slow speed evacuation) vs. routine orthodontic practices without handpiece, but with slow speed evacuation	49.2 (19.4, 79.0)	**0.001**

The minus sign (−) shows better effect for 1st reported group in reducing pathogen load and vice versa. Bold indicate statistically significant comparisons.

[a] In CFUs (colony forming units) as reported in individual studies (no log-transformation of data); CHX, pre-procedural mouthrinse; CIN, cinnamon; DUWL, dental unit waterlines; HRB, herbal; PI, povidone iodine; PMR, pre-procedural mouth rinse.

particulates have long been considered as respiratory system triggering proxies, even making their way deeply within the lungs (Dawson et al. 2016; Napierska et al. 2010; Oberdörster et al. 2005). Aforementioned concerns are augmented by latest awareness of microbial spread, air suspension and stability in aerosols and on surfaces. An up-to-date report, based on experimentally induced simulations, has suggested that stability kinetics of severe acute respiratory-syndrome-related coronaviruses (both SARS-CoV-1 and SARS-CoV-2) may rest them viable in aerosols for at least 3 hours, albeit in reduced infectious titer (van Doremalen et al. 2020). The presence and detectability of SARS-CoV-2 in saliva of infected patients imposes an additional risk for its air-suspension after an aerosol-generating dental procedure (Azzi et al. 2020). To this line, identification of interventions with a refined dynamic of reduction of the microbial load detected after aerosol generating procedures in dental practice environment in general, is considered an important contribution to clinical evidence base. Implications for decision making and safety considerations within high risk occupational environments for patients and healthcare professionals alike are indisputably on the way, their enforcement being particularly necessitated by the existence of seasonal pandemics.

The findings of the present work are framed based on the eligibility and reporting competence of the existing evidence base with regard to aerosol microbial contamination in dentistry as well as in orthodontics. A sound emphasis on interventional designs with an a priori potential of providing minimally biased estimates for efficacy of competing treatments is given. Pre-procedural mouth rinse with tempered CHX 0.2% at 47 °C prevailed as the treatment with the highest probabilities of being opted as the most effective intervention in terms of reducing bacterial counts after ultrasonic scaling in practice, when measured through air sampling within a distance of 90 cm from the dental unit. Other documented intervention alternatives bearing high probabilities of being selected as effective first line treatment alternatives or overall were OZ, standard CHX 0.2% or 0.12%, PI and CIO_2.

6.3.1 Use of Chlorhexine (CHX) as Pre-Procedural Mouth Rinse

Use of chlorhexidine in dentistry has been well-reported mainly as a large-scale disinfectant towards the management of gingival inflammation and plaque control (Al-Maweri et al. 2020), but also as an adjunct to mechanical therapy in chronic periodontitis patients (Herrera et al. 2020). The most recent report from the Cochrane collaboration has identified the use of CHX mouth rinse, irrespective of concentration and as an adjunct to standard mechanical hygiene measures, as particularly effective in terms of dental plaque reduction and management of mild gingivitis. These findings have been supported by high quality evidence (James et al. 2017). However, adverse effects have also been in place, namely, taste disturbance, mucosal ulceration, burning sensation or oral mucosa soreness. To this respect, alternate CHX kinetics have been described early on by König et al. 2002, when testing the use of tempered CHX 0.2% at 47 °C as a mouthrinse for plaque control. Temperature selection was based on safety considerations for preventing any pulpal or mucosal adverse effect, while the tempered solution revealed an increased efficacy against microbial plaque accumulation. Irrigation with tempered CHX solution also demonstrated an increased potential for bacterial counts elimination (König et al. 2002). These early findings on within oral cavity disinfection agents, are in agreement with the results of the first network meta-analysis on the topic (Koletsi et al. 2020), as well as with original clinical reports on reducing aerosol contamination after ultrasonic scaler use (Joshi et al. 2017; Reddy et al. 2012). Notwithstanding this, practical implications may come into light when considering routine use of tempered anti-microbial solutions in dental office. Standard temperature CHX solution should be heated in a thermostatically regulated water bath individually prior to clinical use in order to produce CHX at 47 °C, thus rendering the procedure additionally complicated, as far as practice management is concerned.

6.3.2 Alternative Effects and Actions of Povidone Iodine (PI), Ozone (OZ), and Chlorine Dioxide (ClO_2)

Periodontal research and identification of interventions that could reduce the plaque microbial/bacterial load or act as therapeutic adjuncts to gingival inflammation, has been the backbone of research in aerosolized microbes in dentistry. Povidone Iodine (PI), ozone (OZ), or chlorine dioxide (ClO_2) have been identified by the present NMA as potentially effective agents against bacterial aerosol contamination, while alternative applications of these agents constitute disinfection practices in the treatment of periodontitis (Gandhi et al. 2019; Perrella et al. 2016; Yadav et al. 2015).

Unlike chlorhexidine, PI, OZ, and ClO_2 might be perceived as additionally effective germicides related to certain pathogen types, due to their oxidation potential in reaction with microbial or virus cell structure (Yoo 2018). However, latest FDA release announcements have been particularly critical and alarming against the use of ClO_2 products for disease prevention and treatment, including the novel coronavirus disease 2019 (COVID-19) (FDA 2020). Ozone applications in dentistry have been identified and emerged as promising adjuncts to scaling and root planning in periodontal therapy, either as gaseous compounds or as irrigating substances, but with questionable outcomes (Seydanur Dengizek et al. 2019). Although OZ has been identified as an agent with high probabilities of being effective against aerosolized bacteria, findings indicate a questionable level of confidence to the effect of OZ, raising issues related to within-study bias and imprecision of the estimated effect. Pre-procedural mouthrinse with Povidone Iodine 1% (PI) ranked 4th in terms of probabilities of best treatment of choice for effectiveness related to aerosolized bacteria, according to the results of the network meta-analysis (Koletsi et al. 2020), preceded by chlorhexidine solutions and ozone. Currently, PI (0.2% to 1%) has emerged together with an alternative oxidative agent, namely the hydrogen peroxide 1% (H_2O_2), as prescription solutions, for mouthwash use in dental practice for the management of SARS-CoV-2 diffusion, by two reports (Izzetti et al. 2020; Peng et al. 2020). Both related reports are based on the initial guidance for diagnosis and treatment of novel coronavirus disease 2019, released by the National Health Commission by the People's Republic of China, regarding potential ineffectiveness of CHX against the virus (National Health Commission PRC 2020). There is currently no evidence from clinical trials or relative effectiveness compared to competing interventions, on aerosolized or airborne viral load in dental practice after the use of PI or H_2O_2. However, their use may be reasonable, pertaining to their oxidation potential on viral load in saliva and subsequently in aerosolized compounds of saliva, blood and pathogen following routine dental procedures, especially those implicating high-speed handpiece air-turbine use, including debonding procedures in orthodontics. Inductively, the same goes for the novel SARS-CoV-2. With special interest on PI and implications on its effect on the novel SARS-CoV-2, literature reveals that PI bears the capacity to gradually and slowly release iodine on the lipid shell and the lipid membrane viral pathogens.

Resulting advantage is two-fold: first, lipid shell membrane is destroyed and oxidation of the cellular components renders the virus inactive; second, toxicity and adverse effects are minimized by slow iodine release (Yoo 2018). Up to date, application of H_2O_2 and research in dentistry has been confined to the study of peroxide as mouthwash on the prevention of plaque and gingival inflammation (Hossainian et al. 2011), but mainly as DUWL disinfectant agent, with reported effectiveness in reducing activity of bacterial biofilms within the waterlines (Ditommaso et al. 2016). A pilot study in 2015, reported the use of 1.5% H_2O_2 as a topical agent prior to CHX rinse for pre-procedural ultrasonic scaling and yielded promising results in terms of bacterial reduction in generated aerosol (Ramesh et al. 2015). In addition, calls for the launch of clinical trials to test the effectiveness of flavonoids and/or cyclodextrins against the SARS-CoV-2 viral load in saliva or aerosol expectorations have lately emerged (Carrouel et al. 2020).

6.3.3 Aerosolized Pathogens and Dental Procedures

As most published research on dental aerosols comes from reports on bacterial counts, a fragment of those have examined implication specific species. An array of 38 types of pathogens have been recognized in the latest scoping review in the field (Zemouri et al. 2017). It was interesting that identified micro-organisms included 16 bacterial species and 23 fungal species, while none pertained to parasites or viruses. However, this reflects the simultaneous abundance and scarcity of research paths across different directions. The bulk of currently existing studies focus on a universal identification and assessment of the bacterial load as a whole, with no further perspectives on underlying species. Checkerboard DNA–DNA hybridization technique has been implemented sporadically and solely in two studies (Feres et al. 2010; Retamal-Valdes et al. 2017) to identify microbial composition. A close observation of the microbial complexes, revealed an increased prevalence of species of the "orange complex" in aerosols produced after ultrasonic scaler use, which are mostly represented by the *Fusobacterium* family. The presence of fusobacterium was higher in absence of any active pre-procedural mouthrinse intervention. *Fusobacterium nucleatum* has been implicated in the initiation and progression of periodontitis, while its role has been identified as inhibitory of gingival fibroblast or gingiva-derived mesenchymal cell proliferation, intracellular reactive oxygen species generation, and promotive of cellular apoptosis (Kang et al. 2019); furthermore, *Fusobacterium nucleatum* infection has been linked to other pathologic ophthalmic and respiratory conditions (Bhattacharya et al. 2005). Yet, studies using checkerboard DNA–DNA hybridization are close-ended and can only reveal the absence, presence and levels of the targeted bacterial species, in this instance periodontal pathogens. This does not exclude the possibility that many other species not included in the preselected DNA-probe panel will also be present in the aerosol, but not able to be identified.

The role of DUWLs in the formation of contagious spatter compounds is regarded pivotal and as being the counterpart to patient-related aerosol mixes. Although only one study (Mamajiwala et al. 2018) pertaining to the assessment of effectiveness of different measures of DUWL disinfection, on airborne sampling could be identified, the use of specific add-ins such as CHX as solution extracts, has been proven beneficial in reducing both aerobic and anaerobic bacterial counts originating from aerosols. Furthermore and albeit the fact that the vast majority of research has evaluated microbiota of the waterlines per se, with no speculation about subsequent aerosol formation and its implications, there is increasing awareness regarding the potential health risk problems arising from a contaminated water-supply entry and colonization of pathogenic microbial species. *Mycobacteria, helicobacter pylori, Legionella pneumophilla* as well as *Pseudomonas spp* are some of the implicated species (Castellano Realpe et al. 2020; Giacomuzzi et al. 2019; Tuvo et al. 2020). Water filters installation, shock disinfection of hydrogen peroxide with concentrations ranging from 3% to 6% v/v, chlorhexidine, or specially designed biofilm removing systems have been proposed (Baudet et al. 2020). Such interventions and future planning would prove beneficial for a wide range of dental procedures involving use or spray or high-speed handpiece instrumentation, including the debonding stages of orthodontic treatment.

In all, adoption of occupational measures in dental practice against potentially hazardous aerosol forming procedures should be considered on a universal basis and standard precaution procedures should involve more skeptical application and even reduction in the use of aerosol forming instrumentation in everyday practice. These constitute not only ultrasonic scaling, but also restorative procedures (Purohit et al. 2009), enamel clean-up after fixed appliance orthodontic treatment (Dawson et al. 2016) or massive attachment removal following aligner treatment (Iliadi et al. 2020). To this respect, founding recommendations from the U.S. Centers for Disease Control and Prevention (CDC Report 2016) involve a range of safety considerations, as documented by aerosol and waterline precautions, personal protective equipment and ventilation management.

6.3.4 Strengths and Limitations Stemming from Existing Evidence

The present chapter presents a large-scale assessment of intervention practices to reduce pathogen load of aerosols within dental practice environment. The background information and data is relied upon the first and most rigorous review on the topic since the emergence of the SARS-CoV-2 pandemic and allows for certain advantages to be considered (Koletsi et al. 2020). First, the review involved a priori registration to an open access registry, as well as a reporting framework based on contemporary available guidelines specific for the design of the network meta-analysis, safeguarding against reporting bias. Second, a rigorous approach was followed, involving a network set-up of the existing intervention strategies. Network meta-analysis in general allow for indirect comparisons between pairwise interventions not directly tested across original studies, thus providing additional and potentially more precise information for the estimated effect across treatments (Caldwell et al. 2015). Third, the simultaneous assessment of all available interventions allows for an estimation of their relative ranking for a specific outcome, which is non-applicable for conventional meta-analyses (Chaimani et al. 2019).

Limitations do exist as well, while they are consistently inherent to the contributing primary studies considered. Apart from identified issues with the internal validity over an amount of included studies, aerosolized products were solely considered in terms of bacterial load and their pathogenicity could not be measured. The majority of interventions were also checked under the settings of ultrasonic scaling in practice; however, extrapolation to other spray, or high-speed handpiece comprising settings may be considered feasible, realistic and reasonable.

6.4 Concluding Remarks and Implications for Research

Allowing for all discussed caveats, the existing findings suggest the use of pre-procedural mouthrinse with preferably tempered chlorhexidine as the most effective strategy for the reduction of aerosol related bacterial load in dental practice. In addition, in temporal conditions dictated by seasonal epidemics of other forms of pathogens, mostly represented by oxidative stress-vulnerable viruses, substitute intervention strategies, such as povidone iodine might be considered as viable solutions. In this respect, research towards identification of additionally tested disinfectant agents used as mouthwash rinses should also be endorsed. In the era of SARS-CoV-2 pandemic, the stipulation of a broader evaluation of the aerosolized microbes, including viruses, potentially coupled with disinfectant treatment schemes should be prioritized. However, for all latter approaches, a clear call for robustly conducted and reported clinical trials is indisputable.

References

Al-Maweri, S.A., Nassani, M.Z., Alaizari, N. et al. (2020). Efficacy of aloe vera mouthwash versus chlorhexidine on plaque and gingivitis: a systematic review. *Int. J. Dent. Hyg.* 18 (1): 44–51.

Azzi, L., Carcano, G., Gianfagna, F. et al. (2020). Saliva is a reliable tool to detect SARS-CoV-2. *J. Infect.* S0163-4453 (20): 30213–30219.

Baudet, A., Lizon, J., Martrette, J.-M. et al. (2020). Efficacy of BRS® and Alpron®/Bilpron® disinfectants for dental unit waterlines: a six-year study. *Int. J. Environ. Res. Public Health* 17 (8): 2634.

Bhattacharya, S., Livsey, S.A., Wiselka, M., and Bukhari, S.S. (2005). Fusobacteriosis presenting as community acquired pneumonia. *J. Infect.* 50 (3): 236–239.

Caldwell, D.M., Dias, S., and Welton, N.J. (2015). Extending treatment networks in health technology assessment: how far should we go? *Value Health.* 18 (5): 673–681.

Carrouel, F., Conte, M.P., Fisher, J. et al. (2020). COVID-19: a recommendation to examine the effect of Mouthrinses with β-cyclodextrin combined with Citrox in preventing infection and progression. *J. Clin. Med.* 9 (4): 1126.

Castellano Realpe, O.J., Gutiérrez, J.C., Sierra, D.A. et al. (2020). Dental unit waterlines in Quito and Caracas contaminated with nontuberculous mycobacteria: a potential health risk in dental practice. *Int. J. Environ. Res. Public Health* 17 (7): 2348.

CDC. (2016). Summary of infection prevention practices in dental settings: Basic expectations for safe care.

Chaimani, A., Higgins, J.P.T., Mavridis, D. et al. (2013). Graphical tools for network meta-analysis in STATA. Haibe-Kains B, editor. *PLoS One* 8 (10): e76654.

Chaimani, A., Caldwell, D., Li, T. et al. (2019). Chapter 11: undertaking network meta-analyses. In: *Cochrane Handbook for Systematic Reviews of Interventions* (ed. H. JPT, J. Thomas, J. Chandler, et al.). version 6.0 (updated July 2019). https://training.cochrane.org/handbook/current/chapter-11 (accessed 26 April 2020).

Cokic, S.M., Ghosh, M., Hoet, P. et al. (2020). Cytotoxic and genotoxic potential of respirable fraction of composite dust on human bronchial cells. *Dent. Mater.* 36 (2): 270–283.

Council, A.D.A. (1996). Infection control recommendations for the dental office and the dental laboratory. *J. Am. Dent. Assoc.* (Suppl:1–8).

Dawson, M., Soro, V., Dymock, D. et al. (2016). Microbiological assessment of aerosol generated during debond of fixed orthodontic appliances. *Am. J. Orthod. Dentofacial. Orthop.* 150 (5): 831–838.

Devker, N., Malagi, S., Mohitey, J. et al. (2012). A study to evaluate and compare the efficacy of preprocedural mouthrinsing and high volume evacuator attachment alone and in combination in reducing the amount of viable aerosols produced during ultrasonic scaling procedure. *J. Contemp. Dent. Pract.* 13 (5): 681–689.

Ditommaso, S., Giacomuzzi, M., Ricciardi, E., and Zotti, C.M. (2016). Efficacy of a low dose of hydrogen peroxide (Peroxy Ag^{+}) for continuous treatment of dental unit water lines: challenge test with legionella pneumophila serogroup 1 in a simulated dental unit waterline. *Int. J. Environ. Res. Public Health* 13 (5).

van Doremalen, N., Bushmaker, T., Morris, D.H. et al. (2020). Aerosol and surface stability of SARS-CoV-2 as compared with SARS-CoV-1. *N. Engl. J. Med.* 382 (16): 1564–1567.

FDA. (2020). Coronavirus (COVID-19) update: FDA warns seller marketing dangerous chlorine dioxide products that claim to treat or prevent COVID-19. News release (April 9). https://www.fda.gov/news-events/

press-announcements/coronavirus-covid-19-update-fda-warns-seller-marketing-dangerous-chlorine-dioxide-products-claim (accessed 20 April 2020).

Feres, M., Figueiredo, L.C., Faveri, M. et al. (2010). The effectiveness of a preprocedural Mouthrinse containing Cetylpyridinium chloride in reducing bacteria in the dental office. *J. Am. Dent. Assoc.* 141 (4): 415–422.

Fine, D.H., Mendieta, C., Barnett, M.L. et al. (1992). Efficacy of preprocedural rinsing with an antiseptic in reducing viable bacteria in dental aerosols. *J. Periodontol.* 63 (10): 821–824.

Gandhi, K.K., Cappetta, E.G., and Pavaskar, R. (2019). Effectiveness of the adjunctive use of ozone and chlorhexidine in patients with chronic periodontitis. *BDJ Open.* 5: 17.

Giacomuzzi, M., Zotti, C.M., and Ditommaso, S. (2019). Colonization of dental unit waterlines by helicobacter pylori: risk of exposure in dental practices. *Int. J. Environ. Res. Public Health* 16 (16): 2981.

Gupta, G., Mitra, D., Ashok, K.P. et al. (2014). Efficacy of preprocedural mouth rinsing in reducing aerosol contamination produced by ultrasonic scaler: a pilot study. *J. Periodontol.* 85 (4): 562–568.

Harrel, S.K. and Molinari, J. (2004). Aerosols and splatter in dentistry: a brief review of the literature and infection control implications. *J. Am. Dent. Assoc.* 135 (4): 429–437.

Herrera, D., Matesanz, P., Martín, C. et al. (2020). Adjunctive effect of locally delivered antimicrobials in periodontitis therapy. A systematic review and meta-analysis. *J. Clin. Periodontol.*.

Holloman, J.L., Mauriello, S.M., Pimenta, L., and Arnold, R.R. (2015). Comparison of suction device with saliva ejector for aerosol and spatter reduction during ultrasonic scaling. *J. Am. Dent. Assoc.* 146 (1): 27–33.

Hossainian, N., Slot, D.E., Afennich, F., and Van der Weijden, G.A. (2011). The effects of hydrogen peroxide mouthwashes on the prevention of plaque and gingival inflammation: a systematic review. *Int. J. Dent. Hyg.* 9 (3): 171–181.

Iliadi, A., Koletsi, D., Papageorgiou, S.N., and Eliades, T. (2020). Safety considerations for thermoplastic-type appliances used as orthodontic aligners or retainers. A systematic review and meta-analysis of clinical and in-vitro research. *Materials (Basel).* 13 (8).

Ireland, A.J., Moreno, T., and Price, R. (2003). Airborne particles produced during enamel cleanup after removal of orthodontic appliances. *Am. J. Orthod. Dentofacial. Orthop.* 124 (6): 683–686.

Izzetti, R., Nisi, M., Gabriele, M., and Graziani, F. (2020). COVID-19 transmission in dental practice: brief review of preventive measures in Italy. *J. Dent.* Res.:002203452092058.

James, P., Worthington, H.V., Parnell, C. et al. (2017). Chlorhexidine mouthrinse as an adjunctive treatment for gingival health. *Cochrane Database Syst. Rev.* 3 (CD008676).

Jawade, R., Bhandari, V., Ugale, G. et al. (2016). Comparative evaluation of two different ultrasonic liquid coolants on dental aerosols. *J. Clin. Diagn. Res.* 10: 7, ZC53–57.

Joshi, A.A., Padhye, A.M., and Swatan, H. (2017). Efficacy of two pre-procedural rinses at two different temperatures in reducing aerosol contamination produced during ultrasonic scaling in a dental set-up – a microbiological study. *J. Int. Acad. Periodontol.* 19 (4): 138–144.

Kang, W., Jia, Z., Tang, D. et al. (2019). Fusobacterium nucleatum facilitates apoptosis, ROS generation, and inflammatory cytokine production by activating AKT/MAPK and NF-κB Signaling pathways in human gingival fibroblasts. *Oxid. Med. Cell Longev.* 2019: 1681972.

Kaur, R., Vandana, K., Desai, R., and Singh, I. (2014). Effect of chlorhexidine, povidone iodine, and ozone on microorganisms in dental aerosols: randomized double-blind clinical trial. *Indian J. Dent. Res.* 25 (2): 160–165.

King, T.B., Muzzin, K.B., Berry, C.W., and Anders, L.M. (1997). The effectiveness of an aerosol reduction device for ultrasonic sealers. *J. Periodontol.* 68 (1): 45–49.

Koletsi, D., Belibasakis, G.N., and Eliades, T. (2020). Interventions to reduce aerosolized microbes in dental practice: a systematic review with network meta-analysis of randomized controlled trials. *J. Dent. Res.* 99 (11): 1228–1238.

König, J., Storcks, V., Kocher, T. et al. (2002). Anti-plaque effect of tempered 0.2% chlorhexidine rinse: an in vivo study. *J. Clin. Periodontol.* 29 (3): 207–210.

Laheij, A.M.G.A., Kistler, J.O., Belibasakis, G.N. et al. (2012). Healthcare-associated viral and bacterial infections in dentistry. *J. Oral Microbiol.* 4.

Logothetis, D.D. and Martinez-Welles, J.M. (1995). Reducing bacterial aerosol contamination with a chlorhexidine gluconate pre-rinse. *J. Am. Dent. Assoc.* 126 (12): 1634–1639.

Mamajiwala, A., Sethi, K., Raut, C. et al. (2018). Comparative evaluation of chlorhexidine and cinnamon extract used in dental unit waterlines to reduce bacterial load in aerosols during ultrasonic scaling. *Indian J. Dent. Res.* 29 (6): 749–754.

Mohan, M. and Jagannathan, N. (2016). The efficacy of pre-procedural mouth rinse on bacterial count in dental aerosol following Oral prophylaxis. *Dent. Med. Probl.* 53 (1): 78–82.

Napierska, D., Thomassen, L.C.J., Lison, D. et al. (2010). The nanosilica hazard: another variable entity. *Part. Fibre Toxicol.* 7 (1): 39.

Narayana, T., Mohanty, L., Sreenath, G., and Vidhyadhari, P. (2016). Role of preprocedural rinse and high volume evacuator in reducing bacterial contamination in bioaerosols. *J. Oral Maxillofac. Pathol.* 20 (1): 59.

National Health Commission PRC (2020). *Guidance for Corona Virus Disease 2019. Prevention, Control, Diagnosis and Management*, 5the. National Health Commission by the People's Republic of China http://www.pmph.com.

NCT02319668. (2017). Antimicrobial agent for reducing bacteria in aerosols and oral cavity. https://clinicaltrials.gov/ct2/show/NCT02319668 (accessed 14 April 2020).

Nikolakopoulou, A., Higgins, J.P.T., Papakonstantinou, T. et al. (2020). CINeMA: an approach for assessing confidence in the results of a network meta-analysis. *PLoS Med.* 17 (4): e1003082.

Oberdörster, G., Oberdörster, E., and Oberdörster, J. (2005). Nanotoxicology: an emerging discipline evolving from studies of ultrafine particles. *Environ. Health Perspect.* 113 (7): 823–839.

Papakonstantinou, T., Nikolakopoulou, A., Higgins, J.P.T. et al. (2020). CINeMA: software for semiautomated assessment of the confidence in the results of network meta-analysis. *Campbell Syst. Rev.* 16 (1): e1080.

Paul, B., Baiju, R.P., Raseena, N. et al. (2020). Effect of aloe vera as a preprocedural rinse in reducing aerosol contamination during ultrasonic scaling. *J. Indian Soc. Periodontol.* 24 (1): 37–41.

Peng, X., Xu, X., Li, Y. et al. (2020). Transmission routes of 2019-nCoV and controls in dental practice. *Int. J. Oral Sci.* 12 (1): 9.

Perrella, F.A., da Rovai, E., S., De Marco, A.C. et al. (2016). Clinical and microbiological evaluation of povidone-iodine 10% as an adjunct to nonsurgical periodontal therapy in chronic periodontitis: a randomized clinical trial. *J. Int. Acad. Periodontol.* 18 (4): 109–119.

Purohit, B., Priya, H., Acharya, S. et al. (2009). Efficacy of pre-procedural rinsing in reducing aerosol contamination during dental procedures. *J. Infect. Prevent.* 10 (6): 190–192.

Rajachandrasekaran, Y., Valiathan, M., Jayaraman, B.G. et al. (2019). An herbal alternative to control nosocomial pathogens in aerosols and splatter during ultrasonic scaling. *Pesqui bras odontopediatria clín integr.* 19 (1): 1–9.

Ramesh, A., Thomas, J., Np, M., and Varghese, S. (2015). Efficacy of adjunctive usage of hydrogen peroxide with chlorhexidine as preprocedural mouthrinse on dental aerosol. *Nat. J. Physiol. Pharm. Pharmacol.* 5 (5): 1–5.

Rani, K., Ambati, M., Pinnamaneni, I. et al. (2014). Chemical vs. herbal formulations as pre-procedural mouth rinses to combat aerosol production: a randomized controlled study. *J. Oral Res. Rev.* 6 (1): 9–13.

Reddy, S., Prasad, M.G.S., Satish, K. et al. (2012). Efficacy of 0.2% tempered chlorhexidine as a pre-procedural mouth rinse: a clinical study. *J. Indian Soc. Periodontol.* 16 (2): 213–217.

Retamal-Valdes, B., Soares, G.M., Stewart, B. et al. (2017). Effectiveness of a pre-procedural mouthwash in reducing bacteria in dental aerosols: randomized clinical trial. *Braz. Oral Res.* 31: e21.

Saini, R. (2015). Efficacy of preprocedural mouth rinse containing chlorine dioxide in reduction of viable bacterial count in dental aerosols during ultrasonic scaling: a double-blind, placebo-controlled clinical trial. *Dent. Hypotheses.* 6 (2): 65.

dos Santos, I.R.M., Moreira, A.C.A., Costa, M.G.C., and Barbosa, M. (2014). Effect of 0.12% chlorhexidine in reducing microorganisms found in aerosol used for dental prophylaxis of patients submitted to fixed orthodontic treatment. *Dental Press. J. Orthod.* 19 (3): 95–101.

Sethi, K., Mamajiwala, A., Mahale, S. et al. (2019). Comparative evaluation of the chlorhexidine and cinnamon extract as ultrasonic coolant for reduction of bacterial load in dental aerosols. *J. Indian Soc. Periodontol.* 23 (3): 226–233.

Seydanur Dengizek, E., Serkan, D., Abubekir, E. et al. (2019). Evaluating clinical and laboratory effects of ozone in non-surgical periodontal treatment: a randomized controlled trial. *J. Appl. Oral Sci.* 27: e20180108.

Shetty, S.K., Sharath, K., Shenoy, S. et al. (2013). Compare the efficacy of two commercially available mouthrinses in reducing viable bacterial count in dental aerosol produced during ultrasonic scaling when used as a preprocedural rinse. *J. Contemp. Dent. Pract.* 14 (5): 848–851.

Swahney, A., Venugopal, S., Babu, G. et al. (2015). Aerosols, how dangerous they are in clinical practice. *J. Clin. Diagn. Res.* 9 (4): ZC52–ZC57.

Swaminathan, Y., Thomas, D.J.T., and Muralidharan, N.P. (2014). The efficacy of preprocedural mouth rinse of 0.2% chlorhexidine and commercially available herbal mouth containing salvadora persica in reducing the bacterial load in saliva and aerosol produced during scaling. *Asian J. Pharm. Clin. Res.* 7: 71–74.

Toroglu, M.S., Haytac, M., and Koeksal, F. (2001). Evaluation of aerosol contamination during debonding procedures. *Angle. Orthod.* 71 (4): 299–306.

Tuvo, B., Totaro, M., Cristina, M.L. et al. (2020). Prevention and control of *Legionella* and *Pseudomonas* spp. colonization in dental units. *Pathogens.* 9 (4): 305.

Waghmare, S.V., Srivastava, S., and Kini, V.V. (2018). Comparative evaluation of Colony forming unit count on aerobic culture of aerosol collected following pre-procedural rinses of either 0.2% chlorhexidine gluconate or 1% stabilized chlorine dioxide during ultrasonic scaling: A Clinical and Microbiological Study. *J. Contemp. Dent.* 8 (2): 70–76.

White, I.R. (2015). Network meta-analysis. *Stata J.* 15 (4): 951–985.

World Health Organization. (2020). Coronavirus situation report. https://www.who.int/emergencies/diseases/novel-coronavirus-2019 (accessed 22 April 2020).

Yadav, S.R., Kini, V.V., and Padhye, A. (2015). Inhibition of tongue coat and dental plaque formation by stabilized chlorine dioxide vs chlorhexidine Mouthrinse: A Randomized, Triple Blinded Study. *J. Clin. Diagn. Res.* 9 (9): ZC69–ZC74.

Yoo, J.H. (2018). Review of disinfection and sterilization – back to the basics. *Infect. Chemother.* 50 (2): 101–109.

Zemouri, C., de Soet, H., Crielaard, W., and Laheij, A. (2017). A scoping review on bio-aerosols in healthcare and the dental environment. Zhou D, editor. *PLoS One* 12 (5): e0178007.

7

Future Material Development for Efficient Debonding

Theodore Eliades

Clinic of Orthodontics and Pediatric Dentistry, Center of Dental Medicine, University of Zurich, Zurich, Switzerland

Despite advances in the field of materials, bonding in orthodontics has not been substantially altered during the past three decades. The acid-etching technique is still employed for bonding brackets labially or lingually to enamel, albeit with potential variation such as (i) self-etching, where primers are incorporated into the acid solution; and (ii) moisture-insensitive and moisture-active adhesives, where primers supposedly tolerate the moisture, or a functional component reacts with the moisture present in the surface of the tooth to achieve bonding.

After the initial large-scale application of bonding in orthodontics, various problems gave rise to concerns about the integrity of the enamel. Enamel involvement in etching-mediated bonding takes place at three stages:

1) At the etching stage, the structure and superficial composition of the tissue are permanently altered.
2) During the course of treatment, there is no exchange of ions with the intraoral environment for the enamel portion covered by the adhesive, often with the potential for demineralisation.

Part of this text has previously appeared in the relevant chapter of the book Eliades T, Brantley WA (Eds) Orthodontic Applications of Biomaterials A Clinical Guide 1st Edition, Elsevier 2016.

Debonding and Fixed Retention in Orthodontics: An Evidence-Based Clinical Guide, First Edition. Edited by Theodore Eliades and Christos Katsaros.

3) During debonding, the use of rotary instruments to remove the adhesive results in the development of scratches on the enamel surface, which often outweigh the differences in colour change induced by etching- and non-etching-mediated bonding.

The first category of concern has been long investigated, and efforts to replace etching with another mechanism have taken place with varying degrees of success. Since the mid-1980s, there has been a distinguishable trend in the literature to explore alternative bracket bonding through several mechanisms employing calcium salts or non-etching-mediated bonding. These efforts did not show acceptable results, and no further development on this issue was seen. Glass ionomer cements, with or without the use of polyacrylic acid etching, were adopted to replace orthophosphoric acid etching. Polyacrylic acid induces a significantly shallower depth of penetration (5–7 mm) relative to conventional acid etching; however, the clinical success is still debatable.

To avoid the effects induced by the presence of bonded appliances for an extended time in the oral cavity, several protocols for remineralisation have been developed, including the use of glass ionomers, fluoride-releasing materials and primers.

7.1 Command-Debond Adhesives

The removal of resinous adhesive after debonding is still an issue of interest. The mass of adhesive left on the enamel can be controlled to some extent by altering the adhesive-bracket interfacial characteristics to enhance the interfacial strength by varying the filler content and bracket base retentive characteristics. However, the use of burs has an unfavourable effect on enamel integrity in two ways: (i) the generation of aerosols consisting of particles in the range of 2.5 mm, which can be inhaled and (ii) the potential estrogenic action of these adhesive particles, owing perhaps to the large surface-to-volume ratio and the effect of heat shock on the adhesive, which releases bisphenol A (BPA) under these conditions (as discussed later in this chapter). There is an extensive discussion of BPA in Chapter 11.

A potential solution to this problem may be the development of command-debond adhesives. These are polymers in which the polymerisation can be 'reversed' using the following strategies: (i) irradiation with a specific wavelength capable of drastically lowering the glass transition temperature of the polymer, thereby initiating transformation to a viscous state and allowing for removal of the nonglassy adhesive; or (ii) incorporating a filler that can be employed to cause severe structural alteration of the material upon specific application of a stimulus. For example, ferrous microparticles have been introduced as fillers to allow preferential distribution of the particles within the polymer to improve the mechanical properties predictably to meet service requirements. This is achieved by using magnets to orient the particles in a favourable way. When the polarity of the magnets is reversed, the fillers initiate an internal shock process that destabilises the structural integrity of the polymer, leading to the formation of a network of cracks that in turn can lead to a desirable failure.

7.2 BPA-Free Monomers

The majority of orthodontic adhesive materials are derived from BPA. The BPA configuration assembles a bulky, stiff chain that provides low susceptibility to biodegradation as well as significant strength and rigidity in BPA-derived dimethacrylate polymers based on monomers such as bisphenol A-glycidyl dimethacrylate (BisGMA), its ethoxylated analog (BisEDMA), bisphenol A-dimethacrylate (BisDMA) and urethane-modified BisGMA. Although BPA is not used as a raw material in dental composite resins, it is likely to be present as an impurity from the chemical synthesis procedure.

The unique biologic effects of BPA arise at ranges within the levels of the detection threshold for a majority of analytical techniques and show a nonmonotonic curve pattern on tissues, characterised by intense reactivity at low levels and no response at very high ones. This model of action originates from natural human hormones, such as 17b-estradiol, which can generate effects at concentrations markedly lower than those required to block the specific receptors. BPA and BPA derivatives increase the levels of reactive oxygen species, which are known mediators of signalling cascades under physiological conditions. Elevated levels of such compounds can disrupt the cellular redox equilibrium, causing oxidative DNA damage and apoptosis in mammalian cells.

In orthodontics, BPA dimethacrylate derivatives are mostly used for bonding brackets (bonding resins and composite resins as main adhesives) and lingual retainers, whereas BPA-polycarbonates are used for manufacturing plastic brackets. *In vitro* studies have documented the release of BPA from polycarbonate brackets, orthodontic adhesives and the composite resins that are frequently used for bonding lingual retainers. For traditional and flowable composite resins used as lingual retainers, BPA release was confirmed *in vivo* as well, with the highest values in saliva measured immediately after polymerisation.

Efforts have been undertaken to replace the BPA monomer derivatives with other BPA-free monomers, with the objective of matching the well-established polymer network stiffness, strength, rigidity and low biodegradation susceptibility of BisDMA derivatives. Most alternative approaches included aliphatic comonomers based on triethyleneglycol dimethacrylate, urethane dimethacrylate and cycloaliphatic dimethacrylates, all introduced from restorative composite resin technology, along with proper filler particle reinforcing agents.

Although conventional orthodontic adhesives are mostly used for bonding metallic wires to enamel, several issues remain to be addressed. In retainers, the resinous material is not covered by the brackets, and hence it is directly exposed to the oral environment from all surfaces except the enamel–adhesive interface. Therefore it is more prone to intraoral degradation than adhesives for bracket bonding. In addition, with the current application techniques, the hydrophilic metal surface does not chemically bond with the composite resin, thus creating a weak interface that is exposed intraorally at the mesial and distal margins of the teeth. Moreover, since the retainer wire has no sliding capacity in the manner of the wire in the bracket slots, the modulus of elasticity of the composite resin should have a suitable value to avoid the development of stresses at the weak resin–wire interface.

New monomers have been introduced based on a non-BPA synthesis route. These involve (i) a single-aromatic-ring, highly reactive, multifunctional monomer (phenyl carbamoyloxy-propane dimethacrylate [PCDMA]) that is incorporated along with conventional aliphatic comonomers and glass fillers, or (ii) the use of aromatic-free urethane dimethacrylate monomers.

The two experimental BPA-free materials have demonstrated a better degree of cure and less water plasticisation compared to the control, which was based on a BPA compound (BisGMA). The control demonstrated higher mechanical properties but no statistically significant difference in pullout strength from the two experimental materials. Considering the differences between the two experimental materials, it may be concluded that the material containing the monoaromatic dimethacrylate derivative (PCDMA) with higher hardness and elastic modulus may be used as an alternative to the control.

7.3 Biomimetic Adhesives

The issue of an enamel-friendly bonding mechanism for orthodontic appliances has been the subject of investigations since the original introduction of the acid-etching technique. This intense interest derived from the description of alterations of enamel colour and structure associated with acid-etched-mediated bonding. During the past 15 years, the introduction of a new class of materials that adopt the paradigms of nature has gradually established the category of *biomimetic* materials. This term derives from the Greek ‘bio’ (living) and ‘mimetic’ (imitating or resembling) and refers to how creatures ingenuously employ natural elements to solve problems in the environment.

Geckos, for example, are lizards that belong to the species of *gekkonidae* and are characterised by a remarkable ability to sustain their weight whilst upside down. The strong but temporary adhesion employed by a gecko comes from a mechanical principle known as *contact splitting*. The foot of a gecko has a flat pad that is densely packed with very fine hairs that are split at the ends, resulting in more contact points than if the hairs were not split. More contact points between these hairs and a surface result in a significant increase in adhesion force. Researchers have discovered that this special nature of the foot pads allows the gecko to stick to surfaces through the formation of localised van der Waals forces. This mechanism has been employed for high-friction microfibers or carbon nanotubes sprayed on a surface. Because of the enormous number per unit area, the physical forces developed mimic the ability of a gecko to attach firmly to surfaces without using a chemical substance.

Although this mode of bonding may be suitable for dry environments, it fails to provide reliable performance for wet surfaces. This problem inspired researchers to adopt another natural example of bonding: that of mussels. Combining the important elements of gecko and mussel adhesion, the new adhesive material, called *geckel*, functions like a sticky note and exhibits strong yet reversible adhesion in both air and water. Mussel-mimetic polymers have an amino acid L-3, 4-dihydroxyphenylalanine (DOPA) that is found in high concentrations in the 'glue' proteins of mussels. Analogously to the gecko-based approach, pillar arrays (400–600 nm in diameter and length) coated with the mussel-mimetic polymer improved wet adhesion by 15-fold over uncoated pillar arrays.

The orthodontic application of this innovation is profound. Brackets having bases with pads mimicking the gecko foot and covered with a layer of DOPA would provide adequate bond strength to sound enamel without prior enamel conditioning and with minimal colour and structural alterations to the enamel.

Further Reading

Berengueres, J., Saito, S., and Tadakuma, K. (2007). Structural properties of a scaled-gecko foot hair. *Bioinspir. Biomim.* 2: 1–8.

Eliades, T. (2012). Dental materials in orthodontics. In: *Orthodontics: Current Principles and Techniques*, 5e (ed. L.W. Graber, R.L. Vanarsdall, and K.L. Vig). Philadelphia: Elsevier.

Eliades, T. and Eliades, G. (2014). *Plastics in Dentistry and Estrogenicity*. Heidelberg: Springer.

Eliades, T., Hiskia, A., Eliades, G., and Athanasiou, A.E. (2007). Assessment of bisphenol-A release from orthodontic adhesives. *Am. J. Orthod. Dentofacial Orthop.* 131: 72–75.

Eliades, T., Voutsa, D., Sifakakis, I. et al. (2011). Release of bisphenol-A from a light-cured adhesive bonded to lingual fixed retainers. *Am. J. Orthod. Dentofacial Orthop.* 139: 192–195.

Gioka, C., Eliades, T., Zinelis, S. et al. (2009). Characterization and *in vitro* estrogenicity of orthodontic adhesive particulates produced by simulated debonding. *Dent. Mater.* 25: 376–382.

Iliadi, A., Eliades, T., Silikas, N., and Eliades, G. (2017). Development and testing of novel bisphenol A-free adhesives for lingual fixed retainer bonding. *Eur. J. Orthod.* 39 (1): 1–8.

Kloukos, D., Taoufik, E., Eliades, T. et al. (2013). Cytotoxic effects of polycarbonate-based orthodontic brackets by activation of mitochondrial apoptotic mechanisms. *Dent. Mater.* 29: e35–e44.

Kloukos, D., Sifakakis, I., Voutsa, D. et al. (2015). BPA qualitative and quantitative assessment associated with orthodontic bonding *in vivo*. *Dent. Mater.* 31: 887–894.

Lee, H., Lee, B.P., and Messersmith, P.B. (2007). A reversible wet-dry adhesive inspired by mussels and geckos. *Nature* 448: 338–341.

8

The Use of Attachments in Aligner Treatment: Analyzing the 'Innovation' of Expanding the Use of Acid Etching-Mediated Bonding of Composites to Enamel and Its Consequences

Theodore Eliades[1], Spyridon N. Papageorgiou[1], and Anthony J. Ireland[2]

[1] *Clinic of Orthodontics and Pediatric Dentistry, Center of Dental Medicine, University of Zürich, Zürich, Switzerland*
[2] *Department of Orthodontics, Bristol Dental School, University of Bristol, Bristol, UK*

In the last decade, aligners have become an integral part of orthodontic armamentaria, and their use has been expanded to supposedly manage a wide range of malocclusions. At the same time, there is a populous list of companies offering aligner treatment either to professionals or directly to the public – sometimes even without the direct involvement of a dentist. The establishment of aligners as a treatment modality for malocclusion was made possible with the introduction of bonded attachments, which enhanced the control of the crown's spatial orientation, offering far more possibilities for treatment compared with the initial introduction of aligners when the tooth movement was limited to tipping and a small derotation of anterior teeth. Although the multiplicity of attachment shape and size opened new possibilities in the treatment of rotations, such as buccolingual inclination variations and vertical repositioning of teeth, their use is not free of concerns.

Previously published as Eliades, T., Papageorgiou, S.N., and Ireland, A.J. (2020). The use of attachments in aligner treatment. *American Journal of Orthodontics and Dentofacial Orthopedics* 158 (2): 166–174. Used with permission from Elsevier.

Debonding and Fixed Retention in Orthodontics: An Evidence-Based Clinical Guide, First Edition. Edited by Theodore Eliades and Christos Katsaros.

The purpose of this narrative review is to discuss the concerns arising from the increasing use of composite resins bonded onto the labial surface of teeth, focusing primarily on the biologic and environmental implications of their application.

8.1 Enamel Involvement

One of the main advantages of the early phase of aligners was the absence of any involvement of enamel in the treatment of malocclusions. Although the application spectrum of aligner treatment was limited to Class I crowding cases, the fact that orthodontic treatment of these cases involved no acid etching-mediated bonding offered an advantage owing to the maintenance of the structural integrity of enamel (Brosh et al. 2005; Eliades et al. 2004; Ioannidis et al. 2018; Ireland et al. 2005; Janiszewska-Olszowska et al. 2016; Mohebi et al. 2017), with favorable outcome on the potential for white spot lesions, decalcification (Ogaard et al. 1988), avoidance of the use of rotary instruments to grind the remnants of adhesives after debonding, and essentially a lack of long-term change of the enamel's optical properties (Joo et al. 2011; Karamouzos et al. 2010; Sifakakis et al. 2018), because the absence of resin tags warrants that the surface would be intact.

Expanding the spectrum of indications for aligners to tooth movement in all 3 planes of space necessitated the use of grips bonded onto the enamel to generate buccolingual, mesiodistal, and incisocervical movement, which negated the advantage of an intact enamel surface. Such composite attachments used in conjunction with aligners have dimensions ranging from 2 mm to 5 mm and11 thickness that can exceed well 1 mm (Dasy et al. 2015), are bonded most often on the labial surface of multiple teeth. Moreover, composite attachments used in aligner treatment possess a high surface-area-to-volume ratio, which affects their interaction with the environment.

In orthodontics, specifically in bonding orthodontic brackets, the adhesive application mode effectively alters the exposure pattern of the material to the oral cavity with a potential effect on reducing its reactivity with liquids and other materials. The sandwich pattern of application, where the adhesive is bonded to both enamel and bracket base, allows only the margins of the material to be exposed to the oral cavity. The acid-etched enamel interface on the one side and the morphologic irregularity of bracket base through the welded mesh wire or laser etching on the other side provide a mechanism for the interlocking of the polymeric material in both structures (tooth and bracket) (Kechagia et al. 2015). The average thickness of the adhesive layer between the tooth and bracket has been estimated between 150 and 250 μm, depending on the morphologic condition of the bracket base, with smooth bases resulting in thinner adhesive layers owing to the homogeneous pressure and the lack of retentive sites for the entrapment of the adhesive, whereas rougher bases lead to thicker adhesive layers. Therefore, for a typical bracket with dimensions of 2.5×3.0 mm (height X width) bonded to enamel, the surface of the adhesive layer exposed in the oral cavity can be estimated to be somewhere in the 11-mm perimeter range or $11\,\text{mm} \times 200 \times 10^{-3}$ mm or $2.2\,\text{mm}^2$ adhesive surface area. This multiplied by 20 brackets – the average case – results in a sum of $44\,\text{mm}^2$ of material area exposed to the oral conditions. For wider brackets, which are introduced to provide better rotational and tipping control of teeth, these figures are expected to be higher.

Table 8.1 compares the surface area of adhesives or composites exposed to the oral environment in the routine case of orthodontic bonding and the corresponding values of aligner treatment with the use of attachments (Eliades et al. 1991). The assumption for the aligner scenario was the use of 12 attachments per case with varying shape depending on their position (4 trapezoid, 4 rectangular, and 4 elliptical attachments). However, the actual clinical use of composite for aligner attachments differs vastly from the provided crude theoretical comparison of exposed surfaces because of the following two reasons. First, the adhesive during bracket bonding is applied in a sandwich pattern, which decreases exposed surfaces and its potential reactivity with the oral environment. Second, attachments in aligner treatment possess considerable thickness to assist in tooth positioning, and as such, they are exposed to a daily snagging of the aligner during fitting or mastication. Thus, apart from the larger surface exposed relative to the edges of the adhesive, aligner attachments are also subjected to masticatory stresses during eating and stresses arising from the fitting of the aligner on the teeth multiple times daily, which brings us to the next issue.

Table 8.1 Effective surface exposure area of adhesive in bracket bonding and aligner treatment with attachments.

Procedure	Assumptions	Estimated exposure area
Bracket bonding	• 20 teeth • Brackets 2.5–3.0 mm • Adhesive thickness of 200 μm	Margin exposure: (periphery 11.0 mm) × (thickness 200×10^{-3} mm) (2.2 mm² per tooth) × (20 teeth) Total area = 44 mm²
Attachments with aligners	• 12 teeth with attachments • 4 × beveled attachments 3.0 × 3.0 × 1.5 mm • 4 × rectangular attachments 3.0 × 2.0 × 0.5 mm • 4 × ellipsoid attachments 3.0 × 2.0 × 1.0 mm	Beveled (Exposed surface 11 mm²) × (4 × attachments) = 44 mm² + Rectangular (Exposed surface 11 mm²) × (4 × attachments) = 44 mm² + Ellipsoid (Exposed surface 3.1 mm²) × (4 × attachments) = 12 mm² Total area = 100 mm²

Thickness values for adhesives were derived from Eliades et al. (1991).

8.2 *In Vivo*-Induced Alterations of Aligners and Attachments

Newly delivered aligners that have not been in clinical use have similarly rough surfaces on both sides because of the reproducible industrial manufacturing process of stereolithography, milling, and polishing that does not include much human interference. Intraoral use of aligners during treatment has been reported to reduce the surface roughness of the aligner coming in contact with the composite attachments (Papadopoulou et al. 2019). This can be seen as soon as the first week of service and leads to a decreased coefficient of friction (Kusy and Whitley 1990) and subsequently reduced micromechanical retention of aligners with the tooth and its attachments. In contrast, the lower roughness of as-retrieved aligners after 1- or 2-week exposure could be explained by the intraoral wear of both the aligner attachment and lingual area, with composite and enamel, respectively, indicating a polishing effect from the contact of the aligner with the much harder enamel or composite resin attachment surfaces.

Attachments used for aligner treatment are usually made from composite resins with a hardness of 400–700 N/mm^2 Marten's hardness (HM) (Table 8.2) (Hassan et al. 2019; Sifakakis et al. 2017), whereas human enamel has a hardness of about 2866 N/mm^2 (Ioannidis et al. 2018). This translates to a 6-fold increase of hardness for composite resin and a 23-fold increase for human enamel compared with Invisalign aligners. It can be therefore anticipated that aligners will be subject to severe wear by their contact with the attachments or the labial and/or lingual enamel, leading to smoother surfaces of as-retrieved aligners. In addition, as there is a big difference in HM of composites and enamel, lingual surfaces might present more intense wear, but the surface morphology and

Table 8.2 Mechanical properties of adhesives and composites used for the fabrication of attachments.

Material/manufacturer	Martens hardness (N/mm^2)
Transbond LR (3M, Espe)	785
Transbond XT (3M, Espe)	568
Accolate (Danville materials)	276
IPS Empress direct dentin (Ivoclar Vivadent)	487
ZNano (Danville materials)	375
Brace paste (American Orthodontics)[a]	456
Enlight LV (Ormco Corp)[a]	427
G-aenial (GC Corp)[a]	337
Flow Tain (Reliance Orthodontics)	268
Wave (SDL)[a]	260

Values are indicative-source articles indicate non-statistically significant differences among materials possessing modulus in the range of 6.9–7.4 GPa.
[a] Does not contain 2,2-bis(4-[2-hydroxy-3-methacryloy-loxypropyl]-phenyl)propane (Bis-GMA).

roughness may, in this case, play a more decisive role. In particular, the composite resin attachment area is microscopically characterized by a striation pattern perpendicular to the tooth axis as a positive remnant of the thermoplastic transfer template (Barreda et al. 2017). In contrast, the tooth enamel surface is lacking this abrasive texture and appears to be smoother than the nonpolished composite resin (Botta et al. 2009). Relevant research from Barreda et al. (2017) identified attachment surface alteration depending on the hardness and filler loading of the composite used. Specifically, even if in the majority of patients the shape of the alignments was only slightly changed, noticeable changes were observed in the attachments' texture for most patients, which might include composite cracks or fractures (Barreda et al. 2017). In addition, significantly greater attachment wear was seen with a micro-filled composite with 76% filler content compared with a nano-filled composite with 72.5% filler content.

Intraoral aging likewise has a significant effect on the mechanical properties of orthodontic aligners, which can be seen even after 1 week (Papadopoulou et al. 2019). Invisalign aligners received after periods of 1 or 2 weeks of intraoral use show reduced HM and indentation modulus compared with new aligners, whereas the measured values fall into previously reported ranges (Gerard Bradley et al. 2016). The decrease in hardness indicates a material with reduced wear resistance that is more vulnerable to attrition under occlusal forces. Used Invisalign aligners showed significantly increased relaxation index compared with as-received aligners, which to our knowledge, has not been studied extensively *in vivo* because of the requirement of bulky specimens for relaxation testing (Fang et al. 2013). This finding is associated with material softening or residual stress relaxation and is specifically important for aligners that, like other orthodontic appliances, are preactivated (i.e. prestrained) and then inserted into the mouth to release orthodontic forces. Under constant deformation, the exerted force is lower, whereas under constant strain, the material is relaxed.

Several explanations exist for this deterioration of the mechanical properties of aligners after intraoral use, with the first lying with the material itself. Fourier transform infrared spectroscopies have revealed that Invisalign aligners are made of a polyurethane-based material (Alexandropoulos et al. 2015; Gerard Bradley et al. 2016; Gracco et al. 2009), and thus under clinical conditions, might suffer from a polyurethane softening mechanism (Qi and Boyce 2005). This finding is based on the fact that thermoplastic polyurethane consists of a 2-phase microstructure with hard and soft segments, where the latter tend to be oriented perpendicular to the applied stresses and then break into smaller pieces to receive further deformation. Other factors proposed to be explanatory of the intraoral deterioration of the aligners' mechanical properties include the possibility of residual stresses from by the manufacturing process and the leaching of matrix plasticizers (Gerard Bradley et al. 2016).

According to the results of another study employing mechanical testing of various aligners (Table 8.3) (Alexandropoulos et al. 2015), Invisalign aligners show significantly higher values compared with the other materials used in the laboratory (like A1, Clear Aligner, or Essix ACE Plastic) in terms of hardness, modulus, and elastic index but lower creep resistance. This finding can be ascribed to the different chemical structure between the materials. Significant differences are also seen among different polyethylene terephthalate glycol copolymer (PETG) materials used for in-lab aligners, which might be attributed to 2 factors: (1) different molecular weights of the various PETG polymers and (2) the thermoforming effect on the mechanical properties. Thermoforming may influence the molecular orientation, mean molecular weight, and residual stresses due to rapid cooling of the thermoplastic materials on the stone models (Ryokawa et al. 2006). The HM of commonly used aligner materials varies considerably and lies within the range of 80 to 160 N/mm^2 (Kohda et al. 2013; Kwon et al. 2008). Previous studies have

Table 8.3 Mechanical properties (hardness, indentation modulus) of aligner materials.

Aligner	Martens hardness (N/mm^2)
A1, Dentsply Raintree Essix, Sarasota, Fla	100.0
Clear Aligner, Scheu-Dental GmbH, Iserlohn, Germany	91.8
Essix ACE plastic, Dentsply Raintree Essix, Sarasota, Fla	100.6
Invisalign, Align Technology, San Jose, Calif	117.8

Source: Adapted from Alexandropoulos et al. (2015).

reported that PETG materials have higher wear resistance compared with polypropylene materials (Gardner et al. 2003), but there is no similar comparison between PETG and polyurethane-based materials (like the one Invisalign uses). Likewise, great variability exists in the indentation moduli of aligners, which range between 1500 MPa and 2700 MPa (Kohda et al. 2013). Generally, a higher modulus of elasticity is preferred, because it increases the force delivery capacity of appliances under constant strain. Otherwise, aligners from materials with a higher modulus of elasticity can be constructed with smaller thickness to provide similar forces (Kohda et al. 2013). Invisalign aligners have a significantly higher elastic index than other materials (2467 MPa vs 2112–2374 MPa) (Alexandropoulos et al. 2015), which indicates a slightly more brittle material. At the same time, the higher indentation creep of Invisalign aligners implies that under constant occlusal forces exerted by the occlusion, they are more likely to deform and therefore attenuate the applied orthodontic forces. However, in summary, these data indicate that Invisalign aligners show a preferred combination of higher hardness and higher modulus, but at the same time, higher creep resistance than other aligner materials.

8.3 Release of Compounds

Intraoral aging has been shown to affect the structural integrity and influence an important array of material properties, including mechanical performance (Wu and McKinney 1982), hydrolytic stability (Papagiannoulis et al. 1997; Ruyter and Svendsen 1978), susceptibility to corrosion, and degradation resistance to the intraoral biochemical environment (Munksgaard and Freund 1990; Wu and McKinney 1982) and aggressive chemical stimuli (i.e. fluorides, bleaching agents, alcohol, and so on). As a result, component molecules from orthodontic materials might be released intraorally, with Bisphenol A (BPA) being mostly discussed.

BPA is a chemical substance produced in large quantities for use primarily in the production of polycarbonate plastics, and epoxy resins and diet are the primary source of BPA exposure for most people. In dental materials, BPA is used as a raw material for the formulation of 2,2-bis[4-(2-hydroxy-3-methacryloy-loxypropyl)-phenyl] propane and polycarbonate products;

as a general rule, the estrogenic action is confined to molecules with a double benzoic ring, and its first implication with dental material was reportedly in the saliva of patients with dental sealants (Olea et al. 1996), which however remains disputed (Nathanson et al. 1997; Zampeli et al. 2012). Studies in the late 1990s reported increased prostate weights and other effects on the male reproductive system in mice exposed to levels of BPA below the safety standard (2 and 20 mg/kg) (Soto et al. 1986; Vom Saal et al. 1997). A wide array of other effects were subsequently reported, including increased mammary gland tumors (Muñoz-de-Toro et al. 2005), precancerous lesions in prostates of neonatally exposed animals (Timms et al. 2005), development of hyperglycemia and insulin tolerance (Alonso-Magdalena et al. 2006), elevation of reactive oxygen species (Ooe et al. 2005), and oxidative stress. The resultant turmoil on the hormonal endocrinologic disruptors provoked the investigation of estrogenic action of the full spectrum of polymeric materials used in everyday activities, including plastic utensils and biomaterials for medical and dental applications.

As an empirical rule, the potential of BPA release is restricted to materials that contain BPA as a precursor during the manufacturing process. Any polymer without an aromatic ring in its structure is free of this concern; therefore, acrylic retainers and other linear carbon chain polymers have no known risk for BPA release. Orthodontic materials used in aligner treatment that might be prone to BPA release include thermoformed aligners and composite resins used for attachment fabrication. Even though many manufacturers have reportedly abandoned processes that include 2,2-bis(4-[2-hydroxy-3-methacryloy-loxypropyl]-phenyl]propane) or BPA, assays have found traces of these compounds. In addition, it is important to note here that a BPA release assay may not constitute conclusive evidence in determining the potential of a material to give rise to BPA formation because of the threshold of chromatographic analyses used (Eliades et al. 2007), which means that the release might be undetected.

For aligners, the evidence is contradictory, because BPA's implication in the use of these products has not been conclusive at the cell culture or analytical level. Assessment with immersion analysis of as-received or *in vitro* aged Invisalign aligners failed to demonstrate measurable cytotoxic effects (Eliades et al. 2009) or leaching (Kotyk and Wiltshire 2014; Schuster et al. 2004). The lack of differences among the chemical composition between new and intraorally aged Invisalign aligners (Gerard Bradley et al. 2016) comply with previous results that confirmed no residual monomers and/or byproducts released in artificial saliva (Gracco et al. 2009). This finding might be attributed to the stability of Invisalign aligners, which are polyurethane-derived products. In contrast to the aromatic rings in the configuration of BisGMA, polyether urethanes used as raw materials for aligner manufacturing have short rigid portions (the aromatic rings and the ureas) joined by short flexible hinges (the diamine linker and the methylene group between the aromatic ring) and long flexible portions (the polyether) (Eliades et al. 2005). An *in vivo* study of patients who received after debonding in-lab vacuum-formed retainers and/or aligners (Kotyk and Wiltshire 2014; Raghavan et al. 2017) reported increased salivary BPA levels 1 week after insertion, which was reduced after 1month (Raghavan et al. 2017).

The release potential from adhesives used for aligner attachments is even more unclear as no study up to date has directly assessed the release among patients with attachments bonded on multiple teeth for aligner treatment. Several studies exist assessing qualitative and quantitative parameters of BPA release from adhesives used for bracket bonding, using varying methodologies (Kloukos et al. 2013). Although discrepancies exist between studies, evidence indicates a rise in BPA release immediately after bonding of brackets or lingual retainers (Eliades et al. 2011; Halimi et al. 2016; Kang et al. 2011; Kotyk and Wiltshire 2014; Moreira et al. 2017), whereas an increase of the distance between the light-cure tip and the adhesive introduces a decrease in the degree of conversion of the polymer (Sunitha et al. 2011) that leads to greater BPA release. Furthermore, a clinical study found measurable amounts of BPA released in the saliva after bonding and also that thorough rinsing with water helps return salivary BPA to baseline levels (Kloukos et al. 2015). However, it is important to stress out that release phenomena from bulkier protruding aligner attachments that are under occlusal loads might considerably vary from those of the secluded adhesive layer between tooth and bracket.

8.4 Debonding and Grinding

8.4.1 Aerosol Hazards

At the completion of orthodontic treatment with aligners, it will be necessary to remove the bonded composite attachments. The point has already been made that compared with conventionally bonded fixed appliances, the use of clear aligners with around 3 attachments per quadrant has the potential to require considerably more composite to be removed at the completion of treatment. This finding is not only theoretical as a direct result of the amount of composite used with clear aligner treatments but also because at the removal of conventional fixed appliances the locus of failure is rarely confined to adhesive and/or bracket base interface, meaning that less composite will require removal from the enamel surface. The removal of this residual composite will, in most instances, require the use of rotary instruments, with the inevitable consequence that airborne particulates will be generated, along with the risk of some enamel surface damage directly as a result of contact between the rotary instrument and enamel surface.

Airborne particulates comprise either solid particles produced and emitted directly into the air, known as primary particles or solid particles produced as a result of a chemical reaction between 2 or more gases, known as secondary particles (CONCAWE 2017). Such particulates are of concern if their mass median aerodynamic diameter (MMAD) (which is dependent on their geometric size, mass, and shape) is such that they are likely to be inhaled. Of most concern for health are aerosols in which the MMAD of the particles is <10 µm, known as particulate matter (PM_{10}). It is these which are most likely to be inhaled and deposited within the human respiratory system. The larger of the PM_{10} particles are only likely to reach the pharynx, whereas particles with smaller aerodynamic diameters may be deposited deeper and deeper within the respiratory system. Smaller particles, described as $PM_{2.5}$, in which the MMAD is <2.5 µm, might reach the terminal bronchi of the lungs. Even smaller particles, known as ultrafine particles (MMAD <0.1 µm), might reach as deep as the bronchioles and alveoli of the lungs (Möller et al. 1985). Small particulates, if not immediately inhaled, can also remain airborne almost indefinitely within modest air turbulence, and therefore continue to pose an inhalation risk some considerable time after their production (Hext et al. 1999). In contrast to PM_{10} particulates that are usually quickly cleared by the respiratory mucociliary escalator in 1–2 days, very small particulates, $PM_{2.5}$, and specifically ultrafine particles may take days or months to be cleared from the lungs, as they must first be ingested by alveolar macrophages (Hext et al. 1999). Not only might ultrafine particles penetrate the deeper parts of the lungs, but animal studies have shown them to elicit a greater inflammatory response within the lungs per given mass than larger particles (Borm et al. 2006; Napierska et al. 2010; Oberdörster 2001; Oberdörster et al. 2005).

Following the removal of metallic brackets, bands, and residual adhesive, it is known that both PM_{10} and $PM_{2.5}$ particulates are produced in the air within the clinical environment (Ireland et al. 2003). A laboratory study investigating particulates produced at removal of orthodontic adhesives showed particles less than 0.75 µm in MMAD were produced, irrespective of whether a slow or a high-speed rotary instrument was used, run either dry or under water cooling. However, the greatest quantity of these smaller particles was produced with the highspeed rotary instrument used in combination with water cooling (Day et al. 2008). The same will be true following the use of multiple composite attachments with clear aligners, but potentially to an even greater degree because of the volume of composite requiring removal.

The respirable particulates produced at composite removal have been shown to include the following: calcium and phosphorus, most probably from the tooth enamel; carbon and oxygen most probably from the bonding resin; tungsten from the tungsten carbide debonding bur (Ireland et al. 2003) and iron most probably from the head and bearings of the rotary handpiece. Iron is a highly toxic transition metal, and in the $PM_{2.5}$ fraction will be deposited in the deeper regions of the lung. The most frequently detected particles comprised of silica from the composite bonding resin (Day et al. 2008). Although there are no reported cases of silicosis among orthodontists, there are strict workplace exposure limits (WELs) for silica.

In a combined laboratory and clinical investigation into particulate production at enamel clean up following the use of both conventional metal and flash-free ceramic brackets, silica was identified within the respirable fraction (MMAD\5 µm) of the aerosols generated in all cases (Vig et al. 2019). Although the WEL for dust was not exceeded, the WEL for silica ($0.1\,mg/m^3$) was exceeded in every experiment, but this would only be the case if all the particulates produced were indeed composed of silica, which is unlikely. It was not possible to determine what fraction did comprise silica alone. The WEL for silica is the time-weighted average over 8 hours. Although it is unlikely any single operator would be removing composite continuously for 8 hours, the persistence of airborne particulates generated previously by the same or different operator, or where clinicians work in multi surgery clinical set-ups, could contribute to such an exposure exceeding the WEL. Once again, the same would apply to the composite attachment removal at completion of clear aligner treatment, but possibly to a greater degree, dependent on the number and size of the composite attachments used.

In addition to the particulates so far described, the removal of residual bonding composite at completion of treatment will also lead to the generation of a bioaerosol. It is known that within as little as 5 minutes following fixed appliance removal and enamel clean up, there is a significant increase in the concentration of bioaerosol compared with preoperative resting room levels, with microorganisms derived from the patient's oral cavity (Dawson et al. 2016; Toroğlu et al. 2001). This concentration is likely to be influenced, all other things being equal, on the time taken for composite removal and the surface area of composite previously exposed to the oral environment, and which might, therefore, be contaminated with oral microorganisms. In both cases, this may be greater in the case of multiple attachments used with clear aligners when compared with conventional fixed appliances.

As with conventional fixed appliance composite removal, when removing the composite attachments following clear aligner treatment the operator should make every attempt to minimize the inhalation risk by using a slow speed rotary handpiece and a spiral fluted tungsten carbide bur (Johnston et al. 2009). In this way the risk of enamel damage at composite removal will also be minimized (Ireland et al. 2005). The operator should also wear a facemask, supplemented with the use of a high-volume evacuator held close to the patient's mouth. In addition, the composite removal should not be performed using a water coolant spray as this further increases the aerosol risk (Johnston et al. 2009).

8.4.2 Xenoestrogenic Action (Bulk and Ground Particles) and Other Biologic Effects

As stated earlier, BPA molecules released intraorally might act as an endocrine disruptor because of its similar chemical structure to natural estrogen (17-beta estradiol) (Vom Saal and Hughes 2005). An immersion study with as-received Invisalign aligners measured estrogenicity by the effect on the proliferation of the estrogen-responsive MCF-7 breast cancer cells that are known to express estrogen receptor-α, which is of primary importance for the proliferative effect of estrogens

(Eliades et al. 2009). No significant xenoestrogenic effects were found, which was attributed to the structural stability of these polyurethane-based aligners.

As far as the xenoestrogenicity of orthodontic adhesives is concerned, limited evidence exists, where an *in vitro* assay employing the same MCF-7 breast cancer cells assessing orthodontic adhesives used for simulated bracket bonding found no considerable estrogenic activity (Eliades et al. 2007). In contrast, another potential risk for endocrine disruption lies at the debonding stage, in which the particulate matter produced by grinding of the resin adhesive might have an estrogenic action (Gioka et al. 2009). This finding is of particular interest because greater volumes of adhesive are bonded on the teeth for aligner attachments and must be subsequently removed by grinding. However, no such study has assessed this directly to quantify the underlying risk levels.

Apart from endocrine disruptions, 1 study with eluates obtained from soaking Invisalign plastic in the saline solution used on epithelial cells found some changes in viability, membrane permeability, and adhesion of epithelial cells in a saline-solution environment. The secondary results of compromising epithelial integrity might be microleakage and hapten formation which, in consequence, could lead to isocyanate allergy, either systemic or localized to gingiva (Premaraj et al. 2014). Finally, assessment of the cytotoxicity of various in-lab vacuum-formed aligners found only slight levels of cytotoxicity for human primary gingival fibroblast, whereas the thermoforming process increased the cytotoxicity of Polyethylene terephthalate glycol materials (Martina et al. 2019).

8.5 Concluding Remarks

The application of aligners in the clinical setting introduces a unique scenario of different materials applied in a manner which involves the development of friction and attrition between the attachment and the softer aligner material, all performing in the harsh conditions of the oral environment, which impact on the aging of these materials. The latter may give rise to alterations of the aligners and the composite attachments and potential intraoral release of BPA, a known endocrine disrupting agent.

Because of the extensive enamel involvement in bonding, the release of factors from the attachment aligner complex during service, the aging of these entities in the oral environment, and the laborious debonding and/or composite grinding process coupled with the hazardous nature of aerosol produced during the removal of these bulky specimens, appropriate risk management considerations should be applied. An effort to confine the application of multiple composite specimens bonded to enamel to the absolutely necessary should be pursued.

References

Alexandropoulos, A., Al Jabbari, Y.S., Zinelis, S., and Eliades, T. (2015). Chemical and mechanical characteristics of contemporary thermoplastic orthodontic materials. *Aust. Orthod. J.* 31: 165–170.

Alonso-Magdalena, P., Morimoto, S., Ripoll, C. et al. (2006). The estrogenic effect of bisphenol-A disrupts pancreatic ß-cell function in vivo and induces insulin resistance. *Environ. Health Perspect.* 114: 106–112.

Barreda, G.J., Dzierewianko, E.A., and Mu~noz KA, Piccoli GI. (2017). Surface wear of resin composites used for Invisalign_ attachments. *Acta Odontol. Latinoam.* 30: 90–95.

Borm, P.J., Robbins, D., Haubold, S. et al. (2006). The potential risks of nanomaterials: a review carried out for ECETOC. *Part. Fibre Toxicol.* 3: 11.

Botta, A.C., Duarte, S. Jr., Paulin Filho, P.I. et al. (2009). Surface roughness of enamel and four resin composites. *Am. J. Dent.* 22: 252–254.

Brosh, T., Kaufman, A., Balabanovsky, A., and Vardimon, A.D. (2005). In vivo debonding strength and enamel damage in two orthodontic debonding methods. *J. Biomech.* 38: 1107–1113.

CONCAWE. (2017). An introduction to air quality. https://www.concawe.eu/wp-content/uploads/2017/09/DEF_AQ_AirQuality_digital.pdf (accessed 25 April 2020).

Dasy, H., Dasy, A., Asatrian, G. et al. (2015). Effects of variable attachment shapes and aligner material on aligner retention. *Angle Orthod.* 85: 934–940.

Dawson, M., Soro, V., Dymock, D. et al. (2016). Microbiological assessment of aerosol generated during debond of fixed orthodontic appliances. *Am. J. Orthod. Dentofacial Orthop.* 150: 831–838.

Day, C.J., Price, R., Sandy, J.R., and Ireland, A.J. (2008). Inhalation of aerosols produced during the removal of fixed orthodontic appliances: a comparison of 4 enamel cleanup methods. *Am. J. Orthod. Dentofacial Orthop.* 133: 11–17.

Eliades, T., Viazis, A.D., and Eliades, G. (1991). Bonding of ceramic brackets to enamel: morphologic and structural considerations. *Am. J. Orthod. Dentofacial Orthop.* 99: 369–375.

Eliades, T., Gioka, C., Eliades, G., and Makou, M. (2004). Enamel surface roughness following debonding using two resin grinding methods. *Eur. J. Orthod.* 26: 333–338.

Eliades, T., Eliades, G., Silikas, N., and Watts, D.C. (2005). In vitro degradation of polyurethane orthodontic elastomeric modules. *J. Oral Rehabil.* 32: 72–77.

Eliades, T., Hiskia, A., Eliades, G., and Athanasiou, A.E. (2007). Assessment of bisphenol-A release from orthodontic adhesives. *Am. J. Orthod. Dentofacial Orthop.* 131: 72–75.

Eliades, T., Pratsinis, H., Athanasiou, A.E. et al. (2009). Cytotoxicity and estrogenicity of Invisalign appliances. *Am. J. Orthod. Dentofacial Orthop.* 136: 100–103.

Eliades, T., Voutsa, D., Sifakakis, I. et al. (2011). Release of bisphenol-A from a light-cured adhesive bonded to lingual fixed retainers. *Am. J. Orthod. Dentofacial Orthop.* 139: 192–195.

Fang, D., Zhang, N., Chen, H., and Bai, Y. (2013). Dynamic stress relaxation of orthodontic thermoplastic materials in a simulated oral environment. *Dent. Mater. J.* 32: 946–951.

Gardner, G.D., Dunn, W.J., and Taloumis, L. (2003). Wear comparison of thermoplastic materials used for orthodontic retainers. *Am. J. Orthod. Dentofacial Orthop.* 124: 294–297.

Gerard Bradley, T., Teske, L., Eliades, G. et al. (2016). Do the mechanical and chemical properties of invisalign_ appliances change after use? A retrieval analysis. *Eur. J. Orthod.* 38: 27–31.

Gioka, C., Eliades, T., Zinelis, S. et al. (2009). Characterization and in vitro estrogenicity of orthodontic adhesive particulates produced by simulated debonding. *Dent. Mater.* 25: 376–382.

Gracco, A., Mazzoli, A., Favoni, O. et al. (2009). Short-term chemical and physical changes in Invisalign appliances. *Aust. Orthod. J.* 25: 34–40.

Halimi, A., Benyahia, H., Bahije, L. et al. (2016). A systematic study of the release of bisphenol A by orthodontic materials and its biological effects. *Int. Orthod.* 14: 399–417.

Hassan, M.A., Zinelis, S., Hersberger-Zurfluh, M., and Eliades, T. (2019). Creep, hardness, and elastic modulus of lingual fixed retainers adhesives. *Materials (Basel)* 12: E646.

Hext, P.M., Rogers, K.O., and Paddle, G.M. (1999). The health effects of $PM_{2.5}$ (including ultrafine particles). Report no. 99/60. Brussels: CONCAWE.

Ioannidis, A., Papageorgiou, S.N., Sifakakis, I. et al. (2018). Orthodontic bonding and debonding induces structural changes but does not alter the mechanical properties of enamel. *Prog. Orthod.* 19: 12.

Ireland, A.J., Moreno, T., and Price, R. (2003). Airborne particles produced during enamel cleanup after removal of orthodontic appliances. *Am. J. Orthod. Dentofacial Orthop.* 124: 683–686.

Ireland, A.J., Hosein, I., and Sherriff, M. (2005). Enamel loss at bond-up, debond and clean-up following the use of a conventional light-cured composite and a resin-modified glass polyalkenoate cement. *Eur. J. Orthod.* 27: 413–419.

Janiszewska-Olszowska, J., Tomkowski, R., Tandecka, K. et al. (2016). Effect of orthodontic debonding and residual adhesive removal on 3D enamel microroughness. *Peer J.* 4: e2558.

Johnston, N.J., Price, R., Day, C.J. et al. (2009). Quantitative and qualitative analysis of particulate production during simulated clinical orthodontic debonds. *Dent. Mater.* 25: 1155–1162.

Joo, H.J., Lee, Y.K., Lee, D.Y. et al. (2011). Influence of orthodontic adhesives and clean-up procedures on the stain susceptibility of enamel after debonding. *Angle Orthod.* 81: 334–340.

Kang, Y.G., Kim, J.Y., Kim, J. et al. (2011). Release of bisphenol A from resin composite used to bond orthodontic lingual retainers. *Am. J. Orthod. Dentofacial Orthop.* 140: 779–789.

Karamouzos, A., Athanasiou, A.E., Papadopoulos, M.A., and Kolokithas, G. (2010). Tooth-color assessment after orthodontic treatment: a prospective clinical trial. *Am. J. Orthod. Dentofacial Orthop.* 138 (537): e1–e8. discussion 537.

Kechagia, A., Zinelis, S., Pandis, N. et al. (2015). The effect of orthodontic adhesive and bracket base design in adhesive remnant index on enamel. *J. World Fed. Orthod.* 4: 18–22.

Kloukos, D., Pandis, N., and Eliades, T. (2013). Bisphenol-A and residual monomer leaching from orthodontic adhesive resins and polycarbonate brackets: a systematic review. *Am. J. Orthod. Dentofacial Orthop.* 143 (Suppl): 104–12.e1.

Kloukos, D., Sifakakis, I., Voutsa, D. et al. (2015). BPA qualitative and quantitative assessment associated with orthodontic bonding in vivo. *Dent. Mater.* 31: 887–894.

Kohda, N., Iijima, M., Muguruma, T. et al. (2013). Effects of mechanical properties of thermoplastic materials on the initial force of thermoplastic appliances. *Angle Orthod.* 83: 476–483.

Kotyk, M.W. and Wiltshire, W.A. (2014). An investigation into bisphenol-A leaching from orthodontic materials. *Angle Orthod.* 84: 516–520.

Kusy, R.P. and Whitley, J.Q. (1990). Effects of surface roughness on the coefficients of friction in model orthodontic systems. *J. Biomech.* 23: 913–925.

Kwon, J.S., Lee, Y.K., Lim, B.S., and Lim, Y.K. (2008). Force delivery properties of thermoplastic orthodontic materials. *Am. J. Orthod. Dentofacial Orthop.* 133: 228–234: quiz 328.e1.

Martina, S., Rongo, R., Bucci, R. et al. (2019). D'Ant_o V. in vitro cytotoxicity of different thermoplastic materials for clear aligners. *Angle Orthod.* 89: 942–945.

Mohebi, S., Shafiee, H.A., and Ameli, N. (2017). Evaluation of enamel surface roughness after orthodontic bracket debonding with atomic force microscopy. *Am. J. Orthod. Dentofacial Orthop.* 151: 521–527.

Möller, W., Häussinger, K., Winkler-Heil, R. et al. (1985). Mucociliary and long-term particle clearance in the airways of healthy nonsmoker subjects. *J. Appl. Physiol.* 2004 (97): 2200–2206.

Moreira, M.R., Matos, L.G., de Souza, I.D. et al. (2017). Bisphenol A release from orthodontic adhesives measured in vitro and in vivo with gas chromatography. *Am. J. Orthod. Dentofacial Orthop.* 151: 477–483.

Munksgaard, E.C. and Freund, M. (1990). Enzymatic hydrolysis of (di) methacrylates and their polymers. *Scand. J. Dent. Res.* 98: 261–267.

Muñoz-de-Toro, M., Markey, C.M., Wadia, P.R. et al. (2005). Perinatal exposure to bisphenol-A alters peripubertal mammary gland development in mice. *Endocrinology* 146: 4138–4147.

Napierska, D., Thomassen, L.C., Lison, D. et al. (2010). Thenanosilica hazard: another variable entity. *Part. Fibre Toxicol.* 7: 39.

Nathanson, D., Lertpitayakun, P., Lamkin, M.S. et al. (1997). In vitro elution of leachable components from dental sealants. *J. Am. Dent. Assoc.* 128:1517–1523.

Oberdörster, G. (2001). Pulmonary effects of inhaled ultrafine particles. *Int. Arch. Occup. Environ. Health* 74: 1–8.

Oberdörster, G., Oberdörster, E., and Oberdörster, J. (2005). Nanotoxicology: an emerging discipline evolving from studies of ultrafine particles. *Environ. Health Perspect.* 113: 823–839.

Ogaard, B., Rølla, G., and Arends, J. (1988). Orthodontic appliances and enamel demineralization. Part 1. Lesion development. *Am. J. Orthod. Dentofacial Orthop.* 94: 68–73.

Olea, N., Pulgar, R., Pérez, P. et al. (1996). Estrogenicity of resin-based composites and sealants used in dentistry. *Environ. Health Perspect.* 104: 298–305.

Ooe, H., Taira, T., Iguchi-Ariga, S.M.M., and Ariga, H. (2005). Induction of reactive oxygen species by bisphenol A and abrogation of bisphenol A-induced cell injury by DJ-1. *Toxicol. Sci.* 88: 114–126.

Papadopoulou, A.K., Cantele, A., Polychronis, G. et al. (2019). Changes in roughness and mechanical properties of Invisalign_appliances after one- and two-weeks use. *Materials (Basel)* 12: E2406.

Papagiannoulis, L., Tzoutzas, J., and Eliades, G. (1997). Effect of topical fluoride agents on the morphologic characteristics and composition of resin composite restorative materials. *J. Prosthet. Dent.* 77: 405–413.

Premaraj, T., Simet, S., Beatty, M., and Premaraj, S. (2014). Oral epithelial cell reaction after exposure to Invisalign plastic material. *Am. J. Orthod. Dentofacial Orthop.* 145: 64–71.

Qi, H. and Boyce, M. (2005). Stress–strain behavior of thermoplastic polyurethanes. *Mech. Mater.* 37: 817–839.

Raghavan, A.S., Pottipalli Sathyanarayana, H., Kailasam, V., and Padmanabhan, S. (2017). Comparative evaluation of salivary bisphenol A levels in patients wearing vacuum-formed and Hawley retainers: an in-vivo study. *Am. J. Orthod. Dentofacial Orthop.* 151: 471–476.

Ruyter, I.E. and Svendsen, S.A. (1978). Remaining methacrylate groups in composite restorative materials. *Acta Odontol. Scand.* 36: 75–82.

Ryokawa, H., Miyazaki, Y., Fujishima, A. et al. (2006). The mechanical properties of dental thermoplastic materials in a simulated intraoral environment. *Orthod. Waves* 65: 64–72.

Schuster, S., Eliades, G., Zinelis, S. et al. (2004). Structural conformation and leaching from in vitro aged and retrieved Invisalign appliances. *Am. J. Orthod. Dentofacial Orthop.* 126: 725–728.

Sifakakis, I., Zinelis, S., Patcas, R., and Eliades, T. (2017). Mechanical properties of contemporary orthodontic adhesives used for lingual fixed retention. *Biomed. Technol. (Berlin)* 62: 289–294.

Sifakakis, I., Zinelis, S., Eliades, G. et al. (2018). Enamel gloss changes induced by orthodontic bonding. *J. Orthod.* 45: 269–274.

Soto, A.M., Murai, J.T., Siiteri, P.K., and Sonnenschein, C. (1986). Control of cell proliferation: evidence for negative control on estrogen-sensitive T47D human breast cancer cells. *Cancer Res.* 46: 2271–2275.

Sunitha, C., Kailasam, V., Padmanabhan, S., and Chitharanjan, A.B. (2011). Bisphenol a release from an orthodontic adhesive and its correlation with the degree of conversion on varying light-curing tip distances. *Am. J. Orthod. Dentofacial Orthop.* 140: 239–244.

Timms, B.G., Howdeshell, K.L., Barton, L. et al. (2005). Estrogenic chemicals in plastic and oral contraceptives disrupt development of the fetal mouse prostate and urethra. *Proc. Natl. Acad. Sci. U. S. A.* 102: 7014–7019.

Toroğlu, M.S., Haytaç, M.C., and Köksal, F. (2001). Evaluation of aerosol contamination during debonding procedures. *Angle Orthod.* 71: 299–306.

Vig, P., Atack, N.E., Sandy, J.R. et al. (2019). Particulate production during debonding of fixed appliances: laboratory investigation and randomized clinical trial to assess the effect of using flash-free ceramic brackets. *Am. J. Orthod. Dentofacial Orthop.* 155: 767–778.

Vom Saal, F.S. and Hughes, C. (2005). An extensive new literature concerning low-dose effects of bisphenol a shows the need for a new risk assessment. *Environ. Health Perspect.* 113: 926–933.

Vom Saal, F.S., Timms, B.G., Montano, M.M. et al. (1997). Prostate enlargement in mice due to fetal exposure to low doses of estradiol or diethylstilbestrol and opposite effects at high doses. *Proc. Natl. Acad. Sci. U. S. A.* 94: 2056–2061.

Wu, W. and McKinney, J.E. (1982). Influence of chemicals on wear of dental composites. *J. Dent. Res.* 61: 1180–1183.

Zampeli, D., Papagiannoulis, L., Eliades, G. et al. (2012). In vitro estrogenicity of dental resin sealants. *Pediatr. Dent.* 34: 312–316.

Section B

Fixed Retainer Bonding

9

Composite Resins Used for Retainer Bonding

Iosif Sifakakis

Department of Orthodontics, School of Dentistry, National and Kapodistrian University of Athens, Athens, Greece

9.1 Introduction

The composite resin used for retainer bonding requires specific physical and chemical properties since it is exposed to the oral cavity for the long term. High bond strength is always a key requirement. These materials should be inelastic, with increased hardness and wear resistance, to withstand masticatory forces. Low solubility, water absorption and polymerization shrinkage and a high degree of conversion are also required.

A review of the published scientific literature revealed a lack of consistency in the adhesive type used for bonding retainers. Conventional bracket adhesives have been appropriately modified to improve consistency and viscosity (Årtun et al. 1997; Årtun and Zachrisson 1982; Bearn 1995; Chinvipas et al. 2014). Flowable restorative composite resins have also been used. The filler content of these materials is decreased, and they have lower viscosity. As a result, they flow towards the bulk of the material rather than away from it, and chair time is reduced because trimming and polishing are not required (Elaut et al. 2002; Geserick and Wichelhaus 2004; Radlanski and Zain 2004). Nowadays, most manufacturing companies offer flowable adhesives specifically designed for fixed retainers. However, these composites may exhibit inferior mechanical

Debonding and Fixed Retention in Orthodontics: An Evidence-Based Clinical Guide, First Edition. Edited by Theodore Eliades and Christos Katsaros.

properties compared to conventional and hybrid composites due to their lower filler loading (Asscherickx et al. 1984; Lim et al. 2002). The survival rates of mandibular lingual retainers were similar between chemically and light-cured adhesives (Pandis et al. 2013); however, different bonding guidelines are suggested between these two clinical procedures (Zachrisson and Buyukyilmaz 2005). The use of liquid resin with a conventional adhesive for fixed retainers did not improve the retainer's clinical performance during the first five years post-treatment (Tang et al. 2013). This chapter discusses the physical and chemical properties of the adhesives used to bond lingual retainers.

9.2 Hardness

Hardness is a determinant factor in abrasion by mastication. This property is measured by indentation on a polished flat surface by an indenter, such as a Vickers or Knoop indenter. Several factors may affect traditional Vickers hardness measurements, including the indentation size effect, the operator's perception and the resolution of the optical system magnification system. The Martens test may be advantageous when testing dental materials since it is less influenced by the material's viscoelastic and optical properties. Soft metals have similar Martens and Vickers hardness values, but the comparability fails for materials with high elasticity (Chudoba 2006; Hassan et al. 2019; Shahdad et al. 2007).

The materials used to construct fixed retainers should have high hardness values and thus increased wear resistance. Hardness may differ between commercial brands of composite resins (Table 9.1). Dental composite resins with increased inorganic filler content demonstrate higher hardness and elastic modulus values measured by the dynamic micro-indentation method (Hassan et al. 2019). However, the mechanical properties of the flowable composites are also affected by the properties of the resin matrix (Hirayama et al. 2014; Namura et al. 2020). Clinical manipulation of the material may further affect its properties. Diluting the composite before bonding decreases hardness (Uşümez et al. 2003). High-intensity curing units improve the hardness values of some orthodontic adhesives (Uysal et al. 2008). Ageing may further alter this property: the surface microhardness of two common light-cured retainer adhesives was significantly increased after *in vitro* ageing

Table 9.1 Mean values (± standard deviations) of selected mechanical properties (E_{IT}, ηIT, HV/MH) of common orthodontic adhesives and dental restorative composites.

Adhesive type	E_{IT} (GPa)	ηIT (%)	Hardness HV (or MH)
Transbond LR (3M Unitek)	17.3 ± 0.3 (Iliadi et al. 2017) 22.3 (Hassan et al. 2019)	33.6 ± 1.1 (Iliadi et al. 2017) 32.8 (Hassan et al. 2019)	71.6 ± 2 MPa (MH) (Iliadi et al. 2017) 62.8 before and 79.6 after ageing (Ramoglu et al. 2008) 62–64 (different light sources) (Uşümez et al. 2003)
Transbond XT (3M Unitek)	15.0 ± 0.5 14.8 (Hassan et al. 2019)	30.7 ± 1.7 34 (Hassan et al. 2019)	68.0(Iijima et al. 2010) Cured with quartz tungsten halogen 55.1 (Uysal et al. 2008) Cured with high-intensity quartz tungsten halogen 55.4 (Uysal et al. 2008)
Maximum Cure (Reliance)	8.3 ± 0.7 8.8 ± 1.4(Gugger et al. 2016)	44 ± 2.4 47 ± 3.7 (Gugger et al. 2016)	70 ± 5 79 ± 6.4 (retrieved) (Gugger et al. 2016)
Flow Tain (Reliance)	5.2 ± 0.3 4.7 ± 0.3 (retrieved) (Gugger et al. 2016) 6.5 (Hassan et al. 2019)	45 ± 1.4 46 ± 1.3 (retrieved) (Gugger et al. 2016) 40.9 (Hassan et al. 2019)	37 ± 1.4 36 ± 3.4(retrieved) (Gugger et al. 2016)
Light Bond (Reliance)			Cured with quartz tungsten halogen 92.9 (Uysal et al. 2008) Cured with high-intensity quartz tungsten halogen 95.2 (Uysal et al. 2008)

(*Continued*)

Table 9.1 (Continued)

Adhesive type	E_{IT} (GPa)	ηIT (%)	Hardness HV (or MH)
Light Cure Retainer (Reliance)			40.3 before and 58.3 after ageing (Ramoglu et al. 2008)
			39–42 (different light sources) (Uşümez et al. 2003)
Wave (SDI) flowable	6.9 (Hassan et al. 2019)	38.7 (Hassan et al. 2019)	
Enlight light-cure adhesive (Ormco)	10.1 (Hassan et al. 2019)	43.8 (Hassan et al. 2019)	54.5 (Iijima et al. 2010)
Beauty Ortho Bond (Shofu)			62.3 (Iijima et al. 2010)
Beauty Ortho Bond Salivatect (Shofu)			52.9 (Iijima et al. 2010)
Kurasper F light cure (Kuraray)			75.6 (Iijima et al. 2010)
			Cured with quartz tungsten halogen 67.6 (Uysal et al. 2008)
			Cured with high-intensity quartz tungsten halogen 71.9 (Uysal et al. 2008)
Experimental BPA-free	6.7 ± 0.3	34.9 ± 0.3	30.9 ± 1.1
	12.9 ± 0.5 (Iliadi et al. 2017)	40 ± 2.2 (Iliadi et al. 2017)	53 ± 2 MPa (MH) (Iliadi et al. 2017)
Concise (3M Unitek)			52.4 as received
			46.0 diluted (Uşümez et al. 2003)
IPS Empress Direct (Ivoclar Vivadent)	9.7 ± 0.5	35.7 ± 1.0	50
			26–45 (different irradiation times and storage media) (Bauer and Ilie 2013)
Accolade (Danville Materials)	6.6 ± 0.3	38.1 ± 1.0	35 (Sifakakis et al. 2017)
ZNano (Danville Materials)	9.7 ± 0.3	49.2 ± 0.5	88 (Sifakakis et al. 2017)

(Ramoglu et al. 2008). However, *in vivo* ageing of two other lingual retainer composites did not demonstrate significant differences in Vickers hardness, indentation modulus and elastic index between the reference and long-term retrieved groups (Gugger et al. 2016). IPS Empress Direct, a dimethacrylate resin restoration material, demonstrated even lower indentation modulus and Vickers hardness values than Transbond XT. However, the storage/ageing conditions differed, indicating the effect of these conditions on the mechanical properties of this resin (Bauer and Ilie 2013).

The increase in Martens hardness and indentation modulus is achieved by increasing filler loading, thus decreasing the matrix capacity for plastic deformation. Recent research on seven lingual retainer adhesives demonstrated more than threefold differences between them (Hassan et al. 2019).

Common mechanical properties may differ by twice as much between some commercial products. Transbond LR, an adhesive specially designed for fixed retainers, showed higher modulus (E_{IT}) and hardness (HV) than its counterpart for bracket bonding. Some flowable lingual retainer composites have half the hardness/E_{IT} values of the former material.

9.3 Wear Resistance

This property is very important for the long-term survival of fixed lingual retainers but not for brackets since bracket adhesives are not exposed to wear phenomena. Abrasion may accelerate the detachment of the wire from the surface of the composite (Bearn 1995; Dahl and Zachrisson 1991; Zachrisson 1977) (Figure 9.1). Accordingly, the use of a retainer adhesive with greater abrasion resistance may decrease the failure rate.

Abrasive wear is not the only wear mechanism of the composite of mandibular or maxillary fixed retainers, but it is an important consideration in the total wear process after prolonged retention. Clinical wear is a complex mechanism influenced by several factors related to the properties of the matrix, the filler and the interface. These include the shape, size, content, orientation and distribution of filler; the hardness of the abrasive relative to that of the filler; the wear resistance of the filler relative to that of the matrix; and the loading conditions during

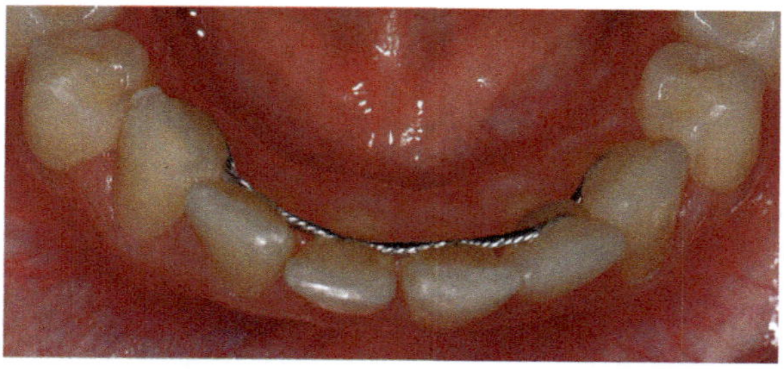

Figure 9.1 Abrasive wear of the composite and microleakage six years post-debonding.

abrasive wear (Turssi et al. 2003). As a result, differences in wear resistance were found between several orthodontic adhesives.

Nowadays, most composite fillers are silicate particles based on oxides of barium, zinc, aluminium, strontium or zirconium, and each filler type has specific advantages and disadvantages. It was demonstrated that increased filler levels resulted in greater hardness, compressive strength and stiffness and decreased water sorption (Li et al. 1985; St Germain et al. 1985). Composites with low filler loading did not show satisfactory abrasion resistance for use in bonded fixed retainers (Bearn et al. 1997; Li et al. 1985; St Germain et al. 1985).

Factors found to affect abrasive wear resistance include shortening of the interparticle filler spacing (Venhoven et al. 1996), finer filler particles (Satou et al. 1992), a higher degree of polymer resin matrix conversion (Ferracane et al. 1997), improvement of the filler/matrix interaction (Manhart et al. 2000) and a more stable silane coupler (Kaway et al. 1998; Turssi et al. 2003). Coarse and angular filler particles produce rougher surfaces and generally more abrasive wear than finer, rounded particles (Söderholm and Richards 1998). However, predicting the wear resistance of a composite based on its physical properties is difficult (Turssi et al. 2003). For instance, high hardness values do not necessarily imply high resistance to abrasive wear (Harrison and Draughn 1976).

A clinical study three to six years after debonding demonstrated considerable abrasion of the retainer composite (Concise: tacking was done with a fast-setting mix of dilute composite) in two-thirds of the sample and wear facets in the retainer wire (0.0195 in. or 0.0215 in.

three- and five-strand stainless steel wires) in one-tenth of the sample. Patients with reduced overbite or anterior open-bite tendencies showed reduced composite wear; however, marked abrasion of the composite was often found among the mandibular retainers. Mechanical factors such as chewing and tooth brushing may contribute to this abrasion, and the authors advise adding a relatively thick layer of composite resin over the mandibular wire or using posterior and light-cured composites, which may have better wear resistance than the chemically cured composite used in this study (Dahl and Zachrisson 1991). A common orthodontic Bis-GMA composite diluted with unfilled resin demonstrated better handling properties for orthodontic bonding; however, it showed a significant decrease in abrasion resistance *in-vitro* (Bearn et al. 1997).

Fibre-reinforced composites (FRCs) covered by flowable resin composites showed some signs of composite wear (with a scanning electron microscope [SEM]) after *in vitro* tooth brushing, but spot-bonded FRCs, i.e. without the cover of a flowable resin composite, showed signs of wear on the FRC and exposed glass fibres from the polymer matrix. Metal specimens (flattened eight-strand braided wire) were not visually affected after tooth brushing (Scribante et al. 2019; Sfondrini et al. 2020). Resistance to abrasive wear of a dental light-cured hybrid composite containing a Bis-GMA/TEGDMA resin and 62vol% strontium glass was improved by increasing the degree of conversion (Ferracane et al. 1997).

9.4 Bond Strength

Failure of mandibular retainers was demonstrated in approximately one-quarter of cases based on observation periods of six months to three years. Interestingly, the duration of follow-up was not significantly associated with the failure rate, at least for that period, suggesting that other factors such as operator technique and experience may override the effects of retainer design or materials (Al-Moghrabi et al. 2016).

Bond failure may occur at the resin–enamel interface, but the most common failure type is detachment at the wire–composite interface (Al-Nimri and Al-Nimri 2015; Bearn 1995; Cooke and Sherriff 2010; Dahl and Zachrisson 1991; Tabrizi et al. 2010). This type of failure is simulated *in vitro* as the wire pullout resistance from the composite material, i.e. the tensile force (Newtons) required to detach the wire from the composite (Bearn et al. 1997). The detachment force is increased by increasing the composite thickness overlying the wire. However, composite thicknesses greater than 1.0 mm offer little clinical advantage. The detachment force is further dependent on the surface characteristics of the wire: flattened wires, more wire strands and a greater diameter positively impact the force required to remove the wire (Baysal et al. 2012; Bearn et al. 1997). Flowable composites demonstrated lower wire pullout resistance than a highly filled, light-cured resin paste (Tabrizi et al. 2010).

Another commonly used laboratory test evaluates the shear bond strength (SBS) of the adhesive on the enamel by recording the shear force applied at the tooth–composite interface during debonding (Baysal et al. 2012; Ulker et al. 2009; Uysal et al. 2009; Veli et al. 2014). Different bonding materials have been evaluated with this test. Lower SBS values were found when the following materials were used: (i) a self-adhering, light-cured flowable composite, with or without acid etching (Veli et al. 2014); (ii) a resin-modified glass ionomer cement (Baysal et al. 2012); (iii) an antibacterial monomer-containing adhesive without prior acid etching (the same adhesive with prior acid etching did not significantly affect shear bond strength) (Ulker et al. 2009); (iv) an adhesive containing amorphous calcium phosphate as a bioactive filler to an etched enamel surface *in vitro* (Uysal et al. 2009); and (v) a conventional bracket composite (Al-Nimri and Al-Nimri 2015). In the studies mentioned, the same adhesive for fixed retainers was used in the control group. Moreover, an amorphous calcium phosphate orthodontic adhesive demonstrated lower SBS values than a conventional orthodontic composite resin for bracket bonding (Baysal et al. 2012). Flowable composites demonstrated SBS values comparable with a highly filled, light-cured resin paste (Tabrizi et al. 2010). Increasing the coaxial wire diameter from 0.0175 in. to 0.0215 in. increased the SBS, but a further increase to 0.032 in. resulted in a lower SBS (Al-Nimri and Al-Nimri 2015).

Sandblasting generally increased SBS for all tested combinations between retainer adhesives and twistflex or glass fibre retainers in bovine incisors (Reicheneder et al. 2014). However, another *in vitro* study evaluating the SBS of bonded twistflex retainers on human premolars did not demonstrate statistically significant differences between etching and sandblasting vs. etching alone (Kilinç and Sayar 2018). A recent systematic review found no evidence to support sandblasting before etching over etching alone with regard to the SBS of orthodontic brackets bonded *in vitro* to lingual enamel surfaces of extracted premolars (Baumgartner et al. 2017).

Another laboratory setting for evaluating the bond strength of a piece of fixed retainer bonded on two teeth uses a universal testing machine to direct the force application along the occlusoapical axis of the incisors until wire pullout from the composite pad (Aldrees et al. 2010; Bryan and Sherriff 1995; Cooke and Sherriff 2010; Reicheneder et al. 2014). Braided wires gave higher results in the tensile tests, and the highest values were recorded in rectangular twisted wires. Lower values were recorded for micro-hybrid composites not designed for retainer bonding (Paolone et al. 2015). Another laboratory test evaluated the tensile strength of different composite/wire combinations by measuring the horizontal force required to remove a wire piece bonded to human teeth (Radlanski and Zain 2004). However, these are variations of the wire pullout resistance test.

Highly filled urethane dimethacrylate adhesives offer greater bond strength between enamel and stainless steel brackets than lower-filled or unfilled resins. The best mechanical properties were achieved by incorporating high concentrations of filler particles of various sizes into the resin (Faltermeier et al. 2007) (Table 9.2).

9.5 Microleakage

Microleakage in fixed retainers may be seen at the composite–enamel or composite–wire interface (Figure 9.2). Only nonclinical papers are available, and most of them evaluated microleakage of 0.0215-in. five-strand stainless steel wire. In these papers, the specimens were sealed with nail varnish and stained with basic fuchsine. After 24 hours, they were sectioned and examined under a stereomicroscope that measured microleakage at the composite–enamel and composite–wire interfaces, distally and mesially (Baysal et al. 2008; Uysal et al. 2009; Uysal et al. 2009; Yagci et al. 2010). These papers concluded that (i) a flowable restorative composite showed significantly greater microleakage at the composite–wire interface than conventional orthodontic composites. Thus, flowable composites may not be appropriate for bonding retainers constructed

Table 9.2 Mean values for shear bond strength (SBS), wire pullout resistance (WPO), and bond strength (BS) for various composite–wire combinations.

Adhesive	SBS (MPa)	WPO (N)	BS (N)
Transbond LR (lingual retainer adhesive)	14.6 24.7 With fibre-reinforced composite (FRC) retainer (after ageing) 8.4 (Brauchli et al. 2009)	19.8 Straight 0.016×0.022 8.6 Round twistflex 9–10 Braided 0.016×0.022 25 (Paolone et al. 2015)	Coaxial 0.0215 in. wire 70.0 3-strand 0.0195 in. wire without sandblasting 63.8 and with sandblasting 146.1 0.016×0.022 in. dead soft 8-braided without sandblasting 73.2 and with sandblasting 156.3
Transbond XT (bracket adhesive)	11.5 Braided 0.010×0.028 6.5 (8.0 if sandblasted) Coaxial retainer 0.0215 7.2 (8.6 if sandblasted) (Kilinç and Sayar 2018)	5-strand 74.7 8-strand 37.9 Coaxial 35.0	3-strand 0.0175 in. 41.4 0.016×0.022-in. dead soft 8-braided 37.7
Light Bond (bracket and lingual retainer adhesive)	19.0	42.4	
Flow Tain (flowable orthodontic adhesive)	14.7	24.0	With gold chain 33.4.
Tetric Flow (flowable restorative composite)	16.8 0.016×0.022 3-braided 13–14 (Foek et al. 2009) With FRC (after ageing) 6.5–7.2 (Brauchli et al. 2009)	33.8	3-strand 0.0195 in. wire without sandblasting 44.8 and with sandblasting 73.3 0.016×0.022 in. dead soft 8-braided without sandblasting 33.5 and with sandblasting 106.5

Filtek Supreme XT (flowable restorative composite)	22.4	26.3	
Vertise Flow (self-adhering flowable composite)	Without acid etching 2.7 With acid etching 8.7 With self-etching bonding agent accompanied by additional acid etching 4.4		
Clearfil Protect: Bond (antibacterial monomer-containing adhesive)	With acid etching 20.2 Without acid etching 12.6		
Fuji Ortho LC (resin-modified glass ionomer cement)	5.9 (enamel surfaces treated with Ortho Conditioner and dried) 10.2 (enamel surfaces acid etched, dried and then moisturized)	11.1 (enamel surfaces acid etched, dried and then moisturized)	
Aegis Ortho (amorphous calcium phosphate–containing adhesive)	8.5		
Concise (chemical cure orthodontic adhesive)	14.9	Various 3-strand and coaxial archwires: 58.7–85.6	
everStick ORTHO (glass fibre reinforced) with StickFLOW (flowable light-cured microhybrid composite)			Without sandblasting 37.0 and with sandblasting 65.6
StickRESIN	With FRC retainers 6.9–8.4 With 0.016 × 0.022 3-braided 10.6–11.7 (Foek et al. 2009)		
Grandio Flow, Synergy Flow	With FRC retainer (after ageing) 8.2–8.5 (Brauchli et al. 2009)		

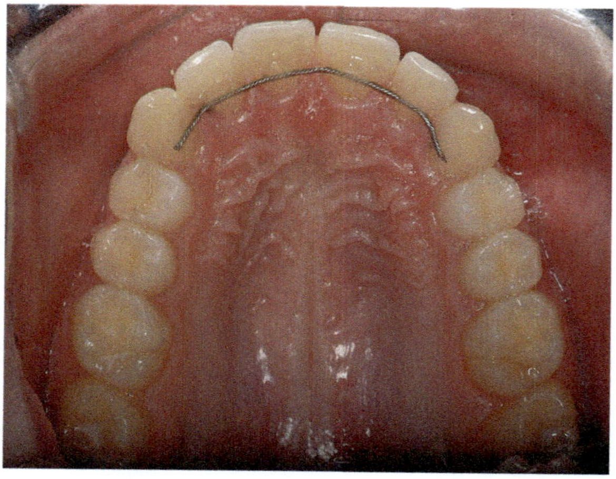

Figure 9.2 Microleakage and abrasive wear of the composite seven years post-debonding.

from multistrand archwires (Uysal et al. 2009). (ii) Greater leakage at the composite–wire interface was demonstrated in an amorphous adhesive containing calcium phosphate compared to a common lingual retainer adhesive. Little or no leakage was observed at the composite–enamel interface for both adhesives (Uysal et al. 2009). (iii) Similar microleakage was observed between an antibacterial monomer-containing adhesive system (with or without acid etching) and a conventional retainer adhesive (Uysal et al. 2009). (iv) Direct vs. indirect retainer bonding procedures did not significantly affect the amount of microleakage at the enamel–composite–wire complex (Yagci et al. 2010). (v) High-intensity light-curing units show statistically significant microleakage at the composite–wire interface and therefore may not be safe for use in bonding retainers (Baysal et al. 2008).

The same research protocol, but with a 0.36 in. stainless steel retainer, showed similar microleakage between conventional adhesives for lingual retainers vs. bracket composites (Uysal et al. 2008). Further research with the same protocol compared a 0.36 in. hard, round stainless steel retainer sandblasted at its ends with a 0.0175 in. multistrand-wire stainless steel retainer and three different composite resins designed for brackets or lingual retainers. The authors concluded that a common adhesive for lingual retainers demonstrated less microleakage at both interfaces (enamel–composite and composite–wire) than conventional bracket adhesives, self- or light-cured (Nimbalkar-Patil et al. 2014).

9.6 Water Sorption

Increased water sorption for two lingual retainer composites was demonstrated after increasing the number of thermal cycles (Catalbas et al. 2010). Moreover, solubility and water sorption of several composites was increased after incomplete light polymerization due to incomplete conversion of the monomer. The marked increase in both properties has a clinical impact on the material's durability (Pearson and Longman 1989). The type of light-curing device may influence water sorption: small increases in water sorption were demonstrated for some orthodontic adhesives cured with a high-intensity quartz tungsten halogen curing unit, compared with a conventional quartz tungsten halogen curing unit (Uysal et al. 2008). The orthodontic adhesives demonstrate various degrees of solubility and sorption, based on the immersion solution (Toledano et al. 2006).

9.7 Ageing

The nature and extent of post-retention change are unknown, so indefinite retention is popular among orthodontists. Lingual fixed retainers remain bonded over many years, even decades, and are exposed to mechanical, thermal, and chemical agents. Bond failures after prolonged intraoral service are often associated with ageing of the wires or adhesive composites caused by the applied stresses. The Fourier transform infrared method has long been considered an appropriate analytical technique in quantifying the % degree of cure (%DC) of resin composites. Intra-orally aged resin composite adhesives showed higher %DC values than water-stored controls, indicating interactions with the oral environment. The authors suggest that retrieval analysis of intra-orally exposed orthodontic specimens may provide a more reliable ageing pattern than *in vitro* water storage. Increased cross-linking or C=C degradation due to ageing may explain the greater degree of cure of the retrieved materials (Iliadi et al. 2014).

Further research on intraoral ageing after prolonged exposure to composites used to bond retainers demonstrated differences in structure and composition, but the bulk of the mechanical properties were unaffected. Secondary electron and backscattered electron images demonstrated a complex surface pattern with microporosity, pitting and cracking in the retrieved specimen (Gugger et al. 2016) (Figures 9.3 and 9.4).

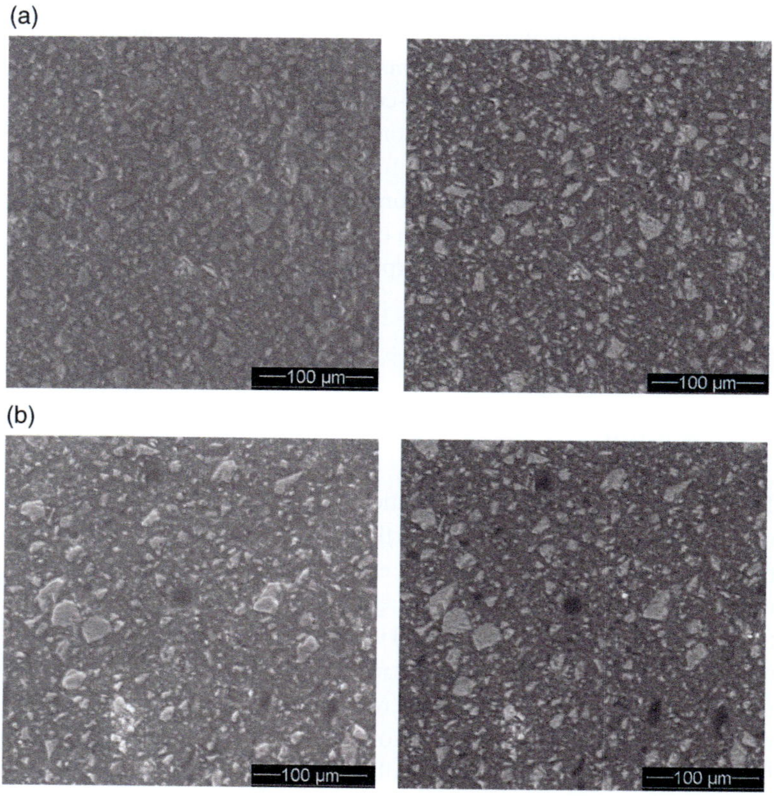

Figure 9.3 Secondary electron and backscattered electron images from the surfaces of control (a) and retrieved (b) specimens of Excel orthodontic adhesive (Reliance Orthodontic Products) (original magnification, 800×; bar 100 µm).

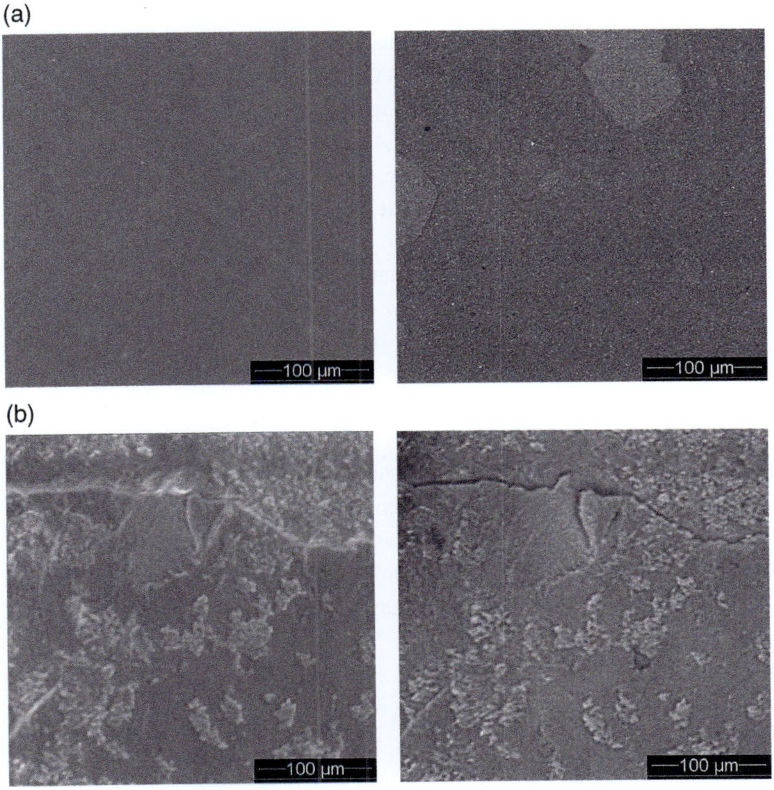

Figure 9.4 Secondary electron and backscattered electron images from the surfaces of control (a) and retrieved (b) specimen of Flow Tain (Reliance Orthodontic Products) (original magnification, 800×; bar 100 µm).

References

Aldrees, A.M., Al-Mutairi, T.K., Hakami, Z.W., and Al-Malki, M.M. (2010). Bonded orthodontic retainers: a comparison of initial bond strength of different wire-and-composite combinations. *J. Orofac. Orthop.* 71: 290–299.

Al-Moghrabi, D., Pandis, N., and Fleming, P.S. (2016). The effects of fixed and removable orthodontic retainers: a systematic review. *Prog. Orthod.* 17 (1): 24.

Al-Nimri, K. and Al-Nimri, J. (2015). Shear bond strength of different fixed orthodontic retainers. *Aust. Orthod. J.* 31 (2): 178–183.

Artun, J. and Urbye, K.S. (1988). The effect of orthodontic treatment on periodontal bone support, in patients with advanced loss of marginal periodontium. *Am. J. Orthod.* 93: 143–148.

Årtun, J. and Zachrisson, B. (1982). Improving the handling properties of a composite resin for direct bonding. *Am. J. Orthod.* 81: 269–276.

Årtun, J., Spadafora, A.T., and Shapiro, P.A. (1997). A 3-year follow-up study of various types of orthodontic canine-to-canine retainers. *Eur. J. Orthod.* 19: 501–509.

Asscherickx, K., Elaut, J., Vande Vannet, B., and Wehrbein, H. (1984). Low viscosity composites as materials for orthodontic bonding [in French]. *Rev. Belge Med. Dent.* 2003 (58): 137–144.

Bauer, H. and Ilie, N. (2013). Effects of aging and irradiation time on the properties of a highly translucent resin-based composite. *Dent. Mater. J.* 32: 592–599.

Baumgartner, S., Koletsi, D., Verna, C., and Eliades, T. (2017). The effect of enamel sandblasting on enhancing bond strength of orthodontic brackets: a systematic review and meta-analysis. *J. Adhes. Dent.* 19 (6): 463–473.

Baysal, A., Uysal, T., Ulker, M., and Usumez, S. (2008). Effects of high-intensity curing lights on microleakage under bonded lingual retainers. *Angle. Orthod.* 78 (6): 1084–1088.

Baysal, A., Uysal, T., Gul, N. et al. (2012). Comparison of three different orthodontic wires for bonded lingual retainer fabrication. *Korean J. Orthod.* 42: 39–46.

Bearn, D.R. (1995). Bonded orthodontic retainers: a review. *Am. J. Orthod. Dentofacial. Orthop.* 108: 207–213.

Bearn, D.R., McCabe, J.F., Gordon, P.H., and Aird, J.C. (1997). Bonded orthodontic retainers: the wire-composite interface. *Am. J. Orthod. Dentofacial. Orthop.* 111: 67–74.

Brauchli, L., Pintus, S., Steineck, M. et al. (2009). Shear modulus of 5 flowable composites to the EverStick ortho fiber-reinforced composite retainer: an in-vitro study. *Am. J. Orthod. Dentofacial Orthop.* 135 (1): 54–58.

Bryan, D.C. and Sherriff, M. (1995). An in vitro comparison between a bonded retainer system and a directly bonded flexible spiral wire retainer. *Eur. J. Orthod.* 17: 143–151.

Catalbas, B., Uysal, T., Nur, M. et al. (2010). Effects of thermocycling on the degree of cure of two lingual retainer composites. *Dent. Mater. J.* 29 (1): 41–46.

Chinvipas, N., Hasegawa, Y., and Terada, K. (2014). Repeated bonding of fixed retainer increases the risk of enamel fracture. *Odontology* 102: 89–97.

Chudoba, T. (2006). Measurement of hardness and Young's modulus by nanoindentation. In: *Nanostructured Coatings* (ed. A. Cabaleiro, J.T. De Hosso, and D.J. Lockwood), 216–260. New York: Springer Science.

Cooke, M.E. and Sherriff, M. (2010). Debonding force and deformation of two multistranded lingual retainer wires bonded to incisor enamel: an in vitro study. *Eur. J. Orthod.* 32: 741–746.

Dahl, E.H. and Zachrisson, B.U. (1991). Long-term experience with direct-bonded lingual retainers. *J. Clin. Orthod.* 25: 619–630.

Elaut, J., Asscherickx, K., Vande Vannet, B., and Wehrbein, H. (2002). Flowable composites for bonding lingual retainers. *J. Clin. Orthod.* 36: 597–598.

Faltermeier, A., Rosentritt, M., Faltermeier, R. et al. (2007). Influence of filler level on the bond strength of orthodontic adhesives. *Angle. Orthod.* 77: 494–498.

Ferracane, J.L., Mitchem, J.C., Condon, J.R., and Todd, R. (1997). Wear and marginal breakdown of composites with various degrees of cure. *J. Dent. Res.* 76: 1508–1516.

Foek, D.L., Ozcan, M., Krebs, E., and Sandham, A. (2009). Adhesive properties of bonded orthodontic retainers to enamel: stainless steel wire vs fiber-reinforced composites. *J. Adhes. Dent.* 11 (5): 381–390.

Geserick, M. and Wichelhaus, A. (2004). A color-reactivated flowable composite for bonding lingual retainers. *J. Clin. Orthod.* 38: 165–166.

Gugger, J., Pandis, N., Zinelis, S. et al. (2016). Retrieval analysis of lingual fixed retainer adhesives. *Am. J. Orthod. Dentofacial Orthop.* 150 (4): 575–584.

Harrison, A. and Draughn, R.A. (1976). Abrasive wear, tensile strength, and hardness of dental composite resins – is there a relationship? *J. Prosthet. Dent.* 36: 395–398.

Hassan, M.N., Zinelis, S., Hersberger-Zurfluh, M., and Eliades, T. (2019 Feb). Creep, hardness, and elastic modulus of lingual fixed retainer adhesives. *Materials (Basel)* 12 (4): 646.

Hirayama, S., Iwai, H., and Tanimoto, Y. (2014). Mechanical evaluation of five flowable resin composites by the dynamic micro-indentation method. *J. Dent. Biomech.* 5: 1758736014533983.

Iijima, M., Muguruma, T., Brantley, W.A. et al. (2010). Effect of mechanical properties of fillers on the grindability of composite resin adhesives. *Am. J. Orthod. Dentofacial. Orthop.* 138: 420–426.

Iliadi, A., Baumgartner, S., Athanasiou, A.E. et al. (2014). Effect of intraoral aging on the setting status of resin composite and glass ionomer orthodontic adhesives. *Am. J. Orthod. Dentofacial Orthop.* 145 (4): 425–433.

Iliadi, A., Eliades, T., Silikas, N., and Eliades, G. (2017). Development and testing of novel bisphenol A-free adhesives for lingual fixed retainer bonding. *Eur. J. Orthod.* 39 (1): 1–8.

Kaway, K., Iwami, Y., and Ebisu, S. (1998). Effect of resin monomer composition on toothbrush wear resistance. *J. Oral Rehabil.* 25: 264–268.

Kilinç, D.D. and Sayar, G. (2018). The effect of prior sandblasting of the wire on the shear bond strength of two different types of lingual retainers. *Int. Orthod.* 16 (2): 294–303.

Li, Y., Swartz, M.L., Phillips, R.W. et al. (1985). Effect of filler content and size on properties of composites. *J. Dent. Res.* 64: 1396–1401.

Lim, B.S., Ferracane, J.L., Condon, J.R., and Adey, J.D. (2002). Effect of filler fraction and filler surface treatment on wear of microfilled composites. *Dent. Mater.* 18 (1): 1–11.

Manhart, J., Kunzelmann, K.H., Chen, H.Y., and Hickel, R. (2000). Mechanical properties and wear behavior of light-cured packable composite resins. *Dent. Mater.* 16: 33–40.

Namura, Y., Takamizawa, T., Uchida, Y. et al. (2020). Effects of composition on the hardness of orthodontic adhesives. *J. Oral Sci.* 62 (1): 48–51.

Nimbalkar-Patil, S., Vaz, A., and Patil, P.G. (2014). Comparative evaluation of microleakage of lingual retainer wires bonded with three different lingual retainer composites: an in vitro study. *J. Clin. Diagn. Res.* 8: ZC83–ZC87.

Pandis, N., Fleming, P.S., Kloukos, D. et al. (2013). Survival of bonded lingual retainers with chemical or photo polymerization over a 2-year period: a single-center, randomized controlled clinical trial. *Am. J. Orthod. Dentofacial. Orthop.* 144: 169–175.

Paolone, M.G., Kaitsas, R., Obach, P. et al. (2015). Tensile test and interface retention forces between wires and composites in lingual fixed retainers. *Int. Orthod.* 13 (2): 210–220.

Pearson, G.J. and Longman, C.M. (1989). Water sorption and solubility of resin-based materials following inadequate polymerization by a visible-light curing system. *J. Oral Rehabil.* 16: 57–61.

Radlanski, R.J. and Zain, N.D. (2004). Stability of the bonded lingual wire retainer – a study of the initial bond strength. *J. Orofac. Orthop.* 65: 321–335.

Ramoglu, S.I., Uşümez, S., and Buyukyilmaz, T. (2008). Accelerated aging effects on surface hardness and roughness of lingual retainer adhesives. *Angle. Orthod.* 78: 140–144.

Reicheneder, C., Hofrichter, B., Faltermeier, A. et al. (2014 Nov). Shear bond strength of different retainer wires and bonding adhesives in consideration of the pretreatment process. *Head Face Med.* 28 (10): 51.

Satou, N., Khan, A.M., Satou, K. et al. (1992). In-vitro and in-vivo wear profile of composite resins. *J. Oral Rehabil.* 19 (1): 31–37.

Scribante, A., Vallittu, P., Lassila, L.V.J. et al. (2019). Effect of long-term brushing on deflection, maximum load, and Wear of stainless steel wires and conventional and spot bonded Fiber-reinforced composites. *Int. J. Mol. Sci.* 20 (23): pii: E6043.

Sfondrini, M.F., Vallittu, P.K., Lassila, L.V.J. et al. (2020). Glass fiber reinforced composite orthodontic retainer: in vitro effect of tooth brushing on the surface wear and mechanical properties. *Materials (Basel)* 13 (5). pii: E1028.

Shahdad, S.A., McCabe, J.F., Bull, S. et al. (2007). Hardness measured with traditional Vickers and martens hardness methods. *Dent. Mater.* 23: 1079–1085.

Sifakakis, I., Zinelis, S., Patcas, R., and Eliades, T. (2017). Mechanical properties of contemporary orthodontic adhesives used for lingual fixed retention. *Biomed. Tech. (Berl).* 62 (3): 289–294.

Söderholm, K.J. and Richards, N.D. (1998). Wear resistance of composites: a solved problem? *Gen. Dent.* 46: 256–263.

St Germain, H., Swartz, M.L., Phillips, R.W. et al. (1985). Properties of microfilled composite resins as influenced by filler content. *J. Dent. Res.* 64: 155–160.

Tabrizi, S., Salemis, E., and Uşümez, S. (2010). Flowable composites for bonding orthodontic retainers. *Angle. Orthod.* 80: 195–200.

Tang, A.T., Forsberg, C.M., Andlin-Sobocki, A. et al. (2013). Lingual retainers bonded without liquid resin: a 5-year follow-up study. *Am. J. Orthod. Dentofacial. Orthop.* 143: 101–104.

Toledano, M., Osorio, R., Osorio, E. et al. (2006). Sorption and solubility testing of orthodontic bonding cements in different solutions. *J. Biomed. Mater. Res. B Appl. Biomater.* 76 (2): 251–256.

Turssi, C.P., De Moraes, P.B., and Serra, M.C. (2003). Wear of dental resin composites: insights into underlying processes and assessment methods--a review. *J. Biomed. Mater. Res. B Appl. Biomater.* 65 (2): 280–285.

Ulker, M., Uysal, T., Ramoglu, S.I., and Ucar, F.I. (2009). Bond strengths of an antibacterial monomer-containing adhesive system applied with and without acid etching for lingual retainer bonding. *Eur. J. Orthod.* 31: 658–663.

Uşümez, S., Büyükyilmaz, T., and Karaman, A.I. (2003). Effects of fast halogen and plasma arc curing lights on the surface hardness of orthodontic adhesives for lingual retainers. *Am. J. Orthod. Dentofacial. Orthop.* 123: 641–648.

Uysal, T., Basciftci, F.A., Sener, Y. et al. (2008). Conventional and high intensity halogen light effects on water sorption and microhardness of orthodontic adhesives. *Angle. Orthod.* 78: 134–139.

Uysal, T., Ulker, M., Baysal, A., and Uşümez, S. (2008). Different lingual retainer composites and the microleakage between enamel-composite and wire-composite interfaces. *Angle. Orthod.* 78 (5): 941–946.

Uysal, T., Ulker, M., Akdogan, G. et al. (2009). Bond strength of amorphous calcium phosphate-containing orthodontic composite used as a lingual retainer adhesive. *Angle. Orthod.* 79: 117–121.

Uysal, T., Baysal, A., Uşümez, S., and Ulker, M. (2009). Microleakage between composite-wire and composite-enamel interfaces of flexible spiral wire retainers. Part 1: comparison of three composites. *Eur. J. Orthod.* 31: 647–651.

Uysal, T., Ulker, M., Baysal, A., and Uşümez, S. (2009). Microleakage between composite-wire and composite-enamel interfaces of flexible spiral wire retainers. Part 2: comparison of amorphous calcium phosphate-containing adhesive with conventional lingual retainer composite. *Eur. J. Orthod.* 31: 652–657.

Uysal, T., Ulker, M., Baysal, A., and Uşümez, S. (2009). Microleakage under lingual retainer composite bonded with an antibacterial monomer-containing adhesive system. *World J. Orthod.* 10: 196–201.

Veli, I., Akin, M., Kucukyilmaz, E., and Uysal, T. (2014). Shear bond strength of a self-adhering flowable composite when used for lingual retainer bonding. *J. Orofac. Orthop.* 75: 374–383.

Venhoven, B.A., de Gee, A.J., Werner, A., and Davidson, C.L. (1996). Influence of filler parameters on the mechanical coherence of dental restorative resin composites. *Biomaterials* 17 (7): 735–740.

Yagci, A., Uysal, T., Ertas, H., and Amasyali, M. (2010). Microleakage between composite/wire and composite/enamel interfaces of flexible spiral wire retainers: direct versus indirect application methods. *Orthod. Craniofac. Res.* 13: 118–124.

Zachrisson, B.U. (1977). Clinical experience with direct-bonded orthodontic retainers. *Am. J. Orthod.* 71: 440–448.

Zachrisson, B.U. and Buyukyilmaz, T. (2005). Bonding in orthodontics. In: *Orthodontics: Current Principles and Techniques*, 4e (ed. T.M. Graber, R.L. Vanarsdall Jr., and K.W.L. Vig), 579–659. Elsevier Mosby, St. Louis.

10

Wires Used in Fixed Retainers

Iosif Sifakakis[1], *Masahiro Iijima*[2], *and William Brantley*[3]

[1] *Department of Orthodontics, School of Dentistry, National and Kapodistrian University of Athens, Athens, Greece*
[2] *Division of Orthodontics and Dentofacial Orthopedics, Department of Oral Growth and Development, Health Sciences University of Hokkaido, Ishikari, Tobetsu, Hokkaido, Japan*
[3] *Division of Restorative and Prosthetic Dentistry, College of Dentistry, The Ohio State University, Columbus, OH, USA*

10.1 Introduction

Most fixed retainers are constructed from a wire piece extending over two or more teeth, bonded on the lingual or labial surfaces of the anterior or posterior teeth. Nowadays, the lower canine-to-canine retainer, bonded on all six lower anterior teeth, is widely accepted by patients and orthodontists after treatment.

The first publications appeared in the orthodontic literature in the 1970s (Kneirim 1973; Rubenstein 1976). These retainers were constructed from plain round (0.032–0.036 in. diameter) or rectangular orthodontic wires with retention loops at each end. Zachrisson preferred multistrand 0.0175 in. diameter wire, bonded on all six anterior teeth, to prevent relapse in 'difficult retention situations', including space closure after a median diastema or multiple diastemas as well as torque of single teeth (Zachrisson 1977). These wires have become the 'gold standard' since they offer increased retention for the adhesive.

Debonding and Fixed Retention in Orthodontics: An Evidence-Based Clinical Guide, First Edition. Edited by Theodore Eliades and Christos Katsaros.

Additionally, it was believed that their flexibility permitted physiologic tooth movements and prevented retainer breakage (Bearn 1995; Tacken et al. 2010).

Later, Årtun and Zachrisson suggested that heavier flexible round multistrand 0.032 in. diameter wire only on the canines could prevent relapse in the anterior teeth. This wire type provided sufficient retention to dispense with the loops. The authors advised bonding additional incisors on the retainer in cases of severe pretreatment rotations. However, this heavier multistrand wire favoured plaque accumulation and reduced wearing comfort (Årtun and Zachrisson 1982).

In 1995, a third-generation retainer wire was introduced, consisting of smooth stainless steel (SS) wire (0.030–0.032 in. diameter) constructed indirectly on a plaster cast. Sandblasting the ends of the wire offered increased composite retention (Watted et al. 2001; Zachrisson 1995). These wires have been used for space maintenance in cases of tooth agenesis until final prosthetic rehabilitation (Zachrisson 2007).

More recently, rectangular 0.016 × 0.022 in. SS archwires, bonded on all six anterior teeth, have been used for fixed retention in patients who require perfect control of the alignment of the mandibular incisors. The 0.022 in. side remains in contact with the tooth surface (Katsaros et al. 2007; Lie Sam Foek et al. 2008). Both the teeth and the wire surface are prepared by sandblasting the area of fixation (Katsaros et al. 2007).

Several design variations of the fixed retainer are described in the literature. Intracoronal or extracoronal wire ligation with composite resin placed over the wires and direct-bonded wire mesh have occasionally been used (Gazit and Lieberman 1976; Greenfield and Nathanson 1980; Stoller and Green 1981). A V-loop bonded lingual retainer (0.016 in. diameter Australian black wire) allows easier access for flossing and sufficient flexibility for independent tooth movement (Lee and Mills 2009). Gold retainer chains (Aldrees et al. 2010), nickel-titanium (NiTi) (Knaup et al. 2019; Liou et al. 2001; Schumacher 2015; Wolf et al. 2015) and beta-titanium (β-Ti) (Kocher et al. 2019) archwires have also been used for fixed retention. A flossable wireless fixed retainer has been developed as an alternative to orthodontic archwire (Amundsen and Wisth 2005).

Polyethylene ribbon-reinforced retainers and glass fibre-reinforced retainers are used occasionally for permanent retention (Diamond 1987;

Karaman et al. 2002; Tacken et al. 2010). These materials blend in with the tooth colour and therefore can be bonded on the labial tooth surfaces. Their properties dictate the bonding of all adjacent anterior teeth on the retainer (canine-to-canine/lateral-to-lateral). These retainers have the disadvantage of creating a rigid splint, limiting physiologic tooth movement, and several authors claim that these characteristics result in a higher failure rate (Bearn 1995; Rose et al. 2002; Tacken et al. 2010). In a recent systematic review, glass fibre-reinforced retainers demonstrated a wider range of bond failures than polyethylene ribbon retainers. This fact may be attributed to the wide variation in their material properties (Iliadi et al. 2015). A further systematic review found no evidence of a difference in failure rates between polyethylene ribbon bonded retainers versus conventional multistrand retainers in the lower or upper arch (Littlewood et al. 2016). Figure 10.1 presents examples of the clinical use of fixed retainers.

(a)

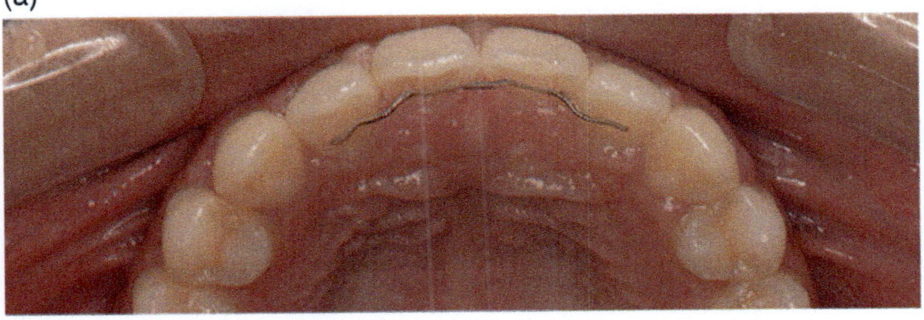

(b)

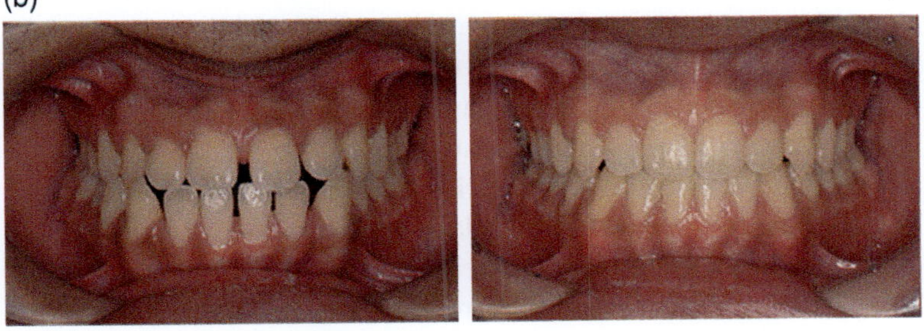

Figure 10.1 Examples of the clinical use of fixed retainers. (a) Multistrand lingual retainer wire bonded to incisors to prevent relapse. (b) Case with median diastemas; after treatment, these diastemas were closed.

10.2 Desirable Properties of Retainer Wires

The orthodontist should consider various factors in selecting wires for fixed retention. These materials should demonstrate excellent biocompatibility since they remain exposed in the oral cavity for long periods. Moreover, they should be able to prevent post-treatment tooth movement and unexpected movements during the retention period.

Unexpected tooth movements in cases of teeth bonded on fixed retainers follow more or less a specific pattern. Torque differences between two adjacent incisors or increased buccal or lingual inclination and/or movement of a canine are more often observed (Katsaros et al. 2007; Sifakakis et al. 2017). A retrospective study with a large sample of patients wearing multistrand flexible spiral-wire canine-to-canine lower retainers, treated in a single private orthodontic practice, demonstrated that in most cases, unexpected movements of the lower anterior teeth were evident in the left canines. This asymmetry among patients suggests that the mechanical properties of retention wires may play a role. These subjects in the unexpected-complications group were significantly younger at debonding and had higher mandibular plane angles and increased pretreatment ventral positions of the lower mandibular incisors (Kucera and Marek 2016). Figures 10.2 and 10.3 present examples of unexpected tooth movement during the retention phase.

10.2.1 Stiffness

The elastic properties of the retainer wire are important if its performance is to be fully described. Stiffness is a measure of resistance to elastic deformation, i.e. of the force required to bend the wire a definitive distance in the elastic range of the wire alloy, but it has nothing to do with how far the wire beam can be bent. The ease of permanent bending depends upon the yield strength of the retainer wire along with its capability to undergo work hardening during manipulation. High stiffness (high modulus of elasticity) implies high resistance to deformation and is desirable for areas where no deflection is preferred. The overall elastic stiffness of a wire is a function of the elastic modulus (material stiffness) and the dimensions of the beam (geometric stiffness). In the orthodontic literature, stiffness is discussed separately regarding bending or torsion.

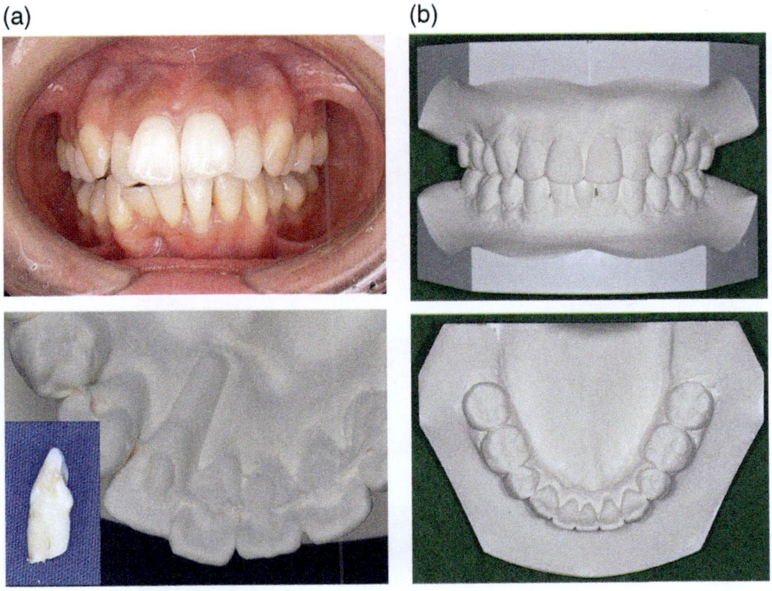

Figure 10.2 (a) An example of unexpected tooth movement during the retention period, where root exposure occurred due to increased root lingual torque of the lateral incisor. (b) The lateral incisor was extracted, and the patient was retreated as a three-lower-incisor case.

The elastic stiffness in bending the retainer is important, especially for the last tooth bonded on the retainer. In that area, usually between the lateral incisor and the canine in a canine-to-canine retainer, the wire may react as a cantilever beam, since the last tooth is supported only at one side, but to a limited extent since this tooth is not free to move. A canine-and-canine retainer may react as a beam supported at both ends. Its stiffness is inversely proportional to the third power of the wire length and has four times the stiffness of the same overhanging beam. With multistrand wires, the strand diameter has the most profound effect on stiffness because it varies with the fourth power of the diameter (Thurow 1982).

Nomograms are available that compare the elastic property ratios between three-strand SS archwires of different cross-sections with selected β-Ti and NiTi archwires (Kusy and Stevens 1987; Rucker and Kusy 2002; Thurow 1982). Increasing the length of the strands of a

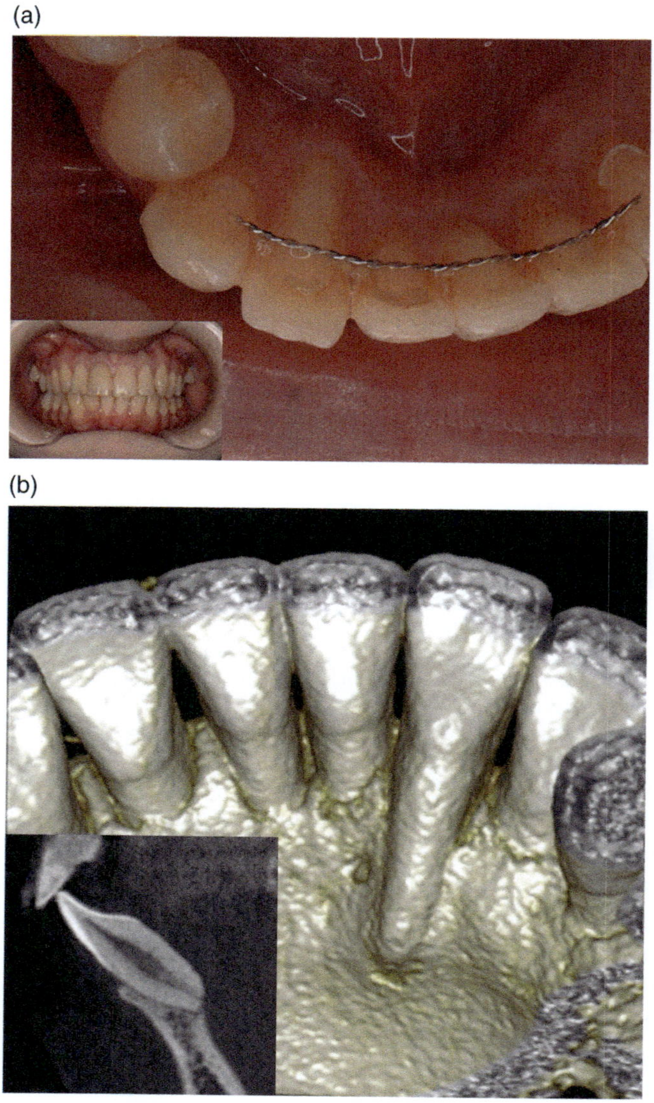

Figure 10.3 (a) Another example of unexpected tooth movement during the retention period, arising again from increased root lingual torque of the lateral incisor. (b) cone-beam computed tomography (CBCT) images.

multistrand archwire decreases its stiffness; however, tight twisting of these strands increases the stiffness. As a result, twisted archwires offer essentially the same stiffness as multiple straight strands but lower stiffness than solid archwires (Kapila and Sachdeva 1989; Rucker and Kusy 2002). Oltjen et al. (1997) have reported the effects of wire size, number of strands and amount of deflection on the stiffness of a variety of multistrand wires.

The retainer wire should be stiff enough to resist twisting/untwisting during its long-term function in the mouth. Stiffness in torsion is a measure of resistance to this deformation. Solid SS wires, used to construct canine-and-canine retainers, resist torsion better than multistrand wires (Ingram Jr et al. 1986; Rucker and Kusy 2002). Stiffness in torsion is proportional to the polar moment of inertia (J), a function of shape. Changes in diameter are more powerful stiffness modifiers than changes in length. For a round beam, the stiffness in torsion is proportional to the fourth power of the wire diameter and inversely proportional to the length of the beam (Thurow 1982). The twist direction of the wire strands (left- or right-handed) could potentially favour a specific rotation, at least for the last tooth bonded on the retainer.

Fixed retainers should be stiff enough to withstand masticatory forces and forces causing relapse, but they should not restrict the physiologic tooth mobility. Unfortunately, it has not been possible to determine the ideal stiffness of the retainer wire since (i) masticatory forces vary considerably between individuals of different ages, sexes and craniofacial morphologies and (ii) the relapse forces have not been quantified.

10.2.2 Strength

Strength is another basic property of elastic materials. It characterizes the maximum possible force that the material can sustain/deliver. This property is important in the resistance to bending by mastication forces of the wires used for fixed retention. Unexpected movements occur several years after debonding, implying plastic deformation of the wire. Strength in torsion and bending for a round wire is proportional to the cube of the diameter. The length of the beam does not affect strength in torsion; however, strength in bending is inversely proportional to the length. Multistrand wires with low stiffness also generally have low strength (Rucker and Kusy 2002).

For rectangular wires, strength has a simple proportional relationship to the width; however, it is proportional to the square of the thickness. This is another reason for bonding the rectangular retainer wires with the thicker side remaining in contact with the tooth surfaces (Katsaros et al. 2007).

10.2.3 Range

Range and strength are measures of the maximum capacity of the archwire. Range describes the maximum possible elastic deformation of the wire, i.e. how much distance can be covered. Regarding the range in bending, the wire supported at both ends by the adhesive has half the range of the same overhanging beam. For a round wire, the range is inversely proportional to its diameter, i.e. reducing the diameter by half; the wire can be bent twice as far without overloading the material. For rectangular wires, the range is inversely proportional to thickness; however, width does not affect the bending range. In torsion, the range is proportional to the diameter of a round wire or the diagonal of a rectangular wire (Thurow 1982).

For a given overall wire diameter and helix angle, the ranges of multistrand wires are independent of wire configurations (Rucker and Kusy 2002; Rucker and Kusy 2002). The range properties of multistrand wires are not influenced to the same extent as in solid wires by the cross-section size and appear to be nearly constant for a particular wire configuration (Oltjen et al. 1997; Rucker and Kusy 2002). The increased length of the strands increases the wire range compared to solid archwires or multistrand archwires with lower pitch (Ingram Jr et al. 1986; Kapila and Sachdeva 1989). Multistrand SS archwires do not match the strength and range of conventional NiTi wires because they are fabricated with SS alloys that have moderately high yield strengths (Kusy and Stevens 1987; Rucker and Kusy 2002).

An *in vitro* experiment evaluated the forces exerted on a lateral incisor or a canine bonded on a canine-to-canine retainer during a vertical or horizontal 0.2 mm tooth displacement. The forces recorded within each wire type were higher during horizontal loading. Moreover, greater forces were recorded on the lateral incisor than on the canine. The wire type significantly affected the force magnitude: thinner or heat-treated wires exerted lower-magnitude forces. Wire displacement was the main determinant of the forces measured in this experiment, which were found to vary between 0.5–1.5 N. This magnitude is high enough to produce unwanted tooth movement during retention. However, this is possible only in cases of wire deformation, and the differences in mean values of the generated forces between the different wire types might not have a definitive clinical effect (Sifakakis et al. n.d.; Sifakakis et al. 2011).

Further *in vitro* experiments with a two- or three-tooth model demonstrated that a tooth attached by a retainer wire to only one neighbouring tooth is less resistant to torque than a tooth connected to two neighbouring teeth. The differences in resistance to torque recorded between different retainers is rather large; however, a high level of torque control can be achieved with a plain 0.016 × 0.016 in. or braided 0.016 × 0.022 in. SS wire (Arnold et al. 2016).

The SS alloys used in orthodontics belong to the 300 series of austenitic SSs and can be hardened by cold working and not by heat treatment. However, the effects of cold working can be eliminated by annealing at high temperatures, and the wire returns to a softer, more workable state (Littlewood et al. 2016). This is the major purpose of heat-treating SS archwires in orthodontics: to minimize breakage by eliminating residual stresses in the material rather than achieve significant decreases in yield strength (Brantley 2001). Heat treatment of austenitic SS wires above 650 °C is not recommended since degradation of their mechanical properties is inevitable because of the loss of their wrought microstructure (Alapati 2012).

Some archwires recommended for fixed retainers are delivered annealed. Annealing is the process of heating the alloy to a particular high temperature (below its melting point) for an extended period. The degree of annealing differs between orthodontic appliances depending on their usage. A wire with a high degree of annealing is often described in the literature as *dead-soft*. Manufacturers claim that these wires are easily adaptable and minimize tooth movement associated with active force wires. However, the increase in the degree of annealing enhances formability at the expense of yield strength (Brantley 2001). Dead-soft archwires can be easily bent at lower force levels but behave identically below the point at which they take a permanent set, in comparison with harder archwires of the same alloy. Unfortunately, in these archwires, the desirable ease of formation becomes an undesirable ease of deformation (Baysal et al. 2012; Brantley and Alapati 2012; Kucera and Marek 2016).

Exposure to the flame of a butane-gas torch for 10 seconds to anneal the wire reduces the stiffness of the retainer wire (Baysal et al. 2012). Heat treatment in air for 10 minutes at 700°, 900° and 1100° F using a conventional dental furnace increased the modulus of elasticity in bending generally by less than 10% compared to the as-received condition. There was little difference between the three temperatures. However, yield strength in bending increased from about 10% to more than 20%, depending on temperature and wire composition (Khier et al. 1988).

A common dead-soft archwire used for fixed retainers was compared *in vitro* with three different types of retainer wires regarding the maximum and residual forces and moments generated on a canine during the intrusive loading of the rest of the anterior teeth. An orthodontic measurement and simulation system (OMSS) was used for this experiment, and the applied load approximated the vertical incisor bite force during mastication. The most interesting finding of this study suggests that canine-to-canine fixed retainers may not be passive after short- or long-term clinical use, especially dead-soft high-formable/low-yield strength archwires (Sifakakis et al. 2015).

An *in vitro* research Investigation compared dead-soft retainers with conventional 0.0215 in. five-strand wire. Greater deformations of the dead-soft wires were seen after debonding of the bonded wire from human incisors by the application of perpendicular forces (Baysal et al. 2012). Figure 10.4 shows a multistrand SS wire and a polyethylene ribbon used for some fixed retainers.

10.3 Clinical Selection of Retainer Wire

There is no agreement in the literature about a uniform retention protocol. It is evident that there is no ideal orthodontic retainer wire; however, each choice has distinct advantages and disadvantages. The major problems related to retainer wire are bond failures, fatigue fracture and unexpected movements during the retention phase. Figures 10.2 and 10.3 show examples of unexpected tooth movement during the retention period in cases from increased root lingual torque of the lateral incisor.

Stainless steel (SS) has higher values of stiffness and modulus of elasticity as well as lower elastic ranges and springback than NiTi and β-Ti alloys. These properties are desirable for fixed retention. Spiral SS wires

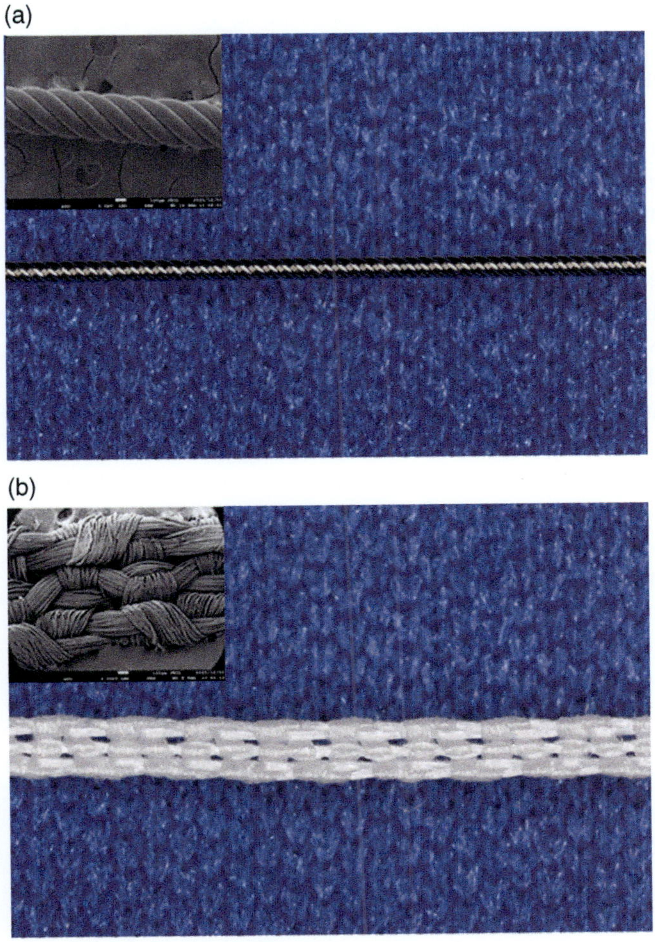

Figure 10.4 Scanning electron microscope images (insets) and photographs of fixed retainer materials: (a) multistrand 0.0175 in. diameter stainless steel wire (Supra-Flex, Rocky Mountain Orthodontics); (b) polyethylene ribbon, 1 mm × 0.4 mm cross-section. *Source:* Ribbond Inc.

may facilitate wire bending (even into complicated configurations), allow physiologic tooth mobility, and are the least expensive of the wire alloys. Therefore, these wires remain the 'gold standard' for fixed retention. Additionally, their susceptibility to fracture is low. Fatigue fractures generally occurred later than loosenings and more often in three-strand than five-strand SS wire (Dahl and Zachrisson 1991). Spiral wires demonstrate lower failure rates. Applying a five-strand wire is suggested to increase the success rate compared to a three-strand wire (Dahl and Zachrisson 1991). Zachrisson recommends a five-strand 0.0215 in. wire (Zachrisson 2015).

A prospective randomized study evaluated dead-soft 0.0195 in. vs. 0.0215 in. (not annealed) six-strand canine-to-canine retainers and found that the latter exhibited a higher detachment rate than the dead-soft 0.0195 in. retainer. This finding was attributed to higher shearing forces at the bonding sites (Störmann and Ehmer 2002). This is in contrast with the findings of an *in vivo* study, which demonstrated decreased failure rates when larger-diameter wires were used and suggested that the limited flexibility of the retainer may be an advantage (Andrén et al. 1998).

A recent systematic investigation concluded that the failure tendency of multistrand retainers decreases with increasing wire diameter, although an actual correlation may not exist (Iliadi et al. 2015). Direct comparison of the results of *in vivo* studies may be misleading. Bias may account for these inconsistencies due to differences in retainer construction/clinical efficacy: the wire may not be properly supported by the teeth surfaces during mastication if it is not closely adapted to the lingual contours of the teeth. Moreover, the distance between the bonding sites and the amount of adhesive determines the length of the free wire and its mechanical properties.

Several clinicians prefer rectangular archwires bonded only on the canines or all six anterior teeth, even in a ribbon-wise configuration (Katsaros et al. 2007; Kocher et al. 2019; Lie Sam Foek et al. 2008; Renkema et al. 2008). They may be superior to the other forms of lingual retainers in the long term; however, evidence regarding these retainer wires is unfortunately scarce. Lee concluded that using rectangular ribbon archwires is recommended for controlling corrected rotations (Lee 1981). No adverse torque changes were observed during 10–15 years in retention if 0.016×0.022 in. eight-strand braided SS canine-to-canine (or solid 0.027-in. round β-Ti canine-and-canine) retainers were used. Rectangular wires are probably more resistant to post-treatment deformation/activation than round flexible wires, however they may demonstrate increased failure rates. Additionally, a more rigid wire may not follow physiologic tooth movements like a multistrand wire. It was shown that the latter decreases tooth mobility depending on the number of teeth to which the retainer is bonded, but mobility remains within the physiologic range (Watted et al. 2001). These concerns may have no basis in fact when we consider the long-term health of multiple splinted prosthetic units; however, further research is needed regarding this issue (Speck 2008).

SS archwires contain substantial amounts of nickel, which has raised some concern among orthodontists about their biocompatibility. Evidence of noteworthy biocompatibility problems in patients because of nickel ion release from SS archwires has not been reported (Brantley et al. 2017). Two different spiral SS wires were found to maintain their mechanical properties (hardness and elastic modulus) and elemental composition, thus showing no evidence of detectable ionic release for service periods up to 14 years (Zinelis et al. 2018).

β-Ti retainers are rarely used, despite their outstanding formability. Fatigue damage is a major clinical drawback of using β-Ti alloys for fixed retainers. Fracture of these wires is caused by degradation under stress in the oral environment, multiple bending or rebending, and hydrogen embrittlement using fluoride-containing products (Brantley 2001; Kaneko et al. 2003; Murakami et al. 2015). A recent study was the first to evaluate canine-and-canine retainers made from round 0.027 in. β-titanium for long-term clinical use (Kocher et al. 2019). No adverse torque changes were observed during 10–15 years in retention when these retainers were used. These archwires are generally more expensive than those manufactured from other popular alloys; however, there is no concern about their biocompatibility since there is no nickel in the alloy composition. Their excellent biocompatibility and corrosion resistance are due to a thin, adherent, passivating surface layer of titanium oxide (TiO_2) (Brantley 2001). Figure 10.5 shows a β-Ti retainer in clinical use.

Preformed NiTi wires should be avoided since permanent bends cannot readily be placed in the wires, which may result in tooth movement if the wire is not bonded passively across the surfaces of the teeth. It is further believed that the low stiffness of NiTi provides inadequate stability after treatment (Kapila and Sachdeva 1989). Moreover, the life expectancy of NiTi retainers may be associated with a higher probability of fatigue fracture of these wires. It was found that retrieved NiTi wires fractured at significantly fewer cycles than their as-received counterparts. An increased chance of failure was documented for larger-diameter wires relative to smaller-diameter wires and square/rectangular

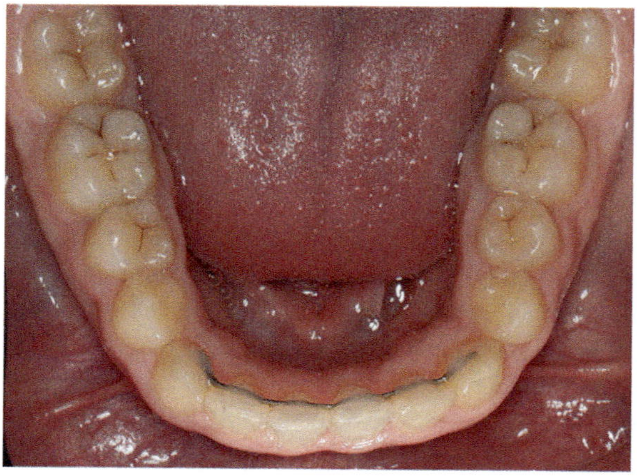

Figure 10.5 Beta-titanium rectangular retainer, with the thicker side remaining in contact with the tooth surfaces.

cross-section wires (Bourauel et al. 2008). Regarding the biocompatibility of these alloys, they achieve corrosion protection from a passivating surface film of TiO_2 similar to β-Ti. Notable biocompatibility problems resulting from *in vivo* Ni release have not been reported (Brantley 2001).

The effects of fixed retainers on magnetic resonance imaging (MRI) distortion should also be considered. Gold retainer chains caused no distortion; however, 0.015–0.018 in. twistflex retainers often caused distortion but only in areas close to the retainer (tongue and jaws). Greater distortions were observed when both maxillary and mandibular retainers were present and with 3 T magnetic fields and T1-weighted spin-echo sequences (Ozawa et al. 2018; Shalish et al. 2015). All non-metallic or NiTi alloy appliances are of little concern regarding MRI image quality, at least for 1.5 T scanners (Wylezinska et al. 2015). Further *in vitro* studies showed that archwires manufactured from nickel-titanium, titanium-molybdenum and cobalt-chromium alloys showed no or negligible forces in the magnetic field of 3 T scanners (Klocke et al. 2006). Moreover, 18-8 SS retainers exposed to 3 T scanners did not cause significant distortion of the cranial MR images except in the intraoral regions close to the retainer (Zhylich et al. 2017). Even with 7 T scanners, *in vitro* simulations demonstrated that several types of fixed retainer wires appear to be MRI-compatible without the risk of enhanced specific absorption rate (Wezel et al. 2014).

10.4 Recent Research

Recent research has focused on the computer-aided design/computer-aided manufacturing (CAD/CAM) fabrication of lingual retainers from zirconium or nickel-titanium. Figure 10.6 shows an example of a fixed retainer fabricated from zirconium. A report described a 1.8 mm thickness CAD/CAM zirconium bar as a bonded mandibular fixed retainer placed on the lingual surface of lower teeth from canine-to-canine with

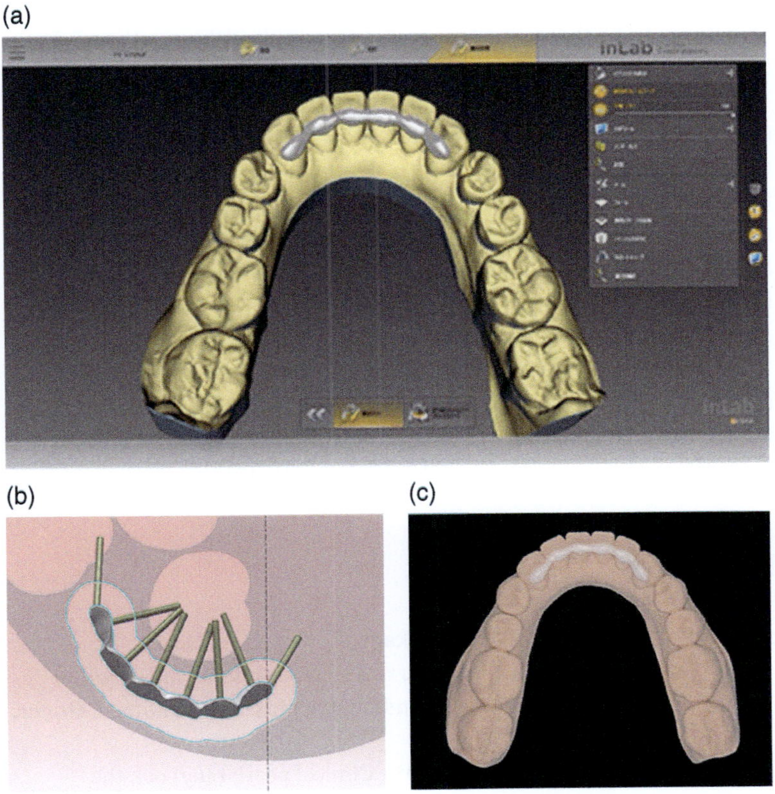

Figure 10.6 (a) Virtual computer-aided design/computer-aided manufacturing (CAD/CAM) zirconium lingual retainer design; (b) connectors designed in a nesting procedure; (c) CAD/CAM zirconium lingual retainer fitted into a 3D printed model.

occlusal rests on mesial sides of first premolars, with a two-year follow-up (Zreaqat et al. 2017).

The CAD/CAM nickel-titanium retainers investigated by another group were not bent but instead were cut from a nickel-titanium sheet in 0.014×0.014 in. rectangular dimensions (Knaup et al. 2019; Schumacher 2015; Wolf et al. 2015). This resulted in a custom-cut wire with smooth curvature and presumably a lower risk of wire fracture compared to retainers constructed by bending. After the construction of the wire, it was electropolished to clean the metallic alloy by electrolysis. This process resulted in slightly rounded corners of the rectangular wire. The intraoral positioning of these retainers was proved to be precise, showing deviations from their planned positions significantly less than 0.5 mm (Wolf et al. 2015).

A retrospective controlled clinical study compared conventional 0.0175 in. SS twistflex and 0.014×0.014 in. CAD/CAM-fabricated retainers regarding the impact of lingual retainers on oral health during the first seven months after debonding. The CAD/CAM-fabricated retainers showed significantly better oral health indices due to the optimal wire fit and bacteria-resistant character of the wire resulting from its electropolished surface. Moreover, lower biofilm formation was detected *in vitro* and after intraoral incubation (Knaup et al. 2019).

A recent article explored *in vitro* the feasibility of yttria-stabilized zirconia (Y-TZP) bars in fixed lingual retention and concluded that this is an adequate material for retention, offering an aesthetic alternative to currently available SS retainers (Stout et al. 2017).

References

Aldrees, A.M., Al-Mutairi, T.K., Hakami, Z.W., and Al-Malki, M.M. (2010). Bonded orthodontic retainers: a comparison of initial bond strength of different wire-and-composite combinations. *J. Orofac. Orthop.* 71: 290–299.

Amundsen, O.C. and Wisth, P.J. (2005). Clinical pearl: LingLock-the flossable fixed retainer. *J. Orthod.* 32: 241–243.

Andrén, A., Asplund, J., Azarmidohkt, E. et al. (1998). A clinical evaluation of long term retention with bonded retainers made from multi-strand wires. *Swed. Dent. J.* 22: 123–131.

Arnold, D.T., Dalstra, M., and Verna, C. (2016). Torque resistance of different stainless steel wires commonly used for fixed retainers in orthodontics. *J. Orthod.* 43: 121–129.

Årtun, J. and Zachrisson, B.U. (1982). Improving the handling properties of a composite resin for direct bonding. *Am. J. Orthod.* 81: 269–276.

Baysal, A., Uysal, T., Gul, N. et al. (2012). Comparison of three different orthodontic wires for bonded lingual retainer fabrication. *Korean J. Orthod.* 42: 39–46.

Bearn, D.R. (1995). Bonded orthodontic retainers: a review. *Am. J. Orthod. Dentofacial Orthop.* 108: 207–213.

Bourauel, C., Scharold, W., Jäger, A., and Eliades, T. (2008). Fatigue failure of as-received and retrieved NiTi orthodontic archwires. *Dent. Mater.* 24: 1095–1101.

Brantley, W.A. (2001). Orthodontic wires. In: *Orthodontic Materials: Scientific and Clinical Aspects* (ed. W.A. Brantley and T. Eliades), 77–103. Stuttgart, New York: Thieme.

Brantley, W.A. and Alapati, S.B. (2012). Heat treatment of dental alloys: A review. In: *Metallurgy – Advances in Materials and Processes* (ed. Y. Pardhi), 1–18. Rijeka: InTech.

Brantley, W., Berzins, D., Iijima, M. et al. (2017). Structure/property relationships in orthodontic alloys. In: *Orthodontic Applications of Biomaterials* (ed. T. Eliades and W. Brantley). UK: Woodhead Publishing.

Dahl, E.H. and Zachrisson, B.U. (1991). Long-term experience with direct-bonded lingual retainers. *J. Clin. Orthod.* 25: 619–632.

Diamond, M. (1987). Resin fiberglass bonded retainer. *J. Clin. Orthod.* 21: 182–183.

Gazit, E. and Lieberman, M.A. (1976). An esthetic and effective retain-er for lower anterior teeth. *Am. J. Orthod.* 70: 91–93.

Greenfield, D.S. and Nathanson, D. (1980). Periodontal splinting with wire and composite resin. A revised approach. *J. Periodontol.* 51: 465–468.

Iliadi, A., Kloukos, D., Gkantidis, N. et al. (2015). Failure of fixed orthodontic retainers: A systematic review. *J. Dent.* 43 (8): 876–896.

Ingram, S.B. Jr., Gipe, D.P., and Smith, R.J. (1986). Comparative range of orthodontic wires. *Am. J. Orthod. Dentofacial Orthop.* 90: 296–307.

Kaneko, K., Yokoyama, K., Moriyama, K. et al. (2003). Delayed fracture of beta titanium orthodontic wire in fluoride aqueous solutions. *Biomaterials* 24: 2113–2120.

Kapila, S. and Sachdeva, R. (1989). Mechanical properties and clinical applications of orthodontic wires. *Am. J. Orthod. Dentofacial Orthop.* 96: 100–109.

Karaman, A.I., Kir, N., and Belli, S. (2002). Four applications of reinforced polyethylene fiber material in orthodontic practice. *Am. J. Orthod. Dentofacial Orthop.* 121: 650–654.

Katsaros, C., Livas, C., and Renkema, A.M. (2007). Unexpected complications of mandibular lingual retainers. *Am. J. Orthod. Dentofacial Orthop.* 132: 838–841.

Khier, S.E., Brantley, W.A., and Fournelle, R.A. (1988). Structure and mechanical properties of as-received and heat-treated stainless steel orthodontic wires. *Am. J. Orthod. Dentofacial Orthop.* 93: 206–212.

Klocke, A., Kahl-Nieke, B., Adam, G., and Kemper, J. (2006). Magnetic forces on orthodontic wires in high field magnetic resonance imaging (MRI) at 3 tesla. *J. Orofac. Orthop.* 67: 424–429.

Knaup, I., Wagner, Y., Wego, J. et al. (2019). Potential impact of lingual retainers on oral health: comparison between conventional twistflex retainers and CAD/CAM fabricated nitinol retainers: A clinical in vitro and in vivo investigation. *J. Orofac. Orthop.* 80: 88–96.

Kneirim, R.W. (1973). Invisible lower cuspid to cuspid retainer. *Angle Orthod.* 43: 218–219.

Kocher, K.E., Gebistorf, M.C., Pandis, N. et al. (2019). Survival of maxillary and mandibular bonded retainers 10 to 15 years after orthodontic treatment: a retrospective observational study. *Prog. Orthod.* 20: 28. https://doi.org/10.1186/s40510-019-0279-8.

Kucera, J. and Marek, I. (2016). Unexpected complications associated with mandibular fixed retainers: A retrospective study. *Am. J. Orthod. Dentofacial Orthop.* 149: 202–211.

Kusy, R.P. and Stevens, L.E. (1987). Triple-stranded stainless steel wires – evaluation of mechanical properties and comparison with titanium alloy alternatives. *Angle Orthod.* 57: 18–32.

Lee, R.T. (1981). The lower incisor bonded retainer in clinical practice: a three year study. *Br. J. Orthod.* 8: 15–18.

Lee, K.D. and Mills, C.M. (2009). Bond failure rates for V-loop vs straight wire lingual retainers. *Am. J. Orthod. Dentofacial Orthop.* 135: 502–506.

Lie Sam Foek, D.J., Ozcan, M., Verkerke, G.J. et al. (2008). Survival of flexible, braided, bonded stain-less steel lingual retainers: a historic cohort study. *Eur. J. Orthod.* 30: 199–204.

Liou, E.J., Chen, L.I., and Huang, C.S. (2001). Nickel-titanium mandibular bonded lingual 3-3 retainer: for permanent retention and solving relapse of mandibular anterior crowding. *Am. J. Orthod. Dentofacial Orthop.* 119: 443–449.

Littlewood, S.J., Millett, D.T., Doubleday, B. et al. (2016). Retention procedures for stabilizing tooth position after treatment with orthodontic braces. *Cochrane Database Syst. Rev.* 1: CD002283. https://doi.org/10.1002/14651858.CD002283.pub4.

Murakami, T., Iijima, M., Muguruma, T. et al. (2015). High-cycle fatigue behavior of beta-titanium orthodontic wires. *Dent. Mater. J.* 34: 189–195.

Oltjen, J.M., Duncanson, M.G. Jr., Ghosh, J. et al. (1997). Stiffness-deflection behavior of selected orthodontic wires. *Angle Orthod.* 67: 209–218.

Ozawa, E., Honda, E.I., Parakonthun, K.N. et al. (2018). Influence of orthodontic appliance-derived artifacts on 3-T MRI movies. *Prog. Orthod.* 19: 7. https://doi.org/10.1186/s40510-018-0204-6.

Renkema, A.M., Al-Assad, S., Bronkhorst, E. et al. (2008). Effectiveness of lingual retainers bonded to the canines in preventing mandibular incisor relapse. *Am. J. Orthod. Dentofacial Orthop.* 134: 179e1–179e8.

Rose, E., Frucht, S., and Jonas, I.E. (2002). Clinical comparison of a multistranded wire and a direct-bonded polyethylene ribbon-reinforced resin composite used for lingual retention. *Quintessence* 33: 579–583.

Rubenstein, B.M. (1976). A direct bond maxillary retainer. *J. Clin. Orthod.* 10: 43.

Rucker, B.K. and Kusy, R.P. (2002). Elastic flexural properties of multistranded stainless steel versus conventional nickel titanium archwires. *Angle Orthod.* 72: 302–309.

Rucker, B.K. and Kusy, R.P. (2002). Theoretical investigation of elastic flexural properties for multistranded orthodontic archwires. *J. Biomed. Mater. Res.* 62: 338–349.

Schumacher, P. (2015). CAD/CAM-fabricated lingual retainers made of nitinol. *Dental Tribune*. https://www.dental-tribune.com/news/cadcam-fabricated-lingual-retainers-made-of-nitinol/ (accessed 1 May 2016).

Shalish, M., Dykstein, N., Friedlander-Barenboim, S. et al. (2015). Influence of common fixed retainers on the diagnostic quality of cranial magnetic resonance images. *Am. J. Orthod. Dentofacial Orthop.* 147: 604–609.

Sifakakis, I., Pandis, N., Eliades, T. et al. (2011). In vitro assessment of the forces generated by lingual fixed retainers. *Am. J. Orthod. Dentofacial Orthop.* 139: 44–48.

Sifakakis, I., Eliades, T., and Bourauel, C. (2015). Residual stress analysis of fixed retainer wires after in vitro loading: can mastication-induced stresses produce an unfavorable effect? *Biomed. Tech. (Berl)* 60: 617–622.

Sifakakis, I., Katsaros, C., and Eliades, T. Fixed retention in orthodontics. In: *Stability, Retention and Relapse in Orthodontics* (ed. C. Katsaros and T. Eliades), 177–187. Berlin: Quintessenz.

Speck, M. (2008). Unexpected complications. *Am. J. Orthod. Dentofacial Orthop.* 133: 484.

Stoller, N.H. and Green, P.A. (1981). A comparison of a composite restorative material and wire ligation as methods of stabilizing excessively mobile mandibular anterior teeth. *J. Periodontol.* 52: 451–454.

Störmann, I. and Ehmer, U. (2002). A prospective randomized study of different retainer types. *J. Orofac. Orthop.* 63: 42–50.

Stout, M.M., Cook, B.K., Arola, D.D. et al. (2017). Assessing the feasibility of yttria-stabilized zirconia in novel designs as mandibular anterior fixed lingual retention after orthodontic treatment. *Am. J. Orthod. Dentofacial Orthop.* 151: 63–73.

Tacken, M.P., Cosyn, J., De Wilde, P. et al. (2010). Glass fibre reinforced versus multistranded bonded orthodontic retainers: a 2 year prospective multi-Centre study. *Eur. J. Orthod.* 32: 117–123.

Thurow, R.R. (1982). *Edgewise Orthodontics*, 4e. St Louis: Mosby.

Watted, N., Wieber, M., Teuscher, T., and Schmitz, N. (2001). Comparison of incisor mobility after insertion of canine-to-canine lingual retainers bonded to two or to six teeth. A clinical study. *J. Orofac. Orthop.* 62: 387–396.

Wezel, J., Kooij, B.J., and Webb, A.G. (2014). Assessing the MR compatibility of dental retainer wires at 7 Tesla. *Magn. Reson. Med.* 72: 1191–1198.

Wolf, M., Schumacher, P., Jäger, F. et al. (2015). Novel lingual retainer created using CAD/CAM technology: evaluation of its positioning accuracy. *J. Orofac. Orthop.* 76: 164–174.

Wylezinska, M., Pinkstone, M., Hay, N. et al. (2015). Impact of orthodontic appliances on the quality of craniofacial anatomical magnetic resonance imaging and real-time speech imaging. *Eur. J. Orthod.* 37: 610–617.

Zachrisson, B.U. (1977). Clinical experience with direct-bonded orthodontic retainers. *Am. J. Orthod.* 71: 440–448.

Zachrisson, B.U. (1995). Geklebter 3-3 Unterkieferlingualretainer der dritten Generation. *Inf. Orthod. Kieferorthop.* 27: 369–379.

Zachrisson, B.U. (2007). Langzeiterfahrungen mit Kleberetainern: Aktueller Überblick und praktische Hinweise. *Inf. Orthod. Kieferorthop.* 39: 92–100.

Zachrisson, B.U. (2015). Multistranded wire bonded retainers: from start to success. *Am. J. Orthod. Dentofacial Orthop.* 148: 724–727.

Zhylich, D., Krishnan, P., Muthusami, P. et al. (2017). Effects of orthodontic appliances on the diagnostic quality of magnetic resonance images of the head. *Am. J. Orthod. Dentofacial Orthop.* 151: 484–499.

Zinelis, S., Pandis, N., Al Jabbari, Y.S. et al. (2018). Does long-term intraoral service affect the mechanical properties and elemental composition of multistranded wires of lingual fixed retainers? *Eur. J. Orthod.* 40: 126–131.

Zreaqat, M., Hassan, R., and Hanoun, A.F. (2017). A CAD/CAM zirconium bar as a bonded mandibular fixed retainer: a novel approach with two-year follow-up. *Case Rep. Dent.* 2017: 1583403.

11

Release of Bisphenol-A from Materials Used for Fixed Retainer Bonding

Iosif Sifakakis

Department of Orthodontics, School of Dentistry, National and Kapodistrian University of Athens, Athens, Greece

11.1 Introduction

Bisphenol A (BPA) is an endocrine-disrupting synthetic compound used in the manufacturing process of plastic products. The increased awareness of the possible risks of BPA among the scientific community is reflected in the recent literature. Several studies have examined specific activities or products for potential human exposure to BPA. These include soft drinks, canned foods, microwave containers, polycarbonate bottles and baby bottles, smoking, alcohol consumption, medical procedures/products including cardiopulmonary bypass and haemodialysis, dental appliances/restorations/sealants, and plastic tubing (Lakind and Naiman 2011). The tolerable daily intake for BPA was established in January 2015 by the European Food Safety Authority (EFSA) at a threshold of 4 micrograms per kg body weight/day. Regarding this aspect, EFSA concludes that BPA poses no health risk to consumers of any age group and that it is virtually impossible to be exposed to the amount of BPA established as a safe limit by European and international authorities via food. However, the tolerable daily intake was made temporary, and EFSA committed to re-evaluating BPA toxicity again after the results of the CLARITY-BPA program, a study by the US National Toxicology Program.

Debonding and Fixed Retention in Orthodontics: An Evidence-Based Clinical Guide, First Edition. Edited by Theodore Eliades and Christos Katsaros.

BPA may have an adverse effect on several physiologic functions in children and adults. Recent data from systematic reviews indicate that BPA can interact with several transcription proliferative/antiproliferative factors and hormonal receptors. It can favour the onset of endometrial cancer with different molecular mechanisms (Caserta et al. 2022). It could potentially elevate the risk of breast cancer (Wan et al. 2021). Another review has shown a potential negative correlation of BPA concentrations with thyroid-stimulating hormone in children, a potential effect on proper neurodevelopment and a gender-specific manner of action (Koutaki et al. 2021).

In dental materials, BPA is used as a raw material for the formulation of BPA glycidyl methacrylate (Bis-GMA) and polycarbonate products; as a general rule, the estrogenic action is confined to molecules with a double benzoic ring (Eliades 2017). Bis-GMA is the reaction product of BPA and glycidyl methacrylate, and is associated with increased levels of reactive oxygen species and DNA damage. It can be released from bonding/restoration biomaterials into the oral cavity either from incomplete polymerization or because of resin degradation due to various chemical or physical mechanisms such as saliva disintegration, mechanical wear, bacterial activity and erosion by food (Romo-Huerta et al. 2021).

Appliances and restorations that remain exposed to the oral cavity over the long term may present an extended and increased BPA release. Many studies have been published on the risk assessment of BPA release from fixed or removable aligners and retainers. This is even more crucial since the demand for and provision of aesthetic orthodontic treatment appliances have recently increased among patients. This trend reflects an acceptance of invisible orthodontic appliances – that is, clear aligners.

One clinical trial measured BPA levels in patients' saliva before and after the placement of different removable retainers. All groups showed increased levels of BPA after placement of the retainer. Higher levels were detected in vacuum-formed retainers and lower levels in heat-cure Hawley-type retainers (Raghavan et al. 2017). The first systematic review from *in vitro* research indicated an absence of an estrogenic or cytotoxic effect of thermoplastic aligners or retainers. According to this review, the evidence from clinical and laboratory studies was inconsistent regarding BPA or monomer release. However, a recent systematic review indicated that 3D-printed aligners may present higher levels of cytotoxicity and genotoxicity when compared to thermoplastic resins, particularly those not subjected to a final surface treatment (Francisco et al. 2022). Another review evaluated the release and toxicity of BPA contained in orthodontic adhesives and concluded that those containing BPA have potential short- and long-term adverse biological effects in humans; however, the level of evidence was low, and the risk of bias ranged from moderate to high (Sabour et al. 2021).

This chapter presents the recent literature data and discusses concerns regarding BPA release from fixed retainers.

11.2 BPA and Fixed Retainers – Clinical Considerations

Fixed retainers in orthodontics are commonly used for an extended period or even permanently, especially in the mandibular arch (Figure 11.1). The main types of mandibular retainers used are large-diameter wires bonded only on the canines and small-diameter wires bonded on six mandibular teeth. Flowable, light-cured adhesives are mainly used for bonding both retainer types, but conventional bracket adhesives and posterior dental composite resins have also been investigated.

The application of orthodontic adhesives as bonding materials for fixed retainers is vastly different from the use of adhesives in bracket bonding. In the former scenario, the adhesive approaches a three-dimensional structure, with a large surface-to-volume ratio, in contrast

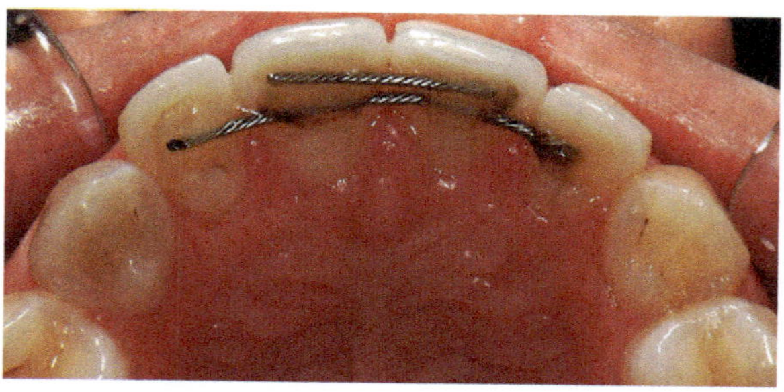

Figure 11.1 Fixed retainers are commonly used for an extended period or even permanently. Microleakage may increase resin degradation and BPA release.

with the exposure of the marginal edges of the material when used as bracket adhesive. This fact increases the adhesive reactivity with the surrounding environment and favours ageing and degradation, with unpredictable BPA release. Retainers bonded on only two instead of six teeth may significantly reduce the amount of adhesive used. A systematic review pointed out that the amounts of BPA released from orthodontic bonding resins were between 0.85 and 20.88 ng per millilitre *in vivo* and from traces to 65.67 ppm *in vitro*. Greater quantities have been detected in saliva one hour after placement (Kloukos et al. 2013, 2015). By having patients rinse thoroughly after bonding, the levels of BPA in their saliva or rinsing medium returned to baseline levels. The different rinsing solutions, i.e. tap water vs. de-ionized water plus absolute ethanol, did not affect BPA levels (Kloukos et al. 2015).

A clinical study evaluated the immediate release of BPA in saliva and the BPA absorbed by the body in urine samples during the first month after bonding of fixed retainers. Two Bis-GMA adhesives were used: a universal restorative and a flowable resin. The only significant high level of BPA was observed in saliva collected just after placement of the lingual bonded retainer, but its maximum level (20.9 ng/ml) was far lower than the reference daily intake dose. Subjects in the restorative resin group had higher BPA levels than those with the flowable adhesive. Decreased BPA levels were found after pumice prophylaxis in the former group. Sex and age did not affect the BPA levels. The authors point out the possibility of underestimating the release of BPA from the one-day-after urine samples because of organ-bound BPA (Kang et al. 2011).

Some authors suggest avoiding liquid resin when using Bis-GMA adhesive materials containing both liquid resin and paste for bonding fixed retainers. A five-year follow-up study showed that the clinical longevity of the retainer is not compromised if bonded without liquid resin. The researchers concluded that this is a more biologic approach to bonding fixed retainers, considering the potential hazards of BPA (Tang et al. 2013).

To this end, the exposure of the operator and staff to BPA is much higher than that of patients since they participate in many bonding and debonding procedures daily. Emphasis should also be placed on protecting the staff from exposure to BPA. Extra care should be taken with masks, fresh air access and surgical suction to minimize the spread of the aerosol in the operatory.

11.3 *In Vitro* Research

The results of *in vitro* studies addressing BPA release from bracket and fixed retainer bonding composites are highly variable because of the diversity of the research protocols and the differences in methods of analysis, immersion media and immersion time. Moreover, a BPA release assay may not constitute conclusive evidence in determining the potential of a material to give rise to BPA formation because of the threshold of chromatographic analyses used. Thus, the amount released could be undetected by instrumental analysis (Eliades 2017). Moreover, the clinical significance of some research protocols evaluating BPA release is questionable. If the specimens are immersed in media immediately after photocuring, this results in a technical increase in the release of unpolymerized species from the material. The same is true when investigating the salivary levels of BPA immediately after bonding orthodontic appliances. In clinical reality, the patient rinses away whatever would later be released in the media as part of the bonding protocol (Eliades 2017).

An initial *in vitro* study evaluated BPA release from small-diameter retainers bonded on human teeth with a common bracket adhesive. The specimens (each retainer was bonded on six human teeth) were immersed in doubled-distilled water, and the BPA concentrations were measured after 10, 20, and 30 days using gas chromatography–mass spectroscopy analysis. Measurable amounts of BPA were detected at all time points, with the most found in the one-month group (2.9 mg/l), whereas the control (tooth storage solution) had only 0.16 mg/l. However, in the clinical setting, BPA release might be higher than that reported in this study, due to the substantially longer expected service life of the retainer, mechanical ageing from masticatory loads and chemical ageing factors (Eliades et al. 2011).

Another *in vitro* evaluation of the same common bracket adhesive with high-performance liquid chromatography detected measurable amounts of BPA in all samples (at 1, 7, 21, and 35 days); the maximum amount was recorded from the specimen light-cured with the greatest light-curing tip distance and reached 65.67 ppm at seven days. An important finding of this research was that BPA release was greater in specimens cured with a greater light-curing tip distance. The degree of conversion decreased with increased light-curing tip distances. A negative correlation was found between BPA release and degree of conversion (Sunitha et al. 2011).

A further study evaluated a standardized specimen of the same bracket adhesive and reported a mean release of 2.75 mg/g of material after three days of immersion in artificial unstimulated saliva. No further BPA release was observed on day 7 or 14 (Kotyk and Wiltshire 2014). Further *in vitro* research failed to detect BPA in standardized samples of the same bracket adhesive, but the detection threshold was not indicated in this study (Małkiewicz et al. 2015).

Gas phase chromatography and mass spectrometry was used in another *in vitro* protocol with a standardized specimen. The quantity of BPA did not exceed the detection threshold of 0.02 ppm (mg/ml) in the first 24 hours. The materials tested included bracket adhesives and a low-viscosity adhesive used for fixed retainers (Bationo et al. 2016).

The most recent *in vitro* study used the same quantitative technique to evaluate the release of monomers from specimens that simulated the six bonding sites of a fixed retainer. No trace of BPA was detected above the detection threshold of 0.02 ppm in the first 24 hours. The materials tested included the same widely used bracket adhesive and a common adhesive for fixed retainers (Pelourde et al. 2018).

11.4 BPA-Free Orthodontic Adhesives

The pervasiveness of BPA-containing adhesives led some researchers to suggest modifications in the synthesis of adhesives to ensure that no BPA is released during use, including ageing (Eliades 2007). In light of these concerns, several BPA-free orthodontic adhesives have been introduced, mainly based on aliphatic dimethacrylates. Two experimental BPA-free resin composite adhesives for retainer bonding have also been developed recently: (E1) a single-aromatic-ring highly reactive multifunctional monomer was incorporated, along with conventional aliphatic co-monomers and glass-fillers (PCDMA, TEGDMA, UEDMA silanated glass [70 wt%], catalysts); (E2) the second was based on aromatic-free urethane dimethacrylate monomers (TEGDMA, UEDMA, silanated glass [60 wt%], catalysts). These experimental adhesives were *in vitro* tested compared to a commercially available adhesive (C) for fixed retainers based on BPA components. For instrumented indentation testing, the ranking of the statistically significant differences in Martens hardness (MH) and indentation modulus (E_{IT}) among the materials tested was C > E1 > E2

Table 11.1 Descriptive statistics for the results of instrumented indentation testing and degree of conversion (DC) of irradiated specimens.

	C	E1	E2
MH (MPa)	71.6 (2.0)	53.0 (2.0)	30.9 (1.1)
E_{IT} (GPa)	17.3 (0.3)	12.9 (0.5)	6.7 (0.3)
n_{IT} (%)	33.6 (1.1)	34.9 (0.3)	40.0 (2.2)
DC	44.1 (4.1)	50.5 (6.6)	63.6 (3.8)

Control: a commercially available adhesive for fixed retainers based on BPA components. E1 and E2: experimental BPA-free adhesives. Mean (SD).

($P < 0.05$). In elastic index (or percentage of the elastic fraction of indentation work, η_{IT}) measurements, E2 showed statistically significant higher values than C and E1 ($P < 0.05$), while no statistically significant difference was found between C and E1 ($P > 0.05$). The degree of convention of the irradiated specimens was also calculated. E2 presented the highest value, with all mean differences being statistically significant ($P < 0.05$) (Table 11.1). Additionally, the effect of prolonged (six months) water storage was evaluated by measuring the changes in Vickers microhardness (VHN). A statistically insignificant interaction was found between material type and storage conditions for both adhesives ($P = 0.074$). Under short (one week) and prolonged (six months) water storage, the ranking in descending VHN order was C, E1 > E2. No statistically significant differences were found in the pullout strength testing employing a multistrand wire.

The authors concluded that the material containing PCDMA, which presented higher hardness and elastic modulus values, may be used as a preferred alternative in clinical retainer bonding (Iliadi et al. 2017; Papadogiannis et al. 2017). Further efforts have been made to replace Bis-GMA with UDMA in orthodontic adhesives. The latter lacks benzoic rings and therefore avoids the potential release of BPA and, concomitantly, its xeno-estrogenic action (Papakonstantinou et al. 2013). Nevertheless, the estrogenic effect of several BPA-free chemicals used as a replacement for BPA-containing resins cannot be excluded (Bittner et al. 2014).

Clinical recommendations for patients are as follows:

1) Optimize polymerization conditions (close proximity of tip to bracket, sufficient light exposure times and adequate light intensity).
2) Pumice prophylaxis after bonding may reduce BPA release.
3) Multiple rinsings after bonding and a suggestion to continue this for some hours may return the initially higher salivary BPA content to baseline levels.
4) The use of liquid resin should be avoided when using Bis-GMA adhesive materials containing both liquid resin and paste.
5) Retainers bonded only on the canines may significantly reduce the amount of adhesive used.
6) It is advisable to use adhesives specially designed for fixed retainers.
7) Sufficient adhesive hardness is essential because of the exposure of the adhesive to masticatory forces.
8) Request details of BPA use at any stage of production by the manufacturer.
9) The benefits and risks of keeping a fixed retainer over long periods should be weighed by the clinician.

11.5 Conclusions

The release of BPA is well-demonstrated after fixed retainer bonding and requires special clinical handling and further research. In most studies, BPA release from fixed retainers is negligible. However, this amount should not be overlooked since the overall health issues attributed to BPA exposure are complex, controversial and not fully understood. Preventive measures for patients and dental staff should be implemented during fixed retainer bonding/debonding to reduce BPA release.

References

Bationo, R., Jordana, F., Boileau, M.J., and Colat-Parros, J. (2016). Release of monomers from orthodontic adhesives. *Am. J. Orthod. Dentofacial Orthop.* 150 (3): 491–498. https://doi.org/10.1016/j.ajodo.2016.02.027. PMID: 27585778.

Bittner, G.D., Yang, C.Z., and Stoner, M.A. (2014). Estrogenic chemicals often leach from BPA-free plastic products that are replacements for BPA-containing polycarbonate products. *Environ. Health.* 13 (1): 41. https://doi.org/10.1186/1476-069X-13-41. PMID: 24886603; PMCID: PMC4063249.

Caserta, D., De Marco, M.P., Besharat, A.R., and Costanzi, F. (2022). Endocrine disruptors and endometrial cancer: molecular mechanisms of action and clinical implications, a systematic review. *Int. J. Mol. Sci.* 23 (6): 2956. https://doi.org/10.3390/ijms23062956. PMID: 35328379; PMCID: PMC8953483.

Eliades, T. (2007). Orthodontic materials research and applications: part 2. Current status and projected future developments in materials and biocompatibility. *Am. J. Orthod. Dentofacial Orthop.* 131 (2): 253–262. https://doi.org/10.1016/j.ajodo.2005.12.029. PMID: 17276868.

Eliades, T. (2017). Bisphenol A and orthodontics: an update of evidence-based measures to minimize exposure for the orthodontic team and patients. *Am. J. Orthod. Dentofacial Orthop.* 152 (4): 435–441. https://doi.org/10.1016/j.ajodo.2017.08.004.

Eliades, T., Voutsa, D., Sifakakis, I. et al. (2011). Release of bisphenol-a from a light-cured adhesive bonded to lingual fixed retainers. *Am. J. Orthod. Dentofacial Orthop.* 139 (2): 192–195. https://doi.org/10.1016/j.ajodo.2009.12.026. PMID: 21300247.

Francisco, I., Paula, A.B., Ribeiro, M. et al. (2022). The biological effects of 3D resins used in orthodontics: a systematic review. *Bioengineering (Basel).* 9 (1): 15. https://doi.org/10.3390/bioengineering9010015. PMID: 35049724; PMCID: PMC8773237.

Iliadi, A., Eliades, T., Silikas, N., and Eliades, G. (2017). Development and testing of novel bisphenol A-free adhesives for lingual fixed retainer bonding. *Eur. J. Orthod.* 39 (1): 1–8. https://doi.org/10.1093/ejo/cjv090. Epub 2015 Dec 11. PMID: 26658921.

Kang, Y.G., Kim, J.Y., Kim, J. et al. (2011). Release of bisphenol a from resin composite used to bond orthodontic lingual retainers. *Am. J. Orthod. Dentofacial Orthop.* 140 (6): 779–789. https://doi.org/10.1016/j.ajodo.2011.04.022. PMID: 22133942.

Kloukos, D., Pandis, N., and Eliades, T. (2013). Bisphenol-a and residual monomer leaching from orthodontic adhesive resins and polycarbonate brackets: a systematic review. *Am. J. Orthod. Dentofacial Orthop.* 143 (4 Suppl): S104–12.e1-2. https://doi.org/10.1016/j.ajodo.2012.11.015. PMID: 23540625.

Kloukos, D., Sifakakis, I., Voutsa, D. et al. (2015). BPA qualtitative and quantitative assessment associated with orthodontic bonding in vivo. *Dent. Mater.* 31 (8): 887–894. https://doi.org/10.1016/j.dental.2015.04.020. Epub 2015 May 19. PMID: 26001991.

Kotyk, M.W. and Wiltshire, W.A. (2014). An investigation into bisphenol-a leaching from orthodontic materials. *Angle. Orthod.* 84 (3): 516–520. https://doi.org/10.2319/081413-600.1.

Koutaki, D., Paltoglou, G., Vourdoumpa, A., and Charmandari, E. (2021). The impact of bisphenol a on thyroid function in neonates and children: a systematic review of the literature. *Nutrients* 14 (1): 168. https://doi.org/10.3390/nu14010168. PMID: 35011041; PMCID: PMC8746969.

Lakind, J.S. and Naiman, D.Q. (2011). Daily intake of bisphenol a and potential sources of exposure: 2005–2006 National Health and nutrition examination survey. *J. Exposure Sci. Environ. Epidemiol.* 21 (3): 272–279. https://doi.org/10.1038/jes.2010.9.

Małkiewicz, K., Turło, J., Marciniuk-Kluska, A. et al. (2015). Release of bisphenol a and its derivatives from orthodontic adhesive systems available on the European market as a potential health risk factor. *Ann. Agric. Environ. Med.* 22 (1): 172–177. https://doi.org/10.5604/12321966.1141390. PMID: 25780850.

Papadogiannis, D., Iliadi, A., Bradley, T.G. et al. (2017). Viscoelastic properties of orthodontic adhesives used for lingual fixed retainer bonding. *Dent. Mater.* 33 (1): e22–e27. https://doi.org/10.1016/j.dental.2016.09.041. Epub 2016 Oct 18. PMID: 27769593.

Papakonstantinou, A.E., Eliades, T., Cellesi, F. et al. (2013). Evaluation of UDMA's potential as a substitute for bis-GMA in orthodontic adhesives. *Dent. Mater.* 29 (8): 898–905. https://doi.org/10.1016/j.dental.2013.05.007. Epub 2013 Jun 17. PMID: 23787036.

Pelourde, C., Bationo, R., Boileau, M.J. et al. (2018). Monomer release from orthodontic retentions: an in vitro study. *Am. J. Orthod. Dentofacial Orthop.* 153 (2): 248–254. https://doi.org/10.1016/j.ajodo.2017.06.021. PMID: 29407502.

Raghavan, A.S., Pottipalli Sathyanarayana, H., Kailasam, V., and Padmanabhan, S. (2017). Comparative evaluation of salivary bisphenol a levels in patients wearing vacuum-formed and Hawley retainers: an in-vivo study. *Am. J. Orthod. Dentofacial Orthop.* 151 (3): 471–476. https://doi.org/10.1016/j.ajodo.2016.07.022. PMID: 28257731.

Romo-Huerta, M.J., Cervantes-Urenda, A.D.R., Velasco-Neri, J. et al. (2021). Genotoxicity associated with residual monomers in restorative dentistry: a systematic review. *Oral Health Prev. Dent.* 19 (1): 471–480. https://doi.org/10.3290/j.ohpd.b2081469. PMID: 34585872.

Sabour, A., El Helou, M., Roger-Leroi, V., and Bauer, C. (2021). Release and toxicity of bisphenol-A (BPA) contained in orthodontic adhesives: A systematic review. *Int. Orthod.* 19 (1): 1–14. https://doi.org/10.1016/j.ortho.2020.11.002. Epub 2020 Dec 8. PMID: 33308954.

Sunitha, C., Kailasam, V., Padmanabhan, S., and Chitharanjan, A.B. (2011). Bisphenol a release from an orthodontic adhesive and its correlation with the degree of conversion on varying light-curing tip distances. *Am. J. Orthod. Dentofacial Orthop.* 140 (2): 239–244. https://doi.org/10.1016/j.ajodo.2010.02.037. PMID: 21803262.

Tang, A.T., Forsberg, C.M., Andlin-Sobocki, A. et al. (2013). Lingual retainers bonded without liquid resin: a 5-year follow-up study. *Am. J. Orthod. Dentofacial Orthop.* 143 (1): 101–104. https://doi.org/10.1016/j.ajodo.2012.09.008. PMID: 23273365.

Wan, M.L.Y., Co, V.A., and El-Nezami, H. (2021). Endocrine disrupting chemicals and breast cancer: a systematic review of epidemiological studies. *Crit. Rev. Food Sci. Nutr.* 5: 1–27. https://doi.org/10.1080/10408398.2021.1903382. Epub ahead of print. PMID: 33819127.

12

Clinical Effectiveness of Bonded Mandibular Fixed Retainers

Thaleia Kouskoura[1], Dimitrios Kloukos[2], Pawel Pazera[2], and Christos Katsaros[2]

[1] *Department of Pediatric Oral Health and Orthodontics, University Center for Dental Medicine, University of Basel, Basel, Switzerland*
[2] *Department of Orthodontics and Dentofacial Orthopedics, School of Dental Medicine/ Medical Faculty, University of Bern, Bern, Switzerland*

12.1 Introduction

Since they were first introduced in the early 1970s, bonded retainers have become an increasingly common means for the post-treatment stabilisation of anterior tooth alignment, and they are used more widely in the mandibular arch (Lai et al. 2014; Meade and Dreyer 2019; Pratt et al. 2011; Wong and Freer 2004). The array of fixed mandibular retainer types available to the orthodontist today is considerable, in terms of both the materials used and the attachment method (Diamond 1987; Kravitz et al. 2017; Liou et al. 2001; Sachdeva 2001; Zachrisson 1995; Zachrisson 2015).

To assist the clinician in making the most appropriate bonded retainer choice for their patients, the best available evidence can provide insight into the clinical effectiveness of the main types of fixed retainers. Factors such as the ability of a bonded retainer to maintain alignment in the short and long terms, its failure rates and its effects on the periodontium are determinants of its clinical effectiveness and have been the subject of both prospective and retrospective studies. Due to the nature of research into

Debonding and Fixed Retention in Orthodontics: An Evidence-Based Clinical Guide, First Edition. Edited by Theodore Eliades and Christos Katsaros.

long-term orthodontic retention, obstacles such as attrition rate and the costs and logistics associated with such studies have limited the number of randomised controlled trials (RCTs) comparing those aspects of different bonded retainers. The merits of well-designed prospective studies employing randomisation are known, and these are the studies that are normally scrutinised and analysed and the conclusions presented/results combined in systematic reviews and meta-analyses. However, in the field of research on retention, some good-quality retrospective and prospective cohort studies with large sample numbers can also add useful information to the pool of available higher levels of evidence.

The main outcome of interest, with respect to clinical effectiveness, is the ability of the different types of bonded retainers to maintain the alignment of the anterior teeth achieved at the conclusion of the orthodontic treatment and prevent post-treatment dental change. The incidence and types of bonded retainer failures are important in terms of both the retainers' ability to fulfil their retentive function and patient satisfaction (cost for repairs and inconvenience caused by additional dental appointments). Given the increasing trend among practitioners to recommend life-long retention, there is also interest in the possible negative effects of long-term use of fixed retainers on gingival and dental tissues, which are also important determinants of their clinical effectiveness. Other factors, such as cost and acceptance (in terms of comfort and aesthetics), have occasionally been investigated but will not be the focus here.

12.2 Short-Term Alignment Stabilisation

There is a general agreement that retention is particularly important in the first year following the completion of orthodontic treatment. Based on an early biological observation, this is when remodelling and stabilisation of the periodontal and gingival tissues occur around the orthodontically moved teeth (Edwards 1968; Reitan 1967).

Bonded retainers are relied on to hold the teeth in the corrected positions during this crucial period without the need for patient cooperation. However, their function can be compromised due to deformation of the retainer wire either before or after bonding or due to undetected fracture or detachment of the wire from tooth unit(s).

A number of studies have examined the extent to which changes in the alignment of the anterior mandibular segment occurred in the short term in the presence of fixed retainers. Two indices are primarily used to assess post-treatment stability: Little's Irregularity Index (LII) (Little 1975) and the peer assessment rating (PAR) index (Richmond et al. 1992). The LII is a straightforward method to assess anterior arch irregularity with the advantage that it is widely used in retention studies, rendering the results comparable. Its limitations lie in (i) providing the sum of point displacements (which may or may not be clinically significant) rather than defining specific point displacements, (ii) not accounting for spacing and other changes (e.g. torque, angulation/inclination, vertical changes), and (iii) potentially unacceptable inter- and intra-examiner variability (Burns et al. 2014; Dowling et al. 2013; Macauley et al. 2012). The PAR index is used much less often in retention studies and includes measurement of tooth alignment irregularities, including spacing. Additional measurements such as intercanine distance, intermolar distance and arch length are also sometimes used to assess the ability of retainers to stabilise post-treatment results.

Large retrospective studies have shown that the failure rate for bonded retainers is highest during the first year of retention (Jin et al. 2018; Lie Sam Foek et al. 2008). This could indicate that alignment changes are likely to occur if such failures are undetected even for a relatively short period, as the teeth are far less stable during this time. Deformation of bonded retainers and changes in the properties of adhesive materials in the oral environment can also affect the ability to maintain tooth alignment.

Different types of wire retainers bonded on all six mandibular anterior teeth were compared in several randomised clinical studies (Adanur-Atmaca et al. 2021; Alrawas et al. 2021; Gelin et al. 2020; Gunay and Alper 2018; Shim et al. 2022). The longest observation period was either six months or a year, while the types of retainers included multistrand retainers of different dimensions (round and rectangular) and computer-aided design/computer-aided manufacturing (CAD/CAM) fabricated retainers (steel or NiTi). None of the studies found a clinically significant difference in irregularity changes between the end of treatment and the end of the observation time. In terms of LII, irregularity changes were also generally small, in most cases less than 1 mm of mean change and in no cases exceeding 2 mm. Attrition rate and lack of blinding were issues in most of the studies, introducing bias to varying degrees.

Experimental arms employing fixed retainers in studies comparing fixed to removable retainers (Atack et al. 2007; Forde et al. 2017; O'Rourke et al. 2016) also indicated that mean changes in tooth alignment for bonded retainers in the short-term are limited (less than 1 mm).

When fixed retainers bonded only on canines were compared to those fixed on all six lower anterior teeth, one study found a significant difference between the two types of retainers (Al-Nimri et al. 2009); the retainer bonded only on the canines performed worse, with a difference of more than 1 mm (LII) after 12 months of retention. The canine-only fixed retainer performed better in a study (Krämer et al. 2020) compared to a removable retainer six months into retention, with an increase in irregularity of 0.3 mm, very similar to the removable retainer.

Although the failure rates of bonded mandibular retainers are reportedly at their highest during the initial period of retention, the levels of increase in tooth irregularity during the same period are, according to the studies mentioned, generally low and clinically not significant. A possible explanation may be that during an initial period after the removal of fixed appliances, patients remain under evaluation by their orthodontist, especially in studies carried out in university settings, and as a result, any retainer failures are detected and rectified promptly before any major changes in tooth alignment occur.

12.3 Long-Term Alignment Stabilisation

The study by Little et al. (1988) showed that post-retention mandibular anterior tooth alignment is the aspect that, in the long-term, shows the most marked deterioration in the absence of retention. A recent systematic review of mainly long-term observational studies (Swidi et al. 2019) found that changes in mandibular alignment post-treatment (with or without retention) are increasing as a function of time and occur to a greater extent at 1–10 years compared to 10–20 years after treatment. A meta-analysis in the same systematic review estimated irregularity changes to be less than 2 mm during the 20-year observation time. The authors reported that their findings were based on studies at high risk of bias, but it can be safely concluded that some post-treatment deterioration in mandibular anterior tooth alignment is a reality regardless of whether some form of retention is employed.

The evidence from studies examining the ability of fixed mandibular retainers to prevent such a post-treatment increase in mandibular irregularity in the long-term is limited. A small number of RCTs (with varying degrees of overall bias) and some retrospective studies have been conducted. The randomised clinical studies by O'Rourke et al. (2016),

Störmann and Ehmer (2002) and Tynelius et al. (2013) had a maximum follow-up time of 1.5–2 years, and all three studies indicated a mean change in LII no greater than 1 mm at the end of the observation time when fixed retainers were used. When comparisons between different fixed retainer types were made in one of the studies (Störmann and Ehmer 2002), the canine-only fixed retainer was found to perform significantly worse than the retainers bonded on all six mandibular anterior teeth. In terms of retrospective studies with longer observation times (up to 20 years post-treatment), one must keep in mind that during such long periods, more retainer failures can occur, and some of them remain undetected. Two retrospective, long-term studies by Renkema et al. (2008, 2011) examined changes in LII when two different types of fixed retainers were used (Figure 12.1). At 5 years post-treatment, the LII for a canine-only retainer increased by a mean value of 0.9 mm for the whole

(a)

(b)

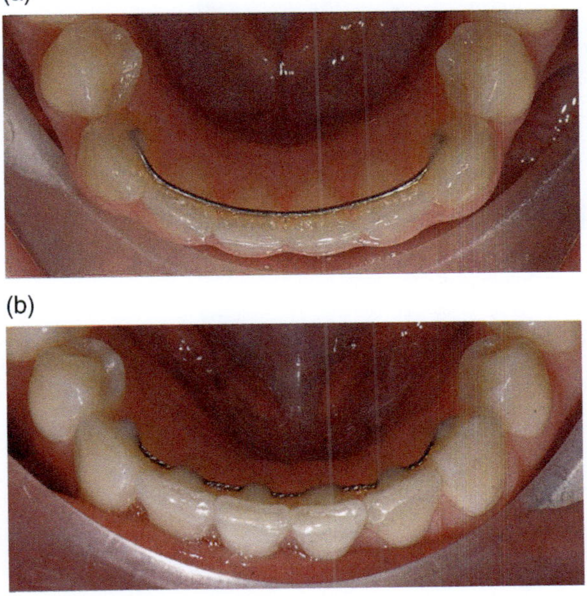

Figure 12.1 The two types of retainers used in the studies by Renkema et al. (2008, 2011). (a) 0.0215 × 0.027-in stainless steel rounded rectangular wire bonded to the mandibular canines only. (b) 0.0195-in three-strand heat-treated twisted wire bonded to all six mandibular anterior teeth. *Source:* Renkema et al. (2013).

sample of patients (Renkema et al. 2008), while for the canine-to-canine retainer, a mean increase of approximately 0.8 mm was measured in the subsample of patients with an increase in irregularity (Renkema et al. 2011). A more recent retrospective study (Kocher et al. 2020) similarly compared two types of retainers (canine-only vs. canine-to-canine) 10–15 years post-treatment. They noted essentially no increase in LII for the canine-to-canine retainer and a mean increase of approx. 0.45 mm for the canine-only retainer. In another study examining canine-only retainers over 20 years post-treatment (Booth et al. 2008), 2% of patients with retainers still in place showed LII greater than 2 mm (Figure 12.2). The results of the retrospective studies show that average changes in LII are well below 2 mm in the even longer term, similar to the randomised clinical studies.

(a)

(b)

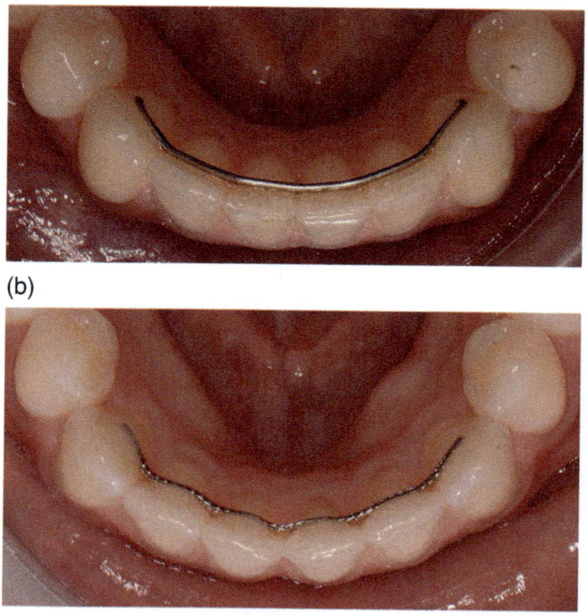

Figure 12.2 The two types of retainers used in the studies by Kocher et al. (2019, 2020). (a) 0.027-in round TMA wire bonded to the mandibular canines only. (b) 0.016 x 0.022-in eight-strand braided SS wire bonded to all six mandibular anterior teeth. *Source:* Kocher et al. (2020).

No safe conclusion can be reached regarding which type of retainer performs better in the long-term. But in general, all retainers examined generally restrict irregularity changes effectively, with a possible tendency of the canine-to-canine retainers to perform better.

12.4 Failure Rates

The failure of different bonded retainers was one of the outcomes examined in recent systematic reviews (Al-Moghrabi et al. 2016; Iliadi et al. 2015; Jedlinski et al. 2021; Littlewood et al. 2016). A common conclusion was the high degree of heterogeneity in the included studies regarding the type of retainer material used, method for attachment to the teeth (adhesive material, number of attachment sites, direct or indirect attachment), operator experience and setting. Large variations in the follow-up periods and outcome measures were also noted. Only a few of the identified studies were judged by all reviewers to be at low risk of bias.

The largest number of prospective high-quality studies examine as part of the outcomes the incidence of failure (localised detachment, wire breakage or complete loss) of multistrand steel retainers bonded on six mandibular anterior teeth. In the available studies, the retainer dimensions of lower arch retainers vary, from the thinnest (0.0175 in.) to thickest (0.039 in.) round wires. More rarely, rectangular stainless steel (SS) wires have been studied. The type of alloys and structure (twisted, coaxial, braided) also vary. The follow-up period ranges from 6 to 24 months. With respect to round wire retainers bonded on all six mandibular anterior teeth, the general conclusion is that the occurrence of any type of failure varies widely between studies.

There is a fair similarity in the outcome of most of the high-quality RCTs using thicker (0.022 in. and 0.0215 in.) multistrand SS retainers bonded with light-cured composite resin and an observation period of 24 months (Egli et al. 2017; Pandis et al. 2013; Wegrodzka et al. 2021). In these studies, failures of 50, 40 and 56%, respectively, were observed in 24 months. When additional prospective studies are considered with less robust designs and more areas that can introduce bias, multistrand retainers with the same dimension (0.0215 in.) showed a risk of failure of 12% in 24 months (Tacken et al. 2010) and 27% in six months (Kartal et al. 2021).

Larger discrepancies exist among the results of studies using thinner multistrand retainers (either 0.0175 in. or 0.0195 in.). For 0.0175 in. retainers, the failure risk was 31.5% and 38% during 18 months in two different high-quality RCT studies (Nagani et al. 2020; Salehi et al. 2013), respectively. In RCTs with a higher potential for introducing bias, the outcome for the 0.0175 in. retainer varied between 7% and 13% risk of failure at 18 months (Gunay and Alper 2018; O'Rourke et al. 2016) and 27% at 24 months (Sobouti et al. 2016). A marked difference between studies was the different bonding material used to attach the retainer and the high attrition in one of the studies (O'Rourke et al. 2016), which could partly account for the discrepancy. In addition, in one study (Gunay and Alper 2018), some retainers reached the first premolars.

When a 6-strand coaxial 0.0195 in. retainer was used in one high-quality RCT, a 4% risk of failure in 24 months was seen (Bazargani et al. 2012), while in another high-quality RCT, a 50% failure risk in 12 months was recorded for a 0.0195 in., three-strand twistflex wire (Forde et al. 2017). The bonding material, the structure of the retainer wire and the operator experience in these two studies differed, but it is unclear the extent to which each could account for the large difference. Another prospective study (Gunay and Alper 2018) using a dead-soft six-strand coaxial 0.0195 in. wire found 19% failure in 12 months of follow-up, including retainers bonded up to the first premolars. Failure rates of 24% in 24 months and 32% in 60 months were recorded in a large retrospective study (Renkema et al. 2011) of patients with a 0.0195 in., three-strand, heat-treated, twist-wire SS retainer.

Rectangular wires were examined in a small number of studies. In a high-quality RCT (Wegrodzka et al. 2021), a 48.5% failure rate in 24 months was recorded for a rectangular 0.0265 × 0.0106 in., eight-strand, braided SS retainer. A very similar failure risk of 47% was found in a non-randomised prospective study of a 0.016 × 0.022 in. eight-strand, braided SS dead-soft wire with a six-month follow-up period (Taner and Aksu 2012). A large retrospective study (Kocher et al. 2020) provided long-term data on the failure risk of 0.016 × 0.022 in. braided SS wire during a mean follow-up period of 12.5 years. The failure risk was 50.5%. Another large retrospective study of 0.016 × 0.022 in. braided SS wire with a maximum follow-up of 3.5 years recorded a failure rate of 32% in the mandibular arch (Lie Sam Foek et al. 2008).

Data on the failure rates of the more recently introduced CAD/CAM fabricated NiTi retainers is limited. These retainers can, in principle, be very closely adapted to the tooth surfaces and interproximal areas, and nickel-titanium wire is used for their fabrication (Kravitz et al. 2017). It has been suggested that the failure rates of these retainers may be lower due to the close adaptation to the contours of the teeth and the precise positioning of these wires regarding occlusal contacts. No significant difference was noted in the failure rates between CAD/CAM NiTi retainers and conventional round SS retainers (0.0175 in. or 0.0215 in.) in the short term in recent studies (Gelin et al. 2020; Kartal et al. 2021). The failure rates reported for this new type of retainer were 23–32% in six months.

Mandibular retainers bonded on all six anterior teeth have been compared to the earlier design of thick wire retainers bonded on the mandibular canines in a few older prospective and some retrospective studies. Canine-only bonded retainers showed significantly lower failure rates in a prospective randomised study (Störmann and Ehmer 2002), with an 18% failure rate in 24 months compared to 29 and 53% for round retainers bonded on all six anterior mandibular teeth in the same study. Similarly, in a retrospective study (Scheibe and Ruf 2010), canine-only retainers showed significantly lower failure rates (22 vs. 35%) compared to canine-to-canine retainers during an observation period of approximately 10–50 months. A retrospective study with a much longer observation time of 10–15 years (Kocher et al. 2019) also found that the rates of different types of failures (including detachment, loss of adhesive or breakages) was also lower for the canine-only bonded retainer compared to the canine-to-canine retainer (approximately 40 vs. 60%), with the type of retainer being the only significant predictor for survival. It was also noted that the average number of failures per patient was higher for canine-to-canine retainers. No significant differences between canine-only and canine-to-canine retainers were reported in non-randomised prospective studies, which recorded failure rates of 21% (vs. 27%) in three years (Årtun et al. 1997) and 13% (vs. 29%) in one to three years (Al-Nimri et al. 2009) for canine-only bonded retainers vs. canine-to-canine retainers. In these studies, canine-only retainers performed better than canine-to-canine retainers. The failure rates of canine-only retainers in longer-term retrospective studies were reported to be approximately 20.5% in 5 years (Renkema et al. 2008) and 25% in 20 years (Booth et al. 2008). However, it must be kept in mind that due to their nature, retrospective studies examining the failure of retainers are subject to several factors (e.g. patient drop-out/loss of or incomplete records, different operators and different materials as time progresses) that are likely to affect the results.

It is likely that an interplay of factors unrelated to the retainer characteristics contributes to the overall failure rate of a fixed wire retainer. Non-patient-related factors may have to do with the clinical performance of the operator, the bonding materials used and the bonding technique employed. There is some indication that operators with more clinical experience may encounter fewer failures (Scheibe and Ruf 2010). *In vitro* studies also show that some bonding materials perform better than others (Aldrees et al. 2010; Papadogiannis et al. 2017; Scribante et al. 2020). The relation between failure rates and bonding method has also been the subject of several comparative studies. The method of indirect bonding of fixed retainers was compared to the conventional method of direct bonding in a small, well-designed RCT with a low risk of bias (Bovali et al. 2014). The same type of retainer (round, six-strand coaxial 0.0215 in. SS) was bonded from canine to canine in the mandibular arch. In the initial short study period of 6 months (Bovali et al. 2014) and in the follow-up longer-term study at 12 and 24 months (Egli et al. 2017), no significant difference in the risk of failure between the two groups was found. A recently published five-year follow-up of the initial RCT population (Cornelis et al. 2022) similarly showed no difference in the survival rate between the indirectly and directly bonded retainers. An interesting finding at the five-year time point was that the incidence of debonding/failure of multiple sites was twice as frequent in the indirectly bonded retainers as the directly bonded ones, which was attributed to the greater risk of salivary contamination of multiple sites when a transfer tray is used during indirect bonding.

Two non-randomised prospective studies (Gökce and Kaya 2019; Taner and Aksu 2012) also found no significant differences in the failure rates between the two bonding techniques. The Taner and Aksu study (2012) used an eight-strand, flattened, SS wire of different dimensions (0.016×0.022 in.) but the same bonding technique and adhesive agents as the RCT studies and a follow-up period of six months, while Gökce and Kaya (2019) used different dimension wires (0.0175 in. and 0.0215 in. multistrand) and different indirect bonding agents and techniques than the RCT studies with a follow-up time of six months. Based on the limited available evidence, it appears neither technique is superior concerning the frequency of bonding failures of these retainers in the short and longer term; this has been the conclusion of a recent systematic review (Ahmed et al. 2021).

The effect of sandblasting tooth surfaces prior to bonding on the failure rate of a mandibular fixed retainer was examined in a single split-mouth RCT with a maximum observation period of one year (Laspos et al. 2023). During this observation period, no difference in the rate of detachment failures or wire breakages of a chairside-made, thin, round, multistrand retainer was observed, indicating that modification of tooth surfaces through sandblasting does not affect the failure rate of this type of retainer in the short-term.

12.5 Periodontal Effects

Various clinical parameters can be examined to determine the negative impact of mandibular fixed retainers on the periodontal tissues in the area where they are attached. In the short term, causative factors of inflammation such as plaque and calculus accumulation and indicators of inflammation such as bleeding on probing (BOP) and gingival inflammation/gingival crevicular fluid volume (GCFV) are measured. In the longer term, clinical outcomes of persistent periodontal inflammation such as increased probing depths, recessions and decreased alveolar bone levels are assessed.

Prospective studies employing randomisation focused primarily on short-term assessment (in most cases, up to 24 months) of periodontal indices (Adanur-Atmaca et al. 2021; Alrawas et al. 2021; Bazargani et al. 2012; Ferreira et al. 2019; Gelin et al. 2020; Kartal et al. 2021; Storey et al. 2018; Störmann and Ehmer 2002; Tacken et al. 2010; Torkan et al. 2014; Wegrodzka et al. 2021). Only a handful of such studies extended the observation time up to four years (Al-Moghrabi et al. 2018; Årtun et al. 1997). There are particular difficulties in conducting high-quality studies of this nature, even if ideal randomisation protocols are employed. For example, the limited feasibility of blinding when clinical measurements are undertaken and the involvement of orthodontists, rather than periodontists, as assessors are likely to introduce considerable detection and performance bias. Attrition bias due to the loss of participants' follow-up in the longer-running studies is an additional area of concern. These concerns have been highlighted in relevant systematic reviews (Al-Moghrabi et al. 2016; Arn et al. 2020).

Comparison between retainers bonded on the lower canines only and those bonded on all six mandibular anterior teeth was made after 6 months (Ferreira et al. 2019), 24 months (Pandis et al. 2013) and 3 years (Årtun et al. 1997). Only one of the studies (Ferreira et al. 2019) detected statistically significant differences in plaque index (PI) and gingival index (GI) at the six-month end point, with canine-only bonded retainers demonstrating reduced plaque accumulation. With respect to loss of attachment, the long-term study detected no differences.

The possibility that factors such as the dimension, structure, material and adaptation of retainers as well as the bonding agents used may affect periodontal parameters was explored for canine-to-canine retainers in several RCT studies (Adanur-Atmaca et al. 2021; Alrawas et al. 2021; Bazargani et al. 2012; Gelin et al. 2020; Kartal et al. 2021; Liu 2010; Rose et al. 2002; Tacken et al. 2010; Torkan et al. 2014; Wegrodzka et al. 2021). The tooth area covered by fixed retainers depends partly on the dimensions of the retainers. Fibre-reinforced composite retainers are larger than metal retainers, and among the metal retainer wires, various dimensions are currently used. The surface characteristics and design of fibre-reinforced composite retainers and wire retainers also differ and could affect the extent of plaque and calculus accumulation. The newly introduced CAD/CAM manufactured NiTi retainers can, in principle, be very closely adapted to the lingual tooth surfaces by virtue of the manufacturing process.

There is currently little evidence that any of these factors lead to significant changes in periodontal health. Fibre-reinforced composite retainers were shown to lead to more plaque and/or gingival inflammation than wire retainers in two of the studies (Tacken et al. 2010, 2014), but no difference in detrimental effects on the periodontium was noted in any of the studies (Liu 2010; Torkan et al. 2014). Similarly, differences in the thickness and configuration of the wire retainers were not associated with significant differences in periodontal indices in any of the relevant studies (Adanur-Atmaca et al. 2021; Wegrodzka et al. 2021). A systematic review of non-randomised studies (Buzatta et al. 2017) also reported no differences between the designs of wire retainers (wave vs. plain) with respect to the assessed indices of periodontal health.

CAD/CAM NiTi retainers were also compared to conventional wire retainers in recent studies (Adanur-Atmaca et al. 2021; Alrawas et al. 2021; Gelin et al. 2020; Kartal et al. 2021). Two studies showed no statistically significant differences in any of the indices (Alrawas et al. 2021; Kartal et al. 2021), while the other two (Adanur-Atmaca et al. 2021; Gelin et al. 2020) identified significant differences in isolated periodontal parameters favouring either standard fixed retainers or CAD/CAM NiTi retainers. However, none noted significant effects on periodontal health.

In research on retention, few studies have examined the long-term periodontal effects of mandibular fixed retainers. Such long-term studies are needed if we are to identify long-term irreversible damage to periodontal tissues, such as a loss of periodontal support or recessions, and available studies are mainly retrospective (Booth et al. 2008; Pandis et al. 2007; Renkema et al. 2013). The quality of these was judged in a systematic review (Wasserman et al. 2016) as moderate, mainly due to the risk of bias introduced by confounders, lack of blinding and detection errors. The studies by Pandis et al. (2007) and Renkema et al. (2013) detected a higher prevalence of mainly labial recession in the mandibular incisor area of orthodontically treated patients with fixed mandibular retainers attached on all six mandibular anterior teeth when these were compared to controls in the long term (6 years and 9.65 years, respectively). The study by Pandis et al. (2007) also noted increased calculus accumulation and probing depths in subjects with retainers. Booth et al. (2008) examined canine-only bonded, thick, round SS retainers 20 years post-treatment. The results indicated no detrimental effects associated with the retainers with respect to the gingival index score. However, no direct correlation could be identified between the presence of retainers and long-term effects on periodontal health, due to the retrospective nature of the studies, which did not account for confounders.

The general conclusion is that although some statistically significant differences in periodontal indices were identified in a few short-term studies, their clinical significance is unclear mainly because no detrimental effects on the periodontium could be detected in the long term. Two recent systematic reviews (Al-Moghrabi et al. 2016; Arn et al. 2020) identified a general lack of high-quality and long-term studies on the subject.

12.6 Side Effects of Fixed Retainers – Unwanted Tooth Movement

Separate from the failure of fixed retainers through breakage, debonding or loss is unwanted movement of the retained tooth unit(s) through the transfer of forces by an active retainer that remains attached and clinically intact. These changes in the position of the retained teeth are distinct from and unrelated to the original malocclusion and cannot be characterised as relapse. They manifest most frequently as inclination and torque changes and are progressive (Figure 12.3). The first published

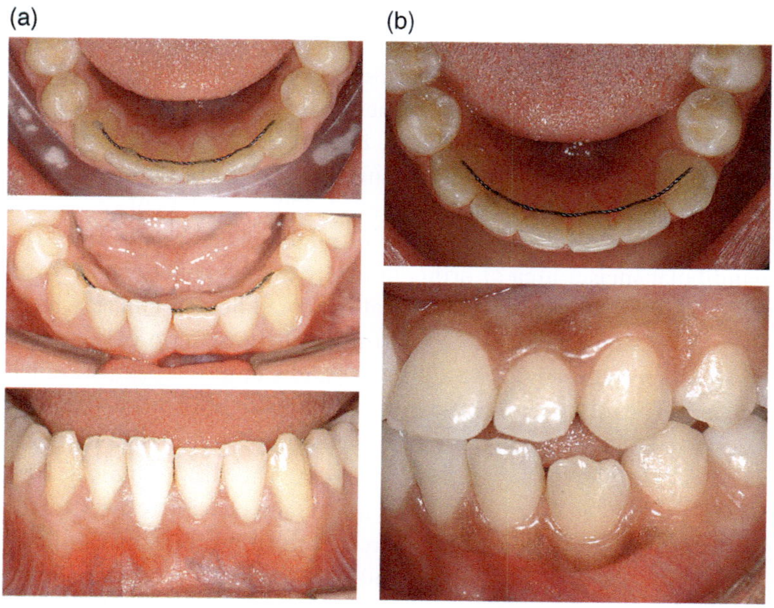

Figure 12.3 (a) Torque difference between the mandibular central incisors at the two-year post-treatment control, due to activation of the .0195-in three-strand heat-treated twist flex retainer; the left central incisor shows excessive lingual root torque, while the right central incisor shows buccal root torque. This difference in torque is also expressed as a difference in the height of the clinical crowns. These tooth movements took place even though the bonded retainer was in situ. (b) Buccal inclination and distobuccal rotation of the left mandibular canine at the one-year posttreatment follow-up, due to activation of the .0195-in three-strand heat-treated twist flex retainer. *Source:* Adapted from Katsaros et al. (2007).

report of such unwanted retainer effects by Katsaros et al. (2007) was followed by a number of others, and a recent systematic review by Charavet et al. (2022) has identified 20 studies, mostly case reports and case series, describing such events. Although re-treatment in these cases is usually possible, permanent damage such as bone dehiscence, gingival recession or loss of tooth vitality due to severe root displacements outside the bony envelope cannot be excluded, particularly if the complications remain undetected at an early stage (Farret et al. 2015; Pazera et al. 2012; Shaughnessy et al. 2016) (Figures 12.4 and 12.5).

Various case-series and retrospective and prospective studies have reported on the prevalence of retainer-related tooth movement in the anterior mandible (Cornelis et al. 2022; Gera et al. 2022; Katsaros et al. 2007; Klaus et al. 2020; Kucera and Marek 2016; Renkema et al. 2011). They reported a prevalence between 1.1% and 17%, with average post-retention times between six months and five years. The sample size, observation time, retainer dimensions and assessment methods differ between the studies and could partly explain the wide range. A single retrospective

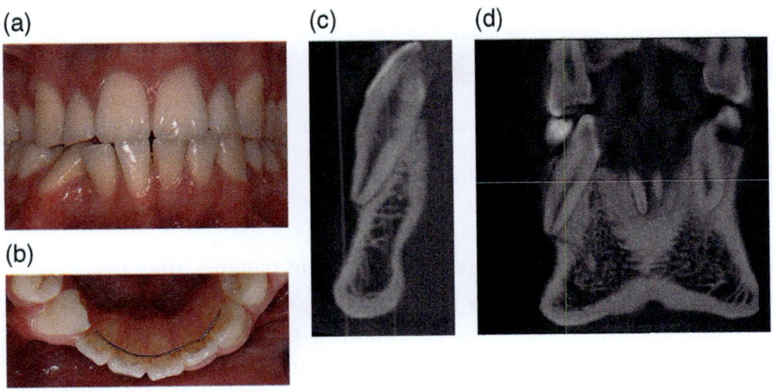

Figure 12.4 (a, b) Excessive torque on the right mandibular canine four years post-treatment. Although the patient had noticed the unusual position of his mandibular right canine, he asked for a clinical check only when his mandibular retainer broke between the mandibular right canine and lateral incisor. Despite the massive buccal position of the root, almost no gingival recession is present. (c, d) Cone-beam computed tomography scan: the root of the canine was completely out of the bone on its buccal side. However, the nerve and the vascular bundle followed the apex, and the tooth's vitality was preserved. *Source:* Adapted from Pazera et al. (2012).

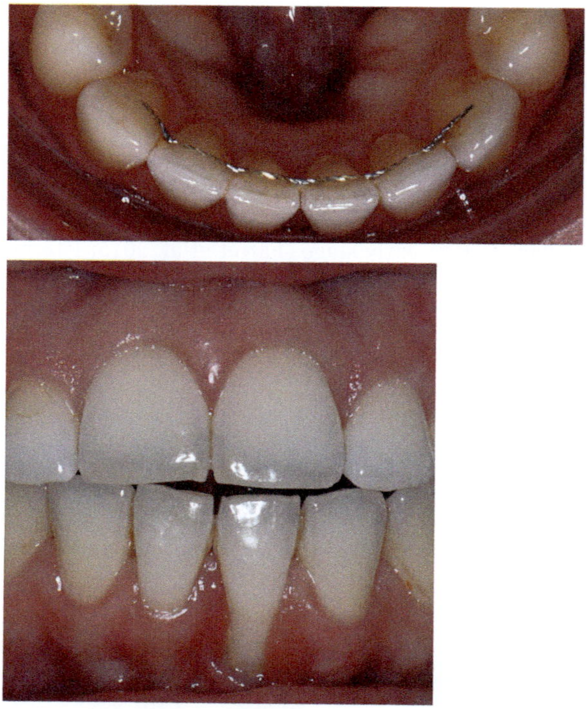

Figure 12.5 Deep labial gingival recession at the mandibular left central incisor resulted from the undetected movement of this tooth due to activation of the bonded flexible round spiral retainer.

study (Kocher et al. 2019) assessed changes in patients after 10–15 years in retention and noted a very small number of cases (less than 0.02% of the patient sample). With the exception of the study by Kocher et al. (2019), the retainers used were round, multistrand SS wires of small dimensions (0.0175–0.0215 in). In the study by Kocher et al. (2019), a 0.016 × 0.022 in. eight-strand, braided SS wire was used.

Observation of these adverse retainer events has led to the suggestion of a number of causes, including the bonding of an already active wire, deformation of the wire during placement, wire distortion during function or professional dental cleaning, change in the mechanical properties of the wire or loss of bonding material with time, and rebonding of an active wire after bond failures.

Despite its relatively low prevalence, unwanted tooth movement due to bonded retainers is an important complication because of the large number of patients having these retainers. Consequently, orthodontists, dentists and dental hygienists must become aware of possible complications of bonded round multistrand retainers to inform and instruct their patients on detecting retainer side effects early.

References

Adanur-Atmaca, R., Cokakoglu, S., and Oztürk, F. (2021). Effects of different lingual retainers on periodontal health and stability. *Angle Orthod.* 91: 468–476.

Ahmed, A., Fida, M., Habib, S. et al. (2021). Effect of direct versus indirect bonding technique on the failure rate of mandibular fixed retainer-a systematic review and meta-analysis. *Int. Orthod.* 19 (4): 539–547.

Aldrees, A.M., Al-Mutairi, T.K., Hakami, Z.W., and Al-Malki, M.M. (2010). Bonded orthodontic retainers: a comparison of initial bond strength of different wire-and-composite combinations. *J. Orofac. Orthop.* 71 (4): 290–299.

Al-Moghrabi, D., Pandis, N., and Fleming, P.S. (2016). The effects of fixed and removable orthodontic retainers: a systematic review. *Prog. Orthodont.* 17 (1): 24.

Al-Moghrabi, D., Johal, A., O'Rourke, N. et al. (2018). Effects of fixed vs removable orthodontic retainers on stability and periodontal health: 4-year follow-up of a randomized controlled trial. *Am. J. Orthod. Dentofac. Orthop.* 154: 167–174.

Al-Nimri, K., Al Habashneh, R., and Obeidat, M. (2009). Gingival health and relapse tendency: a prospective study of two types of lower fixed retainers. *Aust. Orthodont. J.* 25 (2): 142–146.

Alrawas, M.B., Kashoura, Y., Tosun, Ö., and Öz, U. (2021). Comparing the effects of CAD/CAM nickel-titanium lingual retainers on teeth stability and periodontal health with conventional fixed and removable retainers: a randomized clinical trial. *Orthod. Craniofac. Res.* 24 (2): 241–250.

Arn, M.-L., Dritsas, K., Pandis, N., and Kloukos, D. (2020). The effects of fixed orthodontic retainers on periodontal health: a systematic review. *Am. J. Orthod. Dentofac. Orthop.* 157: 156–164.

Årtun, J., Spadafora, A.T., and Shapiro, P.A. (1997). A 3-year follow-up study of various types of orthodontic canine-to-canine retainers. *Eur. J. Orthod.* 19 (5): 501–509.

Atack, N., Harradine, N., and Sandy Ireland, A.J. (2007). Which way forward? Fixed or removable lower retainers. *Angle Orthod.* 77 (6): 954–959.

Bazargani, F., Jacobson, S., and Lennartsson, B. (2012). A comparative evaluation of lingual retainer failure bonded with or without liquid resin. A randomized clinical study with 2-year follow-up. *Angle Orthod.* 82 (1): 84–87.

Booth, F.A., Edelman, J.M., and Proffit, W.R. (2008). Twenty-year follow-up of patients with permanently bonded mandibular canine-to-canine retainers. *Am. J. Orthod. Dentofac. Orthop.* 133 (1): 70–76.

Bovali, E., Kiliaridis, S., and Cornelis, M.A. (2014). Indirect vs direct bonding of mandibular fixed retainers in orthodontic patients: a single-center randomized controlled trial comparing placement time and failure over a 6-month period. *Am. J. Orthod. Dentofac. Orthop.* 146 (6): 701–708.

Burns, A., Dowling, A.H., Garvey, T., and Fleming, G.J.P. (2014). The reliability of Little's irregularity index for the upper dental arch using three dimensional (3D) digital models. *J. Dent.* 42: 1320–1326.

Buzatta, L.N., Shimizu, R.H., Shimizu, I.A. et al. (2017). Gingival condition associated with two types of orthodontic fixed retainers: a meta-analysis. *Eur. J. Orthod.* 39 (4): 446–452.

Charavet, C., Vives, F., Aroca, S., and Dridi, S.-M. (2022). 'Wire Syndrome' following bonded orthodontic retainers: a systematic review of the literature. *Healthcare* 10: 379.

Cornelis, M., Egli, F., Bovali, E. et al. (2022). Indirect vs direct bonding of mandibular fixed retainers in orthodontic patients: comparison of retainer failures and post-treatment stability. A 5-year follow-up of a single-center randomized controlled trial. *Am. J. Orthod. Dentofac. Orthop.* 162 (2): 152–161.

Diamond, M. (1987). Resin fiberglass bonded retainer. *J. Clin. Orthod.* 21: 182–183.

Dowling, A.H., Burns, A., Macauley, D. et al. (2013). Can the intra-examiner variability of Little's irregularity index be improved using 3D digital models of study casts? *J. Dent.* 41: 1271–1280.

Edwards, J.G. (1968). A study of the periodontium during orthodontic rotation of teeth. *Am. J. Orthod. Dentofac. Orthop.* 54: 441–461.

Egli, F., Bovali, E., Kiliaridis, S., and Cornelis, M.A. (2017). Indirect vs direct bonding of mandibular fixed retainers in orthodontic patients: comparison of retainer failures and post-treatment stability. A 2-year follow-up of a single-center randomised controlled trial. *Am. J. Orthod. Dentofac. Orthop.* 151 (1): 15–27.

Farret, M.M., Farret, M.M., da Luz, V.G. et al. (2015). Orthodontic treatment of a mandibular incisor fenestration resulting from a broken retainer. *Am. J. Orthod. Dentofac. Orthop.* 148: 332–337.

Ferreira, L.A., Sapata, D.M., Provenzano, M.A.G. et al. (2019). Periodontal parameters of two types of 3x3 orthodontic retainer: a longitudinal study. *Dental Press J. Orthod.* 24 (3): 64–70.

Forde, K., Storey, M., Littlewood, S.J. et al. (2017). Bonded versus vacuum-formed retainers: a randomized controlled trial. Part 1:stability, retainer survival, and patient satisfaction outcomes after 12 months. *Eur. J. Orthod.* 40 (4): 387–398.

Gelin, E., Seidel, L., Bruwier, A. et al. (2020). Innovative customized CAD/CAM nickel-titanium lingual retainer versus standard stainless-steel lingual retainer: a randomized controlled trial. *Korean J. Orthod.* 50: 373–382.

Gera, A., Gera, S., Cattaneo, P.M., and Cornelis, M.A. (2022). Does quality of orthodontic treatment outcome influence post-treatment stability? A retrospective study investigating short-term stability 2 years after orthodontic treatment with fixed appliances and in the presence of fixed retainers. *Orthod. Craniofac. Res.* 25 (3): 368–376.

Gökce, B. and Kaya, B. (2019). Periodontal effects and survival rates of different mandibular retainers: comparison of bonding techniques and wire thickness. *Eur. J. Orthod.* 41 (6): 591–600.

Gunay, F. and Alper, O.A. (2018). Clinical effectiveness of 2 orthodontic retainer wires on mandibular arch retention. *Am. J. Orthod. Dentofac. Orthop.* 153: 232–238.

Iliadi, A., Kloukos, D., Gkantidis, N., and Katsaros, C. (2015). Failure of fixed orthodontic retainers: a systematic review. *J. Dent.* 43 (8): 876–896.

Jedlinski, M., Grocholewicz, K., Mazur, M., and Janiszewska-Olszowska, J. (2021). What causes failure of fixed orthodontic retention?-systematic review and meta-analysis of clinical studies. *Head Face Med.* 17: 32.

Jin, C., Bennani, F., Gray, A. et al. (2018). Survival analysis of orthodontic retainers. *Eur. J. Orthod.* 40 (5): 531–536.

Kartal, Y., Kaya, B., and Polat-Özsoy, Ö. (2021). Comparative evaluation of periodontal effects and survival rates of Memotain and five-stranded bonded retainers. *J. Orofac. Orthop.* 82 (1): 32–41.

Katsaros, C., Livas, C., and Renkema, A.M. (2007). Unexpected complications of bonded mandibular lingual retainers. *Am. J. Orthod. Dentofac. Orthop.* 132 (6): 838–841.

Klaus, K., Xirouchaki, F., and Ruf, S. (2020). 3D-analysis of unwanted tooth movements despite bonded orthodontic retainers: a pilot study. *BMC Oral Health* 20: 308.

Kocher, K.E., Gebistorf, M.C., Pandis, N. et al. (2019). Survival of maxillary and mandibular bonded retainers 10 to 15 years after orthodontic treatment: a retrospective observational study. *Prog. Orthodont.* 20 (1): 28.

Kocher, K., Gebistorf, M.C., Pandis, N. et al. (2020). Long-term effectiveness of maxillary and mandibular bonded orthodontic retainers. *Oral Health Prev. Dent.* 8 (18): 633–641.

Krämer, A., Sjöström, M., Hallman, M., and Feldmann, I. (2020). Vacuum-formed retainer versus bonded retainer for dental stabilization in the mandible: a randomized controlled trial. Part I: retentive capacity 6 and 18 months after orthodontic treatment. *Eur. J. Orthod.* 42 (5): 551–558.

Kravitz, N.D., Grauer, D., Schumacher, P., and Jo, Y. (2017). Memotain: a CAD/CAM nickel-titanium lingual retainer. *Am. J. Orthod. Dentofac. Orthop.* 151: 812–815.

Kucera, J. and Marek, I. (2016). Unexpected complications associated with mandibular fixed retainers: a retrospective study. *Am. J. Orthod. Dentofac. Orthop.* 149: 202–211.

Lai, C.S., Grossen, J.M., Renkema, A.M. et al. (2014). Orthodontic retention procedures in Switzerland. Swiss. *Dent. J.* 124 (6): 655–561.

Laspos, C., Seehra, J., Katsaros, C., and Pandis, N. (2023). Survival of conventionally bonded mandibular retainers with or without enamel sandblasting in orthodontic patients over a 12-month period. A single-Centre, split-mouth randomized clinical trial. *Eur. J. Orthod.* 45(1):51–57.

Lie Sam Foek, D.J., Özcan, M., Verkerke, G.J. et al. (2008). Survival of flexible, braided, bonded stainless steel lingual retainers: a historic cohort study. *Eur. J. Orthodont.* 30: 199–204.

Liou, E.J.W., Chen, L.I.J., and Huang, C.S. (2001). Nickel-titanium mandibular bonded lingual 3-3 retainer: for permanent retention and solving relapse of mandibular anterior crowding. *Am. J. Orthod. Dentofac. Orthop.* 119: 443–449.

Little, R. (1975). The irregularity index: a quantitative score of mandibular anterior alignment. *Am. J. Orthod. Dentofac. Orthop.* 68: 554–563.

Little, R.M., Riedel, R.A., and Årtun, J. (1988). An evaluation of changes in mandibular anterior alignment from 10 to 20 years postretention. *Am. J. Orthod. Dentofac. Orthop.* 93 (5): 423–428.

Littlewood, S.J., Millett, D.T., Doubleday, B. et al. (2016). Retention procedures for stabilizing tooth position after treatment with orthodontic braces. *Cochrane Database of Syst. Rev.* 2016 (1): CD002283.

Liu, Y. (2010). Application of fibre-reinforced composite as fixed lingual retainer. *Hua Xi Kou Qiang Yi Xue Za Zhi.* 28 (3): 290–293.

Macauley, D., Garvey, T., Dowling, A.H., and Fleming, G.J.P. (2012). Using Little's irregularity index in orthodontics: outdated and inaccurate? *J. Dent.* 40: 1127–1133.

Meade, M.J. and Dreyer, C.W. (2019). A survey of retention and retainer practices of orthodontists in Australia. *Aust. Orthodont. J.* 35 (2): 174–183.

Nagani, N.I., Ahmed, I., Tanveer, F. et al. (2020). Clinical comparison of bond failure rate between two types of mandibular canine-canine bonded orthodontic retainers: a randomized clinical trial. *BMC Oral Health* 20 (1): 180.

O'Rourke, N., Albeedh, H., Sharma, P., and Johal, A. (2016). Effectiveness of bonded and vacuum-formed retainers: a prospective randomized controlled clinical trial. *Am. J. Orthod. Dentofac. Orthop.* 150: 406–415.

Pandis, N., Vlachopoulos, K., Madianos, P., and Eliadis, T. (2007). Long-term periodontal status of patients with mandibular lingual fixed retention. *Eur. J. Orthod.* 29 (5): 471–476.

Pandis, N., Fleming, P.S., Kloukos, D. et al. (2013). Survival of bonded lingual retainers with chemical or photo polymerization over a 2-year period: A single-center, randomized controlled clinical trial. *Am. J. Orthod. Dentofac. Orthop.* 144 (2): 169–175.

Papadogiannis, D., Iliadi, A., Bradley, T.G. et al. (2017). Viscoelastic properties of orthodontic adhesives used for lingual fixed retainer bonding. *Dent. Mater.* 33 (1): e22–e27.

Pazera, P., Fudalej, P., and Katsaros, C. (2012). Severe complication of a bonded mandibular lingual retainer. *Am. J. Orthod. Dentofac. Orthop.* 142: 406–409.

Pratt, M.C., Klümper, G.T., Hartsfield, J.K. Jr. et al. (2011). Evaluation of retention protocols among members of the American Association of Orthodontists in the United States. *Am. J. Orthod. Dentofac. Orthop.* 140 (4): 520–526.

Reitan, K. (1967). Clinical and histological observations on tooth movement during and after orthodontic treatment. *Am. J. Orthod. Dentofac. Orthop.* 53: 721–745.

Renkema, A.-M., Al-Assad, S., Bronkhorst, E. et al. (2008). Effectiveness of lingual retainers bonded to the canines in preventing mandibular incisor relapse. *Am. J. Orthod. Dentofac. Orthop.* 134: 179.e1–179.e8.

Renkema, A.-M., Renkema, A., Bronkhorst, E., and Katsaros, C. (2011). Long-term effectiveness of canine-to-canine bonded flexible spiral wire lingual retainers. *Am. J. Orthod. Dentofac. Orthop.* 139 (5): 614–621.

Renkema, A.-M., Fudalej, P.S., Renkema, A. et al. (2013). Development of labial gingival recessions in orthodontically treated patients. *Am. J. Orthod. Dentofac. Orthop.* 143 (2): 206–12.

Richmond, S., Shaw, W.C., O'Brien, K.D. et al. (1992). The development of the PAR index (peer assessment rating): reliability and validity. *Eur. J. Orthod.* 14: 125–139.

Rose, E., Frucht, S., and Irmtrud, J.E. (2002). Clinical comparison of a multistranded wire and a direct-bonded polyethylene ribbon-reinforced resin composite used for lingual retention. *Quintessence Int.* 33: 579–583.

Sachdeva, R.C.L. (2001). SureSmile technology in a patient-centered orthodontic practice. *J. Clin. Orthod.* 35: 245–253.

Salehi, P., Najafi, H.Z., and Roeinpeikar, S.M. (2013). Comparison of survival time between two types of orthodontic fixed retainer: a prospective randomized clinical trial. *Prog. Orthodont.* 14: 25.

Scheibe, K. and Ruf, S. (2010). Lower bonded retainers: survival and failure rates particularly considering operator experience. *J. Orofac. Orthop.* 71 (4): 300–307.

Scribante, A., Gallo, S., Turcato, B. et al. (2020). Fear of the relapse: effect of composite type on adhesion efficacy of upper and lower orthodontic fixed retainers: in vitro investigation and randomized clinical trial. *Polymers* 12 (4): 963.

Shaughnessy, T.G., Proffit, W.R., and Samara, S.A. (2016). Inadvertent tooth movement with fixed lingual retainers. *Am. J. Orthod. Dentofac. Orthop.* 149: 277–286.

Shim, H., Foley, P., Bankhead, B., and Kim, K.B. (2022). Comparative assessment of relapse and failure between CAD/CAM stainless steel and standard stainless steel fixed retainers in orthodontic retention patients. A randomized controlled trial. *Angle Orthod.* 92 (1): 87–94.

Sobouti, F., Rakhshan, V., Saravi, M.G. et al. (2016). Two-year survival analysis of twisted wire fixed retainer versus spiral wire and fiber-reinforced composite retainers: a preliminary explorative single-blind randomized clinical trial. *Korean J. Orthod.* 46 (2): 104–110.

Storey, M., Forde, K., Littlewood, S.J. et al. (2018). Bonded versus vacuum-formed retainers: a randomized controlled trial. Part 2: periodontal health outcomes after 12 months. *Eur. J. Orthod.* 40 (4): 399–408.

Störmann, I. and Ehmer, U. (2002). A prospective randomized study of different retainer types. *J. Orof. Orthop.* 63 (1): 42–50.

Swidi, A.J., Griffin, A.E., and Buschang, P.H. (2019). Mandibular alignment changes after full-fixed orthodontic treatment: a systematic review and meta-analysis. *Eur. J. Orthod.* 41 (6): 609–621.

Tacken, M.P.E., Cosyn, J., De Wilde, P. et al. (2010). Glass fiber reinforced versus mutlistranded bonded orthodontic retainers: a 2 year prospective multi-center study. *Eur. J. Orthod.* 32 (2): 117–123.

Taner, T. and Aksu, M. (2012). A prospective clinical evaluation of mandibular lingual retainer survival. *Eur. J. Orthod.* 34 (4): 470–474.

Torkan, S., Oshagh, M., Khojastepour, L. et al. (2014). Clinical and radiographic comparison of the effects of two types of fixed retainers on periodontium: a randomized clinical trial. *Prog. Orthodont.* 15 (1): 47.

Tynelius, G.E., Bondemark, L., and Lilja-Karlander, E. (2013). A randomized controlled trial of three orthodontic retention methods in Class I four premolar extraction cases-stability after 2 years in retention. *Orthod. Craniofac. Res.* 16: 105–115.

Wasserman, I., Ferrer, K., Gualdron, J. et al. (2016). Orthodontic fixed retainers: a systematic review. *Rev. Fac. Odontol. Univ. Antioq.* 28 (1): 139–157.

Wegrodzka, E., Kornatowska, K., Pandis, N., and Fudalej, P.S. (2021). A comparative assessment of failures and periodontal health between 2 mandibular lingual retainers in orthodontic patients. A 2-year follow-up, single practice-based randomized trial. *Am. J. Orthod. Dentofac. Orthop.* 160 (4): 494–502.

Wong, P.M. and Freer, T.J. (2004). A comprehensive survey of retention procedures in Australia and New Zealand. *Aust. Orthodont. J.* 20 (2): 99–106.

Zachrisson, B.J. (1995). Third-generation mandibular bonded lingual 3-3 retainer. *J. Clin. Orthod.* 29: 39–48.

Zachrisson, B.J. (2015). Multistranded wire bonded retainers: from start to success. *Am. J. Orthod. Dentofac. Orthop.* 148: 724–727.

13

Masticatory Forces and Deformation of Fixed Retainers

Iosif Sifakakis[1] *and Christoph Bourauel*[2]

[1] *Department of Orthodontics, School of Dentistry, National and Kapodistrian University of Athens, Athens, Greece*
[2] *Department of Oral Technology, School of Dentistry, University Hospital Bonn, Bonn, Germany*

13.1 Introduction

Lingual fixed retainers are designed to remain bonded over many years and even decades. Their long-term effect on the local environment (soft and hard tissues) is more or less evident (Andrén et al. 1998; Arn et al. 2020); however, the effect of the environment on the retainers – the ageing effect – is not often evaluated (Gugger et al. 2016; Zinelis et al. 2018). This effect may compromise the mechanical or chemical properties of the retainer and consequently its efficiency in preventing relapse. It may even induce side effects and unwanted tooth movement. This chapter discusses the possible association between masticatory forces and the mechanical deformation of fixed retainers. This deformation may be responsible for unexpected movement identified after debonding.

13.2 Clinical Observations

Of patients with multistrand wire retainers, 1.15% have unexpected posttreatment changes that could not be explained by the pretreatment malocclusion (Katsaros et al. 2007; Kučera and Marek 2016; Renkema

Debonding and Fixed Retention in Orthodontics: An Evidence-Based Clinical Guide, First Edition. Edited by Theodore Eliades and Christos Katsaros.

et al. 2011), including torque differences between the adjacent incisors and increased buccal or lingual inclination and movement of the canine. However, the aetiology is most likely multifactorial and, unfortunately, not well understood. The changes can probably be attributed to an active component of the wire due to an elastic deflection caused by the clinician or a mechanical deformation from masticatory forces. Even a minimal wire deformation of 0.2 mm can exert forces as high as 1 N on the teeth (Sifakakis et al. 2011).

In a recent retrospective study with a large sample, strong asymmetry of the canine tipping was demonstrated: i.e. in 90% of the patients displaying unexpected inclination of the lower canines, the left one was tipped buccally. Subjects in the unexpected-movement group were significantly younger at debonding and had higher mandibular plane angles. These facts suggest that retainer wires' mechanical properties and use time should be examined (Kučera and Marek 2016). Since facial divergence was identified as a possible predictor, factors associated with this growth pattern should also be examined.

Unwanted tooth movement occurred more often with maxillary than mandibular retainers. Oral dysfunctions or habits before treatment and lack of interincisal contact before or after treatment were also associated with unwanted tooth movement (Klaus et al. 2020). However, the latter research did not find any association between these unintentional tooth movements and the pretreatment mandibular plane angle. Torque discrepancies between adjacent incisors were not evident in cases of larger-diameter canine-and-canine wires secured to the canines only (Shaughnessy et al. 2016).

Recent research demonstrated that all patients with changes in canine inclination were bonded with the direct bonding method; this may support the hypothesis that the indirect bonding technique allows for a more passive bonding of the wire. One could assume that a marginal deflection of the wire resulting in an active force on the left canine was introduced during the direct bonding procedure (Egli et al. 2017). Another research team highly recommended retainer fabrication on a working model to prevent unexpected movement (Shaughnessy et al. 2016). However, this is only an assumption. The active component of a retainer wire is independent of the wire fabrication technique, direct or indirect. It is the bonding technique that may introduce a force in the wire. This could happen when pushing on the wire with a hand instrument or finger pressure during light curing or when elastic deformation of the wire is introduced by the hard pressure of the dental floss used for stabilization. That means even a wire constructed properly in the laboratory could be improperly bonded, introducing an active force. In this case, tooth movement will be evident in the short term after bonding. However, a recent study found that most of these complications are identified within the first five to six years after placement of the bonded retainer, with an average time of occurrence of four years (Kučera and Marek 2016). Unexpected movement evident in the long term after retainer bonding could not be attributed to an active component of the wire due to improper bonding.

The indirect bonding technique may provide better adaptation to the lingual surfaces of the anterior teeth than can be obtained with intraoral fabrication. A wire not perfectly adapted to the lingual surfaces of the teeth, i.e. not touching the lingual surfaces of the teeth, may be more easily deformed after bonding since it is not supported by the tooth surfaces during function. Wire deformation in the posttreatment period could occur from the horizontal labiolingual forces and the vertical masticatory forces, trauma, dental flossing or professional dental cleaning. Bond failures and rebonding or biting habits of the patient could also lead to deflection and distortion of the wire (Egli et al. 2017). There is a lack of consensus about the effect of a repetitive tongue habit on retainer deformation. Although this is described in the literature (Gazit 2005), some authors claim that tongue habits do not play a role in deforming retainer wires (Shaughnessy et al. 2016). The frequency/duration and force magnitude/direction of the habit play pivotal roles in the clinical manifestation of such tooth movement.

A more or less indirect correlation seems to exist between masticatory forces and crowding. A significant correlation was demonstrated between increased occlusal wear and increased bite force or reduced tendency for crowding (Johansson et al. 1993). Further research has shown that the maximum voluntary molar bite force was significantly related to age, sex, lip competency, crowding and other malocclusion parameters (Alam and Alfawzan 2020). Specific crowding patterns were related to large occlusal force, mesial inclination of the first molar and large overjet/overbite (Shigenobu et al. 2007). Even post-retention, a moderate positive correlation was shown between the anterior component of occlusal force and mandibular arch crowding in subjects treated without extractions (Acar et al. 2002). Moreover, after orthognathic surgery, the weakening of masticatory muscle activity by botulinum neurotoxin injection may contribute to mandible stability and prevent open- and deep bite (Seok and Kim 2018).

13.3 Retainer Properties

The clinical behaviour of retainer wire may vary considerably based on the wire dimensions (length and cross-section properties), the alloy type and the dimensions/properties of the composite bulk. The clinical picture is further affected by the properties of the periodontal ligament and the morphology of the bonding area. Recently, *in vitro* research has shown the detrimental effect of high temperature on the reduction of properties of adhesives, which may contribute to a loss of stiffness of the fixed retainer configuration under ordinary clinical conditions with unfavourable effects on tooth position and stability of the orthodontic treatment result (Papadogiannis et al. 2017).

A fixed retainer should have mechanical properties adequate to withstand not only deformation by masticatory and other forces but also forces causing relapse (Figure 13.1). Additionally, it should allow physiologic tooth mobility (Schwarze et al. 1995; Watted et al. 2001). Since the

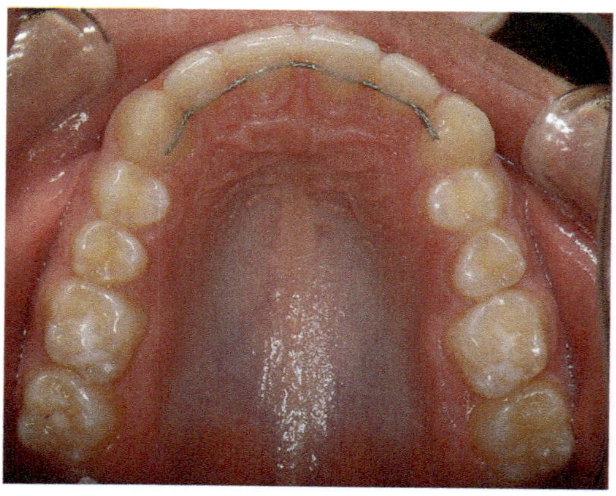

Figure 13.1 Deformation of the dead-soft retainer three years post-debonding, diastema between left lateral incisor/canine and increased inclination of the canine.

forces exerted on the retainer vary considerably between individuals and the relapse forces have not yet been quantified, a determination of the appropriate properties of fixed retainers is still pending.

Among the array of mechanical properties, stiffness, elastic limit (commonly given as yield strength) and range seem to be the most important for the clinical efficacy of fixed retainers. Stiffness is a measure of resistance to deformation in bending and torsion. The latter is especially important for preventing unexpected torque problems from fixed retainers. Stiffness depends on the modulus of elasticity and the wire cross-section and indicates how much force will be applied for a certain deflection. Stiffness is the same for wires of the same alloy, regardless of their hardness. The most potent variable for controlling the stiffness of fixed retainers is size (Thurow 1982); however, the number of strands also affects the stiffness of multistrand archwires (Oltjen et al. 1997). Solid stainless-steel wires offer greater stiffness than multistrand archwires (Ingram Jr et al. 1986; Kapila and Sachdeva 1989). Changes in length do not modify the stiffness as much as changes in diameter. Increasing the length of a cantilever beam reduces the bending strength for a given deflection (Thurow 1982). Recent research demonstrated that unwanted tooth movement occurred more often with maxillary than mandibular retainers (Klaus et al. 2020). Wider upper anterior teeth and increased free interdental wire length reduce wire stiffness and may favour wire deformation.

Yield strength and range are measures of the maximum capacity of the archwire (Thurow 1982). They are important determinants of the clinical performance of fixed retainers since unexpected movement implies a plastic deformation of the wire. A fixed retainer should have adequate yield strength to preserve its shape from permanent plastic deformation during mastication. For a round wire, yield strength in torsion is proportional to the cube of the diameter, as for bending. A multistrand wire with low stiffness generally has low strength (Rucker and Kusy 2002).

Range is the maximum working distance if the archwire is loaded to its elastic limit, i.e. the amount of displacement endured under maximum elastic stress. It is also referred to in the orthodontic literature as range of deflection, working range or maximum elastic deflection. For round solid archwires, range is expected to decrease as size increases. The range of multistrand wires is not influenced to the same extent as solid wires by the cross-section size and remains constant for a particular wire configuration. Round titanium alloy and multistrand stainless steel wires have lower stiffness and higher range compared to solid stainless steel (Ingram Jr et al. 1986).

Hardness is the most dominant factor for wear resistance, as lingual retainers are constantly exposed to abrasion due to mastication, and thus materials with greater hardness are preferable for the construction of these devices (Table 13.1). A high hardness value is desired for materials used intraorally since it reduces abrasive wear due to mastication. The Vickers hardness of commonly used stainless steel wires has been shown to vary within 240–300 kg/mm^2 and for β-Ti within 100–190 kg/mm^2 (Verstrynge et al. 2006). Australian Wire demonstrated increased hardness values and ranged on the order of 660 HV_{500}. The higher hardness values of these wires could be attributed to increased carbon content and the manufacturing process.

High hardness may cause a wire to be more brittle and consequently may adversely affect the wire's ability to withstand bending, a property of primary importance during the loading of the retainer (Pelsue et al. 2009). NiTi archwires have also been used for fixed retention (Knaup et al. 2019; Wolf et al. 2015). Unfortunately, long-term data for this retainer type is unavailable. Some nickel titanium retrieved archwires had much higher fracture incidence than expected in laboratory experiments (Bourauel et al. 2008; Zinelis et al. 2007).

13.4 *In Vitro* Loading of Fixed Retainer Wires

A simulation of anterior biting was conducted in an orthodontic measurement and simulation system (OMSS). This device is widely used to provide insights into several biomechanical issues in dentistry. OMSS allows the complete registration of the force–torque vectors three-dimensionally as well as after simulation of a desirable tooth movement (Figure 13.2). Its applications and setup have been previously described in detail (Bourauel et al. 1992; Drescher et al. 1991). In this simulation, the experimental device exerted an intrusive force on the anterior teeth that approximated the vertical incisor bite force during mastication (Helkimo et al. 1977). Different canine-to-canine retainer types were compared regarding the intrusive forces and labiolingual moments generated on a lower canine during the intrusive loading of the rest of the

Table 13.1 Young's modulus and the Vickers hardness (HV) test results for representative types of orthodontic wires.

Wire type	Young's modulus (GPa)	HV
Australian Wire (A.J. Wilcock)	173–177 (Pelsue et al. 2009)	545 (Zinelis et al. 2015)
Australian Special Plus (T.P. Laboratories)	169 (Kusy and Dilley 1984)	
SuperElastic Regular Force NiTi (Highland Metals)		325–333 (Zinelis et al. 2015)
NiTi	34 (Brantley 2001)	286–428 (Brantley 2001)
Superelastic NiTi	55 (Tonner and Waters 1994)	
β-Titanium (BetaBlue, Highland Metals)		330 ± 9 (Zinelis et al. 2015)
β-Ti (TMA, Ormco)	65 (Kusy and Dilley 1984)	355 ± 4
β-Ti	62–69 (Brantley 2001)	
Solid stainless steel (TruForce, Ortho Technology)		529 (Zinelis et al. 2015)
0.018 solid stainless steel (GAC)	193 (Kusy and Dilley 1984)	
Stainless steel	160–180 (Brantley 2001)	
0.0195 coaxial stainless steel (Respond, Ormco)		488 (Zinelis et al. 2015)
3-strand twisted wire (size 0.0175 in.) (GAC)	199 (Kusy and Dilley 1984)	
0.0155 6-strand stainless steel (Masel)		535 (Zinelis et al. 2015)
Stainless steel alloys and nickel-free (Acme Monaco, Dentaurum, Scheu, Leone)		484–600 (Brüngger et al. 2019)
Nickel-free stainless steel (Dentaurum)		528 (Zinelis et al. 2015)

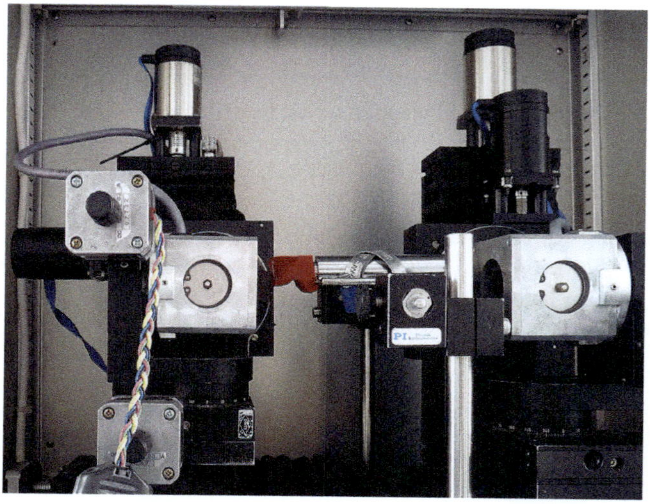

Figure 13.2 The orthodontic measurement and simulation system (OMSS).

anterior teeth (Sifakakis et al. 2015). OMSS recorded the maximum and residual forces and moments after the *in vitro* loading. Four different retainer types were evaluated: Tru-Chrome 7-strand twisted 5 in. 0.027 in. steel wire (RMO) (Andrén et al. 1998), Ortho FlexTech gold chain 0.038×0.016 in. (Reliance) (Arn et al. 2020), Wildcat 0.0175 in. (Gugger et al. 2016) and 0.0215 in. 3-strand twistflex steel wire (GAC) (Zinelis et al. 2018).

Interestingly, the forces and moments after the unloading of the retainer were not zero. This *in vitro* experiment demonstrated that the evaluated fixed flexible retainers may not be passive after short- or long-term clinical use (Table 13.2).

Higher-magnitude residual forces were recorded from twisted arch-wires compared to those exerted from the gold chain. The highest forces were recorded from the seven-strand twisted 0.027 in. steel wire. Additionally, the residual moments recorded from this retainer type were higher than from the other retainer types. This wire is constructed from a high-formable, softer temper than archwire tempers. These residual forces are high enough to induce tooth movement; however, the fixed retainer allows mainly third-order root movement and first/second-order movement of the last tooth bonded on the retainer. These

Table 13.2 Force system during intrusive maximum loading of the anterior teeth and after unloading by type of wire; mean (SD) (Sifakakis et al. 2015).

	Force (N)		Moment (Nmm)	
Retainer type	**Loading**	**After unloading**	**Loading**	**After unloading**
7-strand 0.027 in.	4.4 (0.3)	0.8 (0.1)	13.8 (1.2)	2.2 (0.6)
Ortho FlexTech	2.0 (0.4)	0.1 (0.1)	7.6 (1.5)	0.9 (0.2)
3-strand 0.0195 in.	3.8 (0.3)	0.5 (0.1)	11.5 (1.1)	1.8 (0.4)
3-strand 0.0215-in.	4.8 (0.3)	0.6 (0.1)	15.1 (1.9)	1.8 (0.4)

are usually unexpected post-treatment changes in the position of the mandibular anterior teeth associated with the use of flexible spiral wire retainers (Katsaros et al. 2007).

Several retainer wires are offered with a high degree of annealing and are referred to in the literature as dead-soft. This process eliminates all the effects of cold working, and the wire returns to a softer, more workable state (Thurow 1982). A higher degree of annealing reduces yield strength but allows for better bend formability (Proffit and Fields 2007). Unfortunately, in these archwires, the desirable ease of wire bending becomes an undesirable ease of deformation and even fracture during function (Figure 13.3). Inadvertent tooth movement and loss of alignment are more likely when wires break (Shaughnessy et al. 2016).

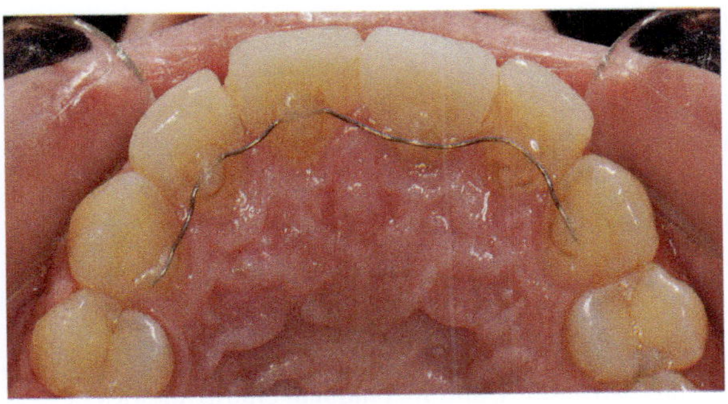

Figure 13.3 Significant deformation of a retainer with a high degree of annealing.

An *in vitro* study concluded that a three-strand 0.036 in. twisted lingual retainer wire had a relatively higher load deflection rate than a stainless steel specimen constructed from custom-made three-strand twisted ligature wires 0.010 in. each or 0.016 × 0.022 in. dead-soft eight-braided wire. According to the authors, this retainer may resist deformation from occlusal forces, thereby reducing inadvertent tooth movement and yet remaining flexible enough to allow physiologic tooth movement (Samson et al. 2018). In conclusion, it is advisable to use archwires with greater bending and torsional stiffness for fixed retention.

References

Acar, A., Alcan, T., and Erverdi, N. (2002). Evaluation of the relationship between the anterior component of occlusal force and postretention crowding. *Am. J. Orthod. Dentofacial Orthop.* 122 (4): 366–370.

Alam, M.K. and Alfawzan, A.A. (2020). Maximum voluntary molar bite force in subjects with malocclusion: multifactor analysis. *J. Int. Med. Res.* 48 (10): 300060520962943.

Andrén, A., Asplund, J., Azarmidohkt, E. et al. (1998). A clinical evaluation of long term retention with bonded retainers made from multistrand wires. *Swed. Dent. J.* 22: 123–131.

Arn, M.L., Dritsas, K., Pandis, N., and Kloukos, D. (2020). The effects of fixed orthodontic retainers on periodontal health: a systematic review. *Am. J. Orthod. Dentofacial Orthop.* 157 (2): 156–164.e17.

Bourauel, C., Drescher, D., and Their, M. (1992). An experimental apparatus for the simulation of three-dimensional movements in orthodontics. *J. Biomed. Eng.* 14: 371–378.

Bourauel, C., Scharold, W., Jäger, A., and Eliades, T. (2008). Fatigue failure of as-received and retrieved NiTi orthodontic archwires. *Dent. Mater.* 24: 1095–1101.

Brantley, W.A. (2001). Orthodontic wires. In: *Orthodontic Materials: Scientific and Clinical Aspects* (ed. W.A. Brantley and T. Eliades), 77–104. Stuttgart: Thieme.

Brüngger, D., Koutsoukis, T., S Al Jabbari, Y. et al. (2019). A comparison of the compositional, microstructural, and mechanical characteristics of ni-free and conventional stainless steel orthodontic wires. *Materials (Basel)* 12 (20): 3424.

Drescher, D., Bourauel, C., and Their, M. (1991). Application of the orthodontic measurement and simulation system (OMSS) in orthodontics. *Eur. J. Orthod.* 13: 169–178.

Egli, F., Bovali, E., Kiliaridis, S., and Cornelis, M.A. (2017). Indirect vs direct bonding of mandibular fixed retainers in orthodontic patients: comparison of retainer failures and posttreatment stability. A 2-year follow-up of a single-center randomized controlled trial. *Am. J. Orthod. Dentofacial Orthop.* 151 (1): 15–27.

Gazit, E. (2005). Ask us. The ultimate retainer? *Am. J. Orthod. Dentofacial Orthop.* 128: 3.

Gugger, J., Pandis, N., Zinelis, S. et al. (2016). Retrieval analysis of lingual fixed retainer adhesives. *Am. J. Orthod. Dentofacial Orthop.* 150 (4): 575–584.

Helkimo, E., Carlsson, G.E., and Helkimo, M. (1977). Bite force and state of dentition. *Acta. Odontol. Scand.* 35: 297–303.

Ingram, S.B. Jr., Gipe, D.P., and Smith, R.J. (1986). Comparative range of orthodontic wires. *Am. J. Orthod. Dentofacial Orthop.* 90: 296–307.

Johansson, A., Kiliaridis, S., Haraldson, T. et al. (1993). Covariation of some factors associated with occlusal tooth wear in a selected high-wear sample. *Scand. J. Dent. Res.* 101 (6): 398–406.

Kapila, S. and Sachdeva, R. (1989). Mechanical properties and clinical applications of orthodontic wires. *Am. J. Orthod. Dentofacial Orthop.* 96: 100–109.

Katsaros, C., Livas, C., and Renkema, A.M. (2007). Unexpected complications of bonded mandibular lingual retainers. *Am. J. Orthod. Dentofacial Orthop.* 132 (6): 838–841.

Klaus, K., Xirouchaki, F., and Ruf, S. (2020). 3D-analysis of unwanted tooth movements despite bonded orthodontic retainers: a pilot study. *BMC Oral Health* 20 (1): 308.

Knaup, I., Wagner, Y., Wego, J. et al. (2019). Potential impact of lingual retainers on oral health: comparison between conventional twistflex retainers and CAD/CAM fabricated nitinol retainers: a clinical in vitro and in vivo investigation. *J. Orofac. Orthop.* 80: 88–96.

Kučera, J. and Marek, I. (2016). Unexpected complications associated with mandibular fixed retainers: a retrospective study. *Am. J. Orthod. Dentofacial Orthop.* 149 (2): 202–211.

Kusy, R.P. and Dilley, G.J. (1984). Elastic modulus of a triple-stranded stainless steel arch wire via three- and four-point bending. *J. Dent. Res.* 63: 1232–1240.

Oltjen, J.M., Duncanson, M.G. Jr., Ghosh, J. et al. (1997). Stiffness-deflection behavior of selected orthodontic wires. *Angle. Orthod.* 67: 209–218.

Papadogiannis, D., Iliadi, A., Bradley, T.G. et al. (2017). Viscoelastic properties of orthodontic adhesives used for lingual fixed retainer bonding. *Dent. Mater.* 33 (1): e22–e27.

Pelsue, B.M., Zinelis, S., Bradley, T.G. et al. (2009). Structure, composition, and mechanical properties of Australian orthodontic wires. *Angle. Orthod.* 79 (1): 97–101.

Proffit, W.R. and Fields, H.W. (2007). *Contemporary Orthodontics*, 4e, 304. St Louis: Mosby.

Renkema, A.M., Renkema, A., Bronkhorst, E., and Katsaros, C. (2011). Long-term effectiveness of canine-to-canine bonded flexible spiral wire lingual retainers. *Am. J. Orthod. Dentofacial Orthop.* 139 (5): 614–621.

Rucker, B.K. and Kusy, R.P. (2002). Theoretical investigation of elastic flexural properties for multistranded orthodontic archwires. *J. Biomed. Mater. Res. Part A* 62: 338–349.

Samson, R.S., Varghese, E., Uma, E., and Chandrappa, P.R. (2018). Evaluation of bond strength and load deflection rate of multistranded fixed retainer wires: an in-vitro study. *Contemp. Clin. Dent.* 9 (1): 10–14.

Schwarze, J., Bourauel, C., and Drescher, D. (1995). The mobility of theanterior teeth after the direct bonding of lingual retainers. A comparison of in-vitro and in-vivo measurements [in German]. *Fortschr. Kieferorthop.* 56: 25–33.

Seok, H. and Kim, S.G. (2018). Correction of malocclusion by botulinum neurotoxin injection into masticatory muscles. *Toxins (Basel).* 10 (1): 27.

Shaughnessy, T.G., Proffit, W.R., and Samara, S.A. (2016). Inadvertent tooth movement with fixed lingual retainers. *Am. J. Orthod. Dentofacial Orthop.* 149 (2): 277–286.

Shigenobu, N., Hisano, M., Shima, S. et al. (2007). Patterns of dental crowding in the lower arch and contributing factors. A statistical study. *Angle. Orthod.* 77 (2): 303–310.

Sifakakis, I., Pandis, N., Eliades, T. et al. (2011). In-vitro assessment of the forces generated by lingual fixed retainers. *Am. J. Orthod. Dentofacial Orthop.* 139: 44–48.

Sifakakis, I., Eliades, T., and Bourauel, C. (2015). Residual stress analysis of fixed retainer wires after in vitro loading: can mastication-induced stresses produce an unfavorable effect? *Biomed. Tech. (Berl).* 60 (6): 617–622.

Thurow, R.C. (1982). *Edgewise Orthodontics*, 4e. St Louis: Mosby.
Tonner, R.I. and Waters, N.E. (1994). The characteristics of super-elastic Ni-Ti wires in three-point bending. Part II: intra-batch variation. *Eur. J. Orthod.* 16: 421–425.
Verstrynge, A., Van Humbeeck, J., and Willems, G. (2006). In-vitro evaluation of the material characteristics of stainless steel and beta-titanium orthodontic wires. *Am. J. Orthod. Dentofacial Orthop.* 130 (4): 460–470.
Watted, N., Wieber, M., Teuscher, T., and Schmitz, N. (2001). Comparison of incisor mobility after insertion of canine-to-canine lingual retainers bonded to two or to six teeth. A clinical study. *J. Orofac. Orthop.* 62: 387–396.
Wolf, M., Schumacher, P., Jäger, F. et al. (2015). Novel lingual retainer created using CAD/CAM technology: evaluation of its positioning accuracy. *J. Orofac. Orthop.* 76: 164–174.
Zinelis, S., Eliades, T., Pandis, N. et al. (2007). Why do nickel-titanium archwires fracture intraorally? Fractographic analysis and failure mechanism of in-vivo fractured wires. *Am. J. Orthod. Dentofacial Orthop.* 132 (1): 84–89.
Zinelis, S., Al Jabbari, Y.S., Gaintantzopoulou, M. et al. (2015). Mechanical properties of orthodontic wires derived by instrumented indentation testing (IIT) according to ISO 14577. *Prog. Orthod.* 16: 19. https://doi.org/10.1186/s40510-015-0091-z.
Zinelis, S., Pandis, N., Al Jabbari, Y.S. et al. (2018). Does long-term intraoral service affect the mechanical properties and elemental composition of multistranded wires of lingual fixed retainers? *Eur. J. Orthod.* 40: 126–131.

Index

Debonding and Fixed Retention in Orthodontics: An Evidence-Based Clinical Guide, First Edition. Edited by Theodore Eliades and Christos Katsaros.

x

y

z

Printed and bound by CPI Group (UK) Ltd, Croydon, CR0 4YY

14/09/2023

08114786-0001